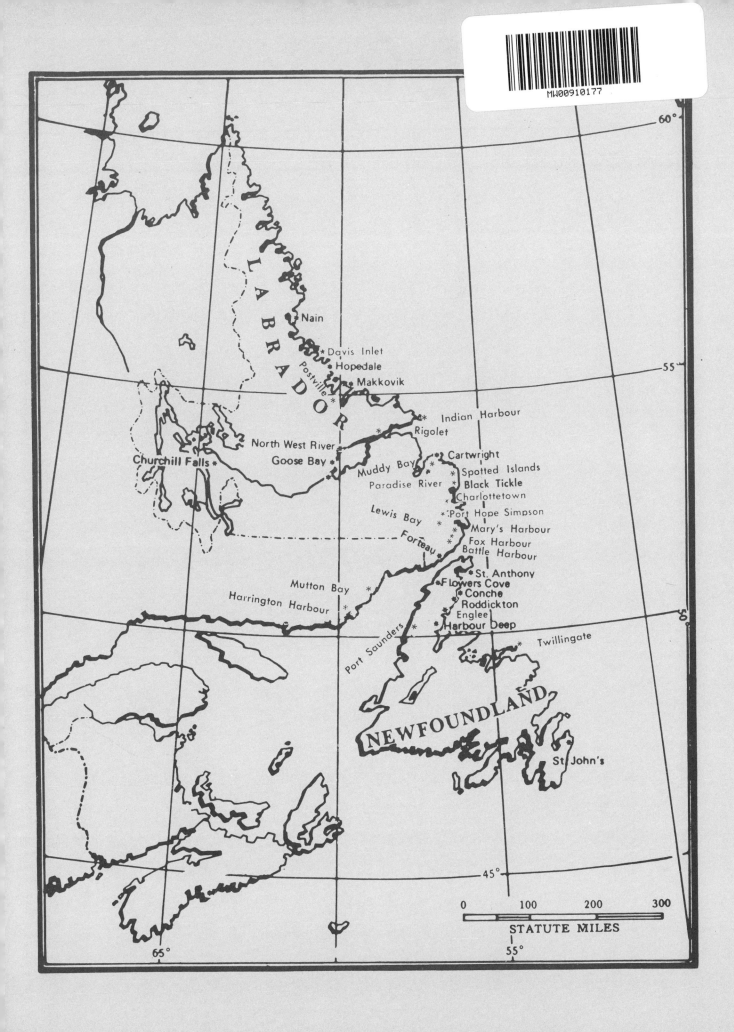

LABRADOR

*Nain
*Davis Inlet
Postville *Hopedale
*Makkovik

*Indian Harbour
Rigolet
North West River
Churchill Falls* Goose Bay
Muddy Bay *Cartwright
Paradise River *Spotted Islands
*Black Tickle
Charlottetown
Lewis Bay *Port Hope Simpson
*Mary's Harbour
Forteau Fox Harbour
Battle Harbour
*St. Anthony
Mutton Bay *Flowers Cove
*Conche
Harrington Harbour Roddickton
Englee
*Harbour Deep
Port Saunders *Twillingate

NEWFOUNDLAND

St. John's

60°
55°
50°
45°

65°
55°

0   100   200   300
STATUTE MILES

The GRENFELL OBSESSION
An Anthology

Patricia O'Brien

The GRENFELL OBSESSION
An Anthology

Patricia O'Brien

Creative Publishers
St. John's, Newfoundland
1992

Cover: Janice Udell

Published by
CREATIVE PUBLISHERS

A Division of Robinson-Blackmore Printing & Publishing Ltd.
P.O. Box 8660, St. John's, Newfoundland A1B 3T7

All reasonable efforts have been made to acquire relevant reprint permission for this publication. In some cases the publisher of record had ceased operations or the rights had reverted to the author. In the latter case, where an address was available, attempts were made to reach the author or designated copyright holder. In some cases, where we were unsuccessful in this endeavour, we have chosen to reprint the excerpt in the belief that the author or heirs would wish the article to be included in this anniversary anthology.
THE PUBLISHER

Royalties are assigned to
THE INTERNATIONAL GRENFELL ASSOCIATION

∝ Printed on recycled, acid-free Eco Matte offset paper

Printed in Canada by:

ROBINSON-BLACKMORE PRINTING & PUBLISHING LTD.
P.O. Box 8660, St. John's, Newfoundland A1B 3T7

Canadian Cataloguing in Publication Data

The Grenfell obsession

Includes bibliographical references.
ISBN 1-895387-08-6

1. Grenfell, Wilfred Thomason, Sir, 1865–1940.
2. Grenfell Labrador Medical Mission — History.
3. Missions, Medical — Newfoundland — History.
4. Missionaries, Medical—Newfoundland—Biography.
5. Physicians — Newfoundland — Biography.
I. O'Brien, Patricia Ruth, 1946–

FC2193.3.G74G74 1992   610.69'5'092   C92-098686-2
F1137.G74G74 1992

Photograph Acknowledgements

Photographs are courtesy of the Sir Wilfred Thomason Grenfell Historical Society, St. Anthony, Newfoundland, with the following exceptions in the Public Archives of Newfoundland and Labrador (PANL), International Grenfell Association (IGA) collection:

p. 1: VA 91 25-1;
p. 3 at bottom: 26-112;
p. 4 top to bottom: VA 91 9-3, 23-107;
p. 5: 25-135;
p. 6: 26-112;
p. 7: 22-76;
p. 8: 27-60;
p. 9 at bottom: 24-452;
p. 11 at bottom: 23-496;
p. 13 top to bottom: 27-12, 24-371;
p. 15 top to bottom: Magic lantern 1-317, 17-30;
p. 16: 14-178;
p. 21: 15-87;
p. 23 at top: 26-73;
p. 24: 26-88;
p. 25 at bottom: 25-124;
p. 29 at bottom: 22-30;
p. 30 at bottom: 18-94;
p. 34: 25-169;
p. 35: 18-158;
p. 37 at bottom: 17-23;
p. 38 top to bottom: Magic lanterns 1-348, 1-226;
p. 39 top to bottom: 18-106, 24-463;
p. 40: 18-60;
p. 41 at bottom: 18-270;
p. 43 at top: 25-12;
p. 47: 28-46;
p. 48: 25-17;
p. 49: 17-25;
p. 57 at top: 24-314;
p. 58 at bottom: 18-74;
p. 59 1st at top, bottom right: 15-131, 14-213;
p. 60 at bottom: 24-317, 17-325;
p. 61: 25-134;
p. 62 at top: 27-22;
p. 63: 25-180;
p. 64: 15-197;
p. 67 top & bottom: 14-367, 25-5;
p. 68: 23-501;
p. 70 top to bottom: 18-175, 25-168;
p. 73 top to bottom: 18-49, Magic lantern 1-321;
p. 75: 25-186;
p. 77 at top: 15-242;
p. 79 at top: 23-481;
p. 80 at top: 23-51;
p. 82: 28-34;
p. 83: 16 50;
p. 84 at top: 24-379;
p. 85 top to bottom: 15-36, 23-427;
p. 86 at top: 15-266;
p. 88 at top: 24-439;
p. 89: 18-56;
p. 90: 19-5;
p. 92 top to bottom: 17-328, 23-363;
p. 93 top to bottom: 25-206, magic lantern 1-225;
p. 94: 18-54;
p. 95: 25-79; p. 97: 23-141;
p. 98: 18-164;
p. 99 top to bottom: 25-150, 14-157;
p. 100: 15-296;
p. 103: 23-457;
p. 104 top to bottom: 25-8, 18-288;
p. 106: 22-42;
p. 107: 24-175;
p. 110 1st & 2nd top: 16-32, 24-124;
p. 111 left to right, top to bottom, excluding top left: 14-27, 25-193, 25-3, 19-31;
p. 114 at top: 15-124;
p. 120: 25-307;
p. 121 top to bottom: 24-390, 24-168;
p. 124 at top: 17-214;
p. 125 at top: 22-93;
p. 126 at bottom: 24-205;
p. 127 top to bottom: 26-108, 24-236;
p. 128 top to bottom: 24-185, 23-278;
p. 129: 25-225;
p. 131 at bottom, left to right: 23-10, 17-57;
p. 132 1st top, 1st middle: 23-15, 23-8;
p. 133 left to right, top to bottom: 25-14, 17-3, 14-470, 24-335, 23-23;
p. 135: 14-141;
p. 137 top to bottom: 25-229, 23-467;
p. 138 at bottom: 23-119;
p. 140: 18-8;
p. 141 at bottom: 15-129;
p. 143: 24-434;
p. 145 top to bottom: 22-24, 18-221;
p. 146: 14-227;
p. 147: 14-67;
p. 148 top to bottom: 23-476, 14-423;
p. 150: 17-440;
p. 151: 22-18;
p. 152 top & bottom: 24-350, 24-399;
p. 153 top to bottom: 17-419, 22-21;
p. 155: 14-168;
p. 156: 18-193.

Additional photographs—p. 2, p. 11 at top: Norman Duncan, *Dr. Grenfell's Parish*; p. 28: Alfreda Withington, *My Eyes Have Seen*, frontispiece; p. 65: Rosalie Slaughter Morton, *A Woman Surgeon*, frontispiece; p. 71: Elizabeth Goudie, *Woman of Labrador*, back cover; p. 84 at bottom: Anne Grenfell & Katie Spalding, *Le Petit Nord*; p. 149: Anne E. Carney, *Harrington Harbour*; p. 157: Peter Roberts; back cover: PANL IGA VA-111-10. End maps from *Among the Deep Sea Fishers*, 1928, 1981.

For Grenfell Staff
Past and Present

Whatsoever is not simple, whatsoever is affected, boastful, and wilful—covetous—tarnishes, even destroys, the heroic character of a deed; because all these faults spring out of self. On the other hand, whenever you find a perfectly simple, frank, unconscious character, there you have the possibility at least of heroic action.

Charles Kingsley, 1819-1875

There is a difference between theology and religion: theology is what one comprehends, religion what one does.

Wilfred T. Grenfell

A Grenfell worker, on being asked if she had found Labrador a healthful climate, replied: "Yes, but there is one thing we all get—something incurable which gets into your system and keeps returning, but which is never fatal. It is called 'Grenfellitis,' and its most dangerous symptoms is a lasting enthusiasm for the north!"

Grenfell Worker 1934

Table of Contents

Preface – ix

The Mission's Early Years

The Middle Years

The Mission After Grenfell

Preface

High on a hill overlooking the town of St. Anthony in northern Newfoundland, at the end of a long path that winds through the woods, there is a small clearing. At the centre of that clearing stands a large boulder in which six cavities have been hollowed out. On the boulder are six brass plaques bearing the names of the three men and three women whose ashes are sealed within—Wilfred Grenfell; his wife Anne; his first surgeon, Dr John Mason Little; his successor, Dr Charles Curtis; Curtis' wife Harriot; and Curtis' head nurse, Selma Carlson. Silent tribute is thus paid to an era when missions played an important role in most parts of the colonial and post-colonial world; when the degree of control they exercised over people's lives was not regarded with mistrust; when health care, education and social services were a function of disjointed, often unintelligible, forces that frequently failed to deliver the needed benefits; and when the actions of a single individual could still make a difference. How came these six people—missionaries in a sense, American and British—to find their final resting place in this spot, overlooking where once stood the headquarters of a northern frontier?

St. Anthony itself, near the tip of the Great Northern Peninsula, is today an ordinary town of about 3,100 people. Once, before Dr Wilfred Grenfell's time, it was a collection of about fifteen houses. Then its sole purpose was as a staging point for hundreds of vessels that late each spring headed out from the bays of eastern Newfoundland, to cross the Strait of Belle Isle and fish the cod-rich waters of Labrador until mid-autumn. The spirit of this fishery, in which some 20,000 to 25,000 Newfoundland men, women and children were seasonally engaged either as 'floaters' (fishing from schooners) or as 'stationers' (working from small boats and fixed locations), has been brilliantly captured by the journalist Norman Duncan in his 1905 essay, "With the Fleet."* Duncan called it "a great lottery of hope and fortune." And lottery it was, in the sense that in some years it provided the Newfoundlanders with the means to carry themselves through to the next fishing season in a reasonably comfortable style, while in other years it did not.

In addition to these annual migrants, Labrador a century ago was home to 4,000 permanent residents, or 'liveyers' (a corruption of 'live here'). They had developed a multitude of technical skills, a store of knowledge and a complex pattern of seasonal mobility that enabled them to live off land and sea through a combination of fishing, trapping and hunting, both for subsistence and trade. For most of the year they lived in secluded homesteads situated up the sheltered bays, isolated from the rest of the world and from each other. In summer they took to their fishing stations on the ruthless North Atlantic coast to join the "lottery." In many cases the men were the descendants of hardy British pioneers who had come to Labrador to fish, trap and trade as much as a century earlier, and who had married native, usually Inuit, women. Others were Newfoundlanders who chose to settle permanently 'on the Labrador,' either bringing their wives or finding wives there. By 1892 most of the fully Inuit had left the southern Labrador coast to these settlers and now lived on mission stations established by the Moravian Church north of Hamilton Inlet, in coastal communities like Nain, Hopedale, Okak and Hebron. The Labrador Innu, the Naskapi and Montagnais Indians, for the most part lived inland, pursuing vast caribou herds that roamed the interior. They came to the coast only for trade.

Labrador was thus a culturally mixed community of people—seasonal fishermen and their families, settlers, Inuit and Innu—attempting to make the most of a harsh environment, surviving in an unpredictable, largely fishing, economy. They were governed from St. John's, the capital of Newfoundland, but had few services provided. They had no doctors (save for a single physician sent north each summer on the government's coastal steamer/mail vessel), no nurses, no magistrates or policemen or other government officials. There was little or no schooling, though there were a few Church-employed itinerant teachers. Because fishing and trapping operated on the credit system, there were few opportunities for wage-labour. Agriculture for all intents and purposes did not exist.

These, then, were the people to whom Wilfred Grenfell (1865-1940) came in the hospital vessel *Albert* a century ago. A young English doctor in the employ of the Mission to Deep Sea Fishermen, a charitable association founded in England in 1884 to provide physical and spiritual care to fishermen in the North Sea, he came because to the Mission's ears had come tales of crying need amongst another group of fishermen—those on the Labrador coast, to the north of Newfoundland. What he found on that first visit, in August 1892, was sufficient to draw him back to Labrador, still working for the Mission to Deep Sea Fishermen, again and again. He established hospitals and brought other people, British

---

* Norman Duncan, *Dr. Grenfell's Parish* (New York: Fleming H. Revell 1905): pp. 83-102

doctors and nurses, to work with him. Soon dissatisfied with merely healing bodies and saving souls, the normal job of a medical missionary, Grenfell quickly branched out into other fields. To sustain his endeavours he began raising funds not only in Great Britain and Newfoundland, but in Canada and the United States, and there tapped into a brand new source of contributors, workers and patrons. They formed supporting committees in various American and Canadian cities. Grenfell's Labrador territory included a section of the coast falling within the boundaries of Canada, and in 1899–1900 he extended his sphere to embrace the coast of northern Newfoundland, establishing his main base at St. Anthony.

This anthology seeks to tell the story of what to its participants seemed like a remarkable adventure—the Grenfell Mission. Those who worked for the Mission as well as those who observed it are for the most part allowed to speak for themselves, with editorial comment restricted to an introduction to each selection. The material has been chosen from an astonishing variety of first-hand accounts, an embarrassment of riches, all previously published with the exception of one piece—Grenfell's letter to the colonial secretary, a minister of the Newfoundland government, written in August 1919. Grenfell alone produced thirty-three books and scores of articles, not including his regular contributions to *Toilers of the Deep*, the monthly journal of the Mission (later, Royal National Mission) to Deep Sea Fishermen, as well as to *Among the Deep Sea Fishers*, a quarterly magazine devoted exclusively to the Labrador and Newfoundland work. As well there was Grenfell's 'Log,' occasional reports of his activities distributed to newspapers in Newfoundland, the United States and Canada. Many of his staff were prolific writers. And this does not take into account the seemingly endless flow of words stemming from the pens of those who served the Mission as volunteers—doctors, nurses, dentists, teachers, artists, craftspeople, nutritionists, horticulturists, people skilled in all professions and trades, not to mention university students (known as 'Wops') bent on excitement. The Mission's workers—salaried staff and volunteers—numbered around five thousand (5000!) between the 1920s and 1950s alone, and many more came before them. They came north in droves and formed the Grenfell 'alumni.' In addition to sending students and staff, American universities, colleges and medical schools financed hospitals, nursing stations, vessels and schools.

From the Table of Contents it may be seen that as far as possible, the selections are arranged chronologically to correspond with three time periods: the Mission's early years (1892 to roughly 1914); its middle years (1915 to 1939); and the Mission after Grenfell (1940 to present). In the text, in introductions to the text, and in photo captions and margin notes, the words "served" and "service" crop up frequently. The words are not mine but reflect the way the Mission and its workers saw themselves. Editing has been limited mostly to the standardization of capitalization and spelling.

For an overview of Grenfell's career, the reader is referred to Ronald Rompkey's *Grenfell of Labrador: A Biography*, published in 1991 by the University of Toronto Press. It covers his early years in particular and explores the forces, spiritual and otherwise, that motivated his initial decision to work as a doctor in the North Sea, among fishermen. Grenfell idealized fishermen, regarding them as a special breed of people—paragons of daring and resourcefulness, virtue and romance—the qualities he admired most. Rompkey provides the background of Grenfell's altered role within the Deep Sea Mission, of how he transformed his own personal field of action from adjacent British seas to the coasts of Labrador and northern Newfoundland, and traces the growth of the International Grenfell Association. In 1914 the International Grenfell Association (IGA) was formally created, to include five associated bodies: the Royal National Mission to Deep Sea Fishermen; the Grenfell Association of America; the New England Grenfell Association; the Grenfell Medical Mission (of Canada); and the Grenfell Association of Newfoundland. Their job was to raise the money enabling the IGA to administer and direct all the various enterprises associated with the name 'Grenfell' in Labrador and Newfoundland, hiring staff and allocating funds. The IGA was managed by a board of ten directors, each of the associated or subscribing associations nominating two; its main office was in St. John's, Newfoundland, but most business was conducted from New York. Grenfell was superintendent of the IGA, even though by the 1920s he spent most of his time on tour, lecturing on his Mission's behalf at churches, clubs and halls in order to create an endowment fund of $1.5 million, maintaining an arduous speaking schedule while drawing only a modest income for himself. In 1926 Grenfell formed the Grenfell Association of Great Britain and Ireland and gradually severed his ties with the Deep Sea Mission. The number of Newfoundlanders fishing coastal Labrador had by this time sharply dropped in response to poor fish markets, and the Grenfell Mission was serving an increasingly settler clientele living further up the bays, away from the headlands. Communities like Cartwright and St. Mary's Harbour replaced those like Indian Harbour and Battle Harbour as centres for medical, educational and social services, and for agricultural and industrial development.

The twenty-three-year-old American Anne MacClanahan married Wilfred Grenfell (aged forty-four) in 1909. In the following pages she remains a shadowy figure, but her Mission role was hardly inconsequential. She was college educated, well connected and, unlike her husband, a born organizer with good business sense. Her contribution to the Mission's industrial department, its child welfare department and its educational fund were enormous. She handled arrangements for volunteer workers. As her husband's secretary she worked endlessly on his manuscripts, in some cases virtually producing them herself. And she brought the semblance of order to his near-chaotic life. Anne Grenfell was also effective in the 1920s in reorganizing the Mission's various departments and placing efficient women the likes of Harriot P. Houghteling (who married Charles Curtis), Dorothy Stirling and Marion R. Mosley—all friends of hers—in charge. Many of the Mission's larger benefactors, such as Louie A. Hall, were her friends as well.

Wilfred Grenfell worked like a man obsessed, but obsessed by what? A passion for the north? A love of Christ? A need to be useful? A desire to control? The romance and adventure of it all? Commentators have ascribed varying motives to Grenfell's particular version of practical, 'muscular,' Christianity, his creed of action, courage and achievement. But that he fostered a legend and left a mark none would dispute. In the following pages many traits of Grenfell's character emerge clearly—his love of physical activity and the outdoors, his dedication, his personal magnetism, his infectious vitality and above all, his understanding that the problems of the north were long-term and structural and that life could be improved by an onslaught on several fronts—health, educational, social, economic and industrial. Other less attractive traits surface more obliquely—his insensitivity, his Anglo-Saxon ethnocentricity, his vagueness, his impatience and his intolerance of authority and detail, even though he exercised the former with an indomitable sway. The Grenfell Mission was in every sense colonial, being almost entirely financed, staffed and run by foreigners, foreigners who furthermore had a particular conception of how society should operate. So it is not difficult to sympathize with the Mission's detractors in St. John's, the capital of Newfoundland, which from 1855 to 1934 enjoyed not only Responsible Government but full Dominion status, yet saw a large part of its territory controlled by people from away. What annoyed the opposition most was the general tone of Mission publicity: benevolent but condescending, always concentrating on extremes.

After Grenfell the Mission persevered, if not prospered. Just as workers had come in his lifetime they continued to come after his death, propelled, one can assume, by many of the same forces that had propelled him. The IGA itself had grown into an efficient business organization controlled by powerful directors. Grenfell 'alumni' had always provided considerable sums of money and gradually they had taken over the boards of the supporting associations. But directors were aloof and far from the field. The Mission's workers on site, moreover, no matter how well prepared in advance or how committed they might be, could never fully make common cause with local people, from whom they were distanced by culture, experience and background. So the Mission remained forever caught on the edge of a precipice—seeking to foster independence on the one hand but creating dependence on the other; never able to make the transition from mission to community service. Local people were continually overwhelmed by the presence of outsiders, permitted little or no say in the formulation of policies and programs designed ostensibly for them.

Acknowledgements

A number of people have been instrumental in the production of this book. My chief thanks are due to Dr Peter Roberts of Grenfell Regional Health Services (GRHS) whose support for the project has been unstinting, and without whose encouragement the work would not have taken its present shape. At St. Anthony other staff, past and present, manifest a degree of kindness and good-will for which I have every reason to be grateful, not least for having provided me with insight into the way the Grenfell tradition has translated into the present. I appreciate the support of those associated with the IGA and the Grenfell Centennial Committee, whose members have coordinated this year's events. The assistance of Gillian Hillyard of the Grenfell Historical Society warrants particular mention. Staff at the Centre for Newfoundland Studies of Memorial University have been helpful in various ways. Tor Fosnaes of Mobilewords has provided me with editorial advice; Joan Morgan and Susan Meyers with typing assistance; Ann Devlin-Fischer of the Provincial Archives of Newfoundland and Labrador with access to photographs (see p. iv for an identifying list); and Janice Udell with the print appearing on the front cover. To publisher Don Morgan I owe a special thanks for his unfailing patience and good humour.

P.O'B

BE YOU A REAL DOCTOR?*

*On 15 June 1892, on board the hospital vessel Albert, Dr Wilfred Thomason
Grenfell set sail from Great Yarmouth, England, on the first leg of his voyage
to Labrador. Departing on 2 August from St. John's, Newfoundland, he arrived
at Domino Run in southern Labrador, his first anchorage. The following is his
account of what followed.*

At last we came to anchor among many schooners in a wonderful natural
harbour called Domino Run, so named because the northern fleets all pass
through it on their way north and south. Had we been painted scarlet, and
flown the Black Jack instead of the Red Ensign, we could not have attracted
more attention. Flags of greeting were run up to all mastheads, and boats from
all sides were soon aboard inquiring into the strange phenomenon. Our object
explained, we soon had calls for a doctor, and it has been the experience of
almost every visitor to the coast from that day to this that he is expected to have
a knowledge of medicine.

One impression made on my mind that day undoubtedly influenced all my
subsequent actions. Late in the evening, when the rush of visitors was largely
over, I noticed a miserable bunch of boards, serving as a boat, with only a dab
of tar along its seams, lying motionless a little way from us. In it, sitting silent,
was a half-clad, brown-haired, brown-faced figure. After long hesitation,
during which time I had been watching him from the rail, he suddenly asked:

"Be you a real doctor?"

"That's what I call myself," I replied.

"Us hasn't got no money," he fenced, "but there's a very sick man ashore, if
so be you'd come and see him."

A little later he led me to a tiny sod-covered hovel, compared with which the
Irish cabins were palaces. It had one window of odd fragments of glass. The
floor was of pebbles from the beach; the earth walls were damp and chilly. There
were half a dozen rude wooden bunks built in tiers around the single room,
and a group of some six neglected children, frightened by our arrival, were
huddled together in one corner. A very sick man was coughing his soul out in
the darkness of a lower bunk, while a pitiably covered woman gave him cold
water to sip out of a spoon. There was no furniture except a small stove with
an iron pipe leading through a hole in the roof.

My heart sank as I thought of the little I could do for the sufferer in such
surroundings. He had pneumonia, a high fever, and was probably tubercular.
The thought of our attractive little hospital on board at once rose to my mind;
but how could one sail away with this husband and father, probably never to
bring him back. Advice, medicine, a few packages of food were only temporiz-
ing. The poor mother could never nurse him and tend the family. Furthermore,
their earning season, 'while the fish were in,' was slipping away. To pray for
the man, and with the family, was easy, but scarcely satisfying. A hospital and
a trained nurse was the only chance for this bread-winner—and neither was
available.

I called in a couple of months later as we came south before the approach of
winter. Snow was already on the ground. The man was dead and buried; there
was no provision whatever for the family, who were destitute, except for the
hollow mockery of a widow's grant of twenty dollars a year [from the New-

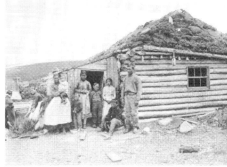

A Labrador home and family

The caption in Grenfell's album reads,
'Widow Thomas and her family of which
two are away.'

---

* Wilfred T. Grenfell, *A Labrador Doctor: The Autobiography of Wilfred Thomason Grenfell, M.D.*
(*Oxon.*), *C.M.G.* (Boston and New York: Houghton and Mifflin 1919)

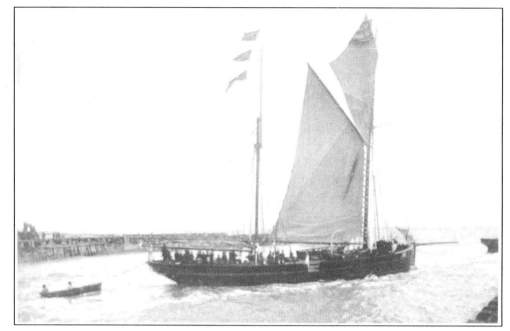

The *Albert* sets sail from Great Yarmouth on the first leg of its voyage to Labrador

A hospital vessel belonging to the Mission to Deep Sea Fishermen, the *Albert* was 155 gross tons and roughly 100 feet in length. From its spacious hold Grenfell distributed used clothing, Bibles, books and religious tracts, and as well held religious services on board.

foundland government]. This, moreover, had to be taken up in goods at a truck store, less debts *if* she owed any.

Among the nine hundred patients that still show on the records of that long-ago voyage, some stand out more than others for their peculiar pathos and their utter helplessness. I shall never forget one poor Eskimo. In firing a cannon to salute the arrival of the Moravian Mission ship, the gun exploded prematurely, blowing off both the man's arms below the elbows. He had been lying on his back for a fortnight, the pathetic stumps covered only with far from sterile rags dipped in cold water. We remained some days, and did all we could for his benefit; but he too joined the great host that is forever 'going west,' for want of what the world fails to give them.

… One mere boy came to me with necrosis of one side of his lower jaw due to nothing but neglected toothache. It had to be dug out from the new covering of bone which had grown up all around it. The whimsical expression of his lop-sided face still haunts me.

Deformities went untreated. The crippled and blind halted through life, victims of what 'the blessed Lord saw best for them.' The torture of an ingrowing toe-nail, which could be relieved in a few minutes, had incapacitated one poor father for years. Tuberculosis and rickets carried on their evil work unchecked. Preventable poverty was the efficient handmaid of these two latter diseases.

There was also much social work to be done in connection with the medical. Education in every one of its branches—especially public health—was almost non-existent—as were many simple social amenities which might have been so easily induced.…

Obviously the coast offered us work that would not be done unless we did it. Here was real need along any line on which one could labour, in a section of our own Empire, where the people embodied all our best sea traditions. They exhibited many of the attractive characteristics which, even when buried beneath habits and customs the outcome of their environment, always endear men of the sea to the genuine Anglo-Saxon. They were uncomplaining, optimistic, splendidly resourceful, cheerful and generous.

After our first cruise of three months in a small schooner, without power, the freezing sea drove us out, and I found myself sailing back across the Atlantic, studying my records of over 900 cases, which included almost every kind of surgical need, and arrears of medical neglect that were challenge enough for any one man's life.

W. Grenfell 1930 (2)

IT WAS A MEMORABLE DAY*

John Thomas Richards (1875-1958), a native of Bareneed, Conception Bay, was among the hundreds of Newfoundland fishermen encountered by Grenfell during the course of his trip along the coast, when initial impressions were formed on both sides. Encouraged by the Grenfell medical missionary Dr Graham Aspland, Richards in 1899 entered teachers' training in St. John's and then studied to become an Anglican minister. In 1904 he achieved his ambition when appointed to the Mission of Flowers Cove: it encompassed some 120 miles of coast on both sides of the Strait of Belle Isle, in the heart of Grenfell's territory. Richards remained at this post until 1945, an able cleric, a regular contributor to Among the Deep Sea Fishers, *and a staunch supporter of Grenfell and his Mission.*

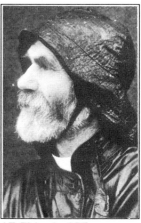

J.T. Richards, OBE

Time: August, 1892. He sat on a log and talked to the fishermen at Indian Tickle, Labrador. It was early morning and the fishers awaited the return of the bait boat with its load of shining caplin, their bait, before sailing away to the fishing grounds.

I drew near, and, for the first time, saw him and heard his voice. That face, that form, that voice, I should never more forget. With slouched hat, light home-spun suit, and thigh rubbers, he sat there and held those fishermen spellbound, as he broke the news of the great fire at St. John's, and recounted the destruction of the various parts of the city in detail.

I was a lad of seventeen. My father, a planter, who took a crew from the south of Newfoundland to fish cod every summer, had taken me with him at the age of nine.

He had died in May, and my three brothers and I assumed control of the summer fishery. My education had been thus interrupted at a very early age, and whilst a great desire for knowledge possessed my soul, I could only hope to acquire such odds and ends as could be gleaned from the scant supply of

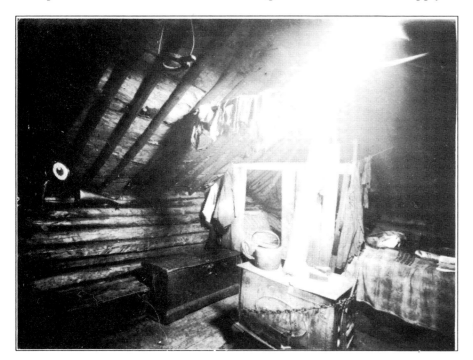

Interior of a Labrador home

* J.T. Richards, *Snapshots of Grenfell*, Irving Letto, intro. (St. John's: Creative Publishers 1989). Copyright, Irving Letto

reading matter one could procure. To meet an educated Englishman who, at once, took so great an interest in us fishermen, was an outstanding event in my life.

A little later he went outside the harbour and brought in his mission-ship, a sloop with a spanker. We fishermen had never seen a vessel so rigged before, and were greatly interested. Dr Grenfell was himself a navigator, but had with him a captain. At present he must sail cautiously. Charts of the day did not locate all shoals, as he was to find out by experience. Fishermen of that day were not a godless lot. True, we were, on the whole, illiterate; but we had kindly hearts, and we said our prayers. Sunday was a day of rest, and, from experience, I can testify that six consecutive days arising at two in the morning and toiling until ten, eleven, and sometimes midnight, made the Sabbath morn, especially for sleepy youths, a time of unconscious joy and gladness. A nice spacious building had been built by the summer fishermen, and here we assembled on Sunday evenings for prayers. If, by chance, an itinerant missionary came along we would crowd this Bethel; otherwise a local lay reader would officiate. When it was announced that this strange doctor would hold a service on Sunday, and in the night display a magic lantern, something extremely rare in those days, the building was literally crammed. I can see him now standing there, and in the simplest language, telling the old, old story. We were used to it in our services at our various real homes in south Newfoundland.

There was something unusually attractive, however, in the voice, the fervour and the personality of this young English doctor. When he threw on the screen that beautiful picture "The Rock of Ages," with a figure clinging to its base, as the waves dashed around it, there was a real hush in the audience, as in clear-cut, simple phrase, he proclaimed Christ as the Rock, the sure Refuge, the Shelter in time of stress and temptation.

I have never forgotten, simply because I could not forget, the text of the first address I heard him give.

"Noah was a just man and perfect in his generations, and Noah walked with God." Genesis VI:9.

That Sunday was a memorable day with us fishermen at Indian Tickle, Labrador.

Here was a medical doctor to heal our sick, to cure our festered fingers, chafed by the fishing line, or torn by the barbed trawl hook; but here, too, was a man of God, whose simple Christ-like spirit was to make him beloved by the fishermen of Labrador, as Jesus, whom he then and always preached to be the eternal Son of God, was followed and beloved two thousand years before by the humble fishermen of the Sea of Galilee.

As I watched his crew pulling on board his sloop after service that Sunday, and heard their sweet English voices singing "Throw out the life line," I longed, as I had never longed for anything before, to be one of his crew and help, even in that humble way, to carry this great medical missionary and his ministrations to the thousands of my fellow fishermen, scattered along the ironbound coast of Labrador.

Splitting fish at Blanc Sablon, 1892

Battle Harbour, Labrador

In the foreground nets are spread to dry; in the background, the 'fields of fish.'

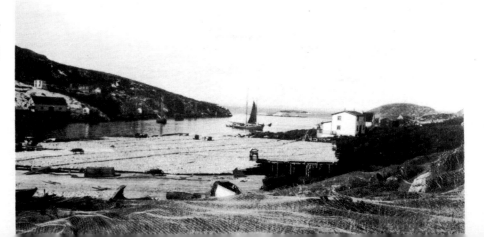

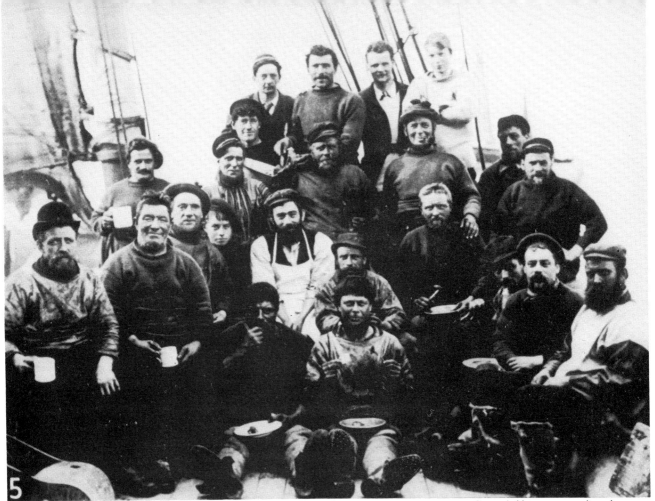
Several skippers come aboard

THEM ARE GOOD MEN*

The Reverend John Sidey, resident Methodist minister in southern Labrador, was witness to the unexpected arrival of the Albert *at Red Bay as the vessel headed south on its return voyage that first fall. His following description appeared in the* Methodist Monthly Greeting *towards the end of 1892.*

All through the summer we had heard about it; many vessels, either trading or fishing, had visited our harbour, and the friendly crews had aroused our curiosity by their recitals of the work being done by the Mission ship and its crew. "Them are good men, whomever they be," said one, while another expatiated, with all a sailor's delight to sailors equally delighted, upon the size and rig and sailing powers of the vessel, until we were all hoping she would pay us a visit. The probability of this latter question was very freely discussed among our fishermen, who, now the season was well-nigh over and no more fish to be caught, were to be found daily sitting about in small groups, smoking and talking with that peculiar gravity which belong to the liveyers of the coast.... Would she come here? Many shook their heads, "No" ... "But why?" Then followed an argument on the pros and cons in fisherman fashion, with sundry allusions to the weather, the rough harbours, strong tides and the lateness of the season....

A strange-looking vessel was slowly making her way round the point. Two flags were flying, and, as she dropped anchor, we were able to read the insignia of the Mission plainly.... We decided to go on board. Boats filled with fishermen

* John Sidey quoted in J. Lennox Kerr, *Wilfred Grenfell: His Life and Work* (New York: Dodd, Mead 1959)

were already on the way out. We were just ready for a start when a sharp knock came on the door and on opening it we were greeted with "I am George Stoney [a member of the *Albert*'s crew], and this is Doctor Grenfell." Not much time did the worthy doctor give us for fraternal chat. He was soon asking us about the sick and the needy, and, with a promptness that was calculated to teach us a lesson, the three of us were out visiting the poorest of the families.

VIKINGS OF TODAY*

Frederick Treves (1853-1923), the eminent anatomist and surgeon, was an instructor at the London Hospital when Grenfell was a medical student. A highly motivated man, possessed of great energy and considerable persuasive powers, the young Wilfred found in him a sympathetic teacher and good role model. Treves loved the sea, held a master's certificate, and was chairman of the hospital committee of the Mission to Deep Sea Fishermen. It was he who suggested Grenfell take up mission work in the North Sea.

Treves published widely on medical and other topics; he served in the Boer War and during the First World War; he was surgeon extraordinary to Queen Victoria and Edward VII, and was knighted in 1902. For many years Treves remained a director of the Deep Sea Mission and a powerful influence in Grenfell's life.

In his following preface to Grenfell's first book, Vikings of Today, *Treves evokes a number of the themes and images—the Oxford athlete, the seafaring adventurer, the pluck, the daring and the manliness—that would become part of the Grenfell mythology.*

At the present time—near to the close of the nineteenth century—we are being constantly reminded, with somewhat unpleasant persistence, that the human race is degenerating and that the changes of decay are most marked among the most civilized people. It is among the young men especially that these unwelcome signs of the times are assumed to be the more noticeable. It is claimed that the splendid physique and the heroic courage of the British race are both deteriorating, and that those who seek for the time of noble deeds and sturdy hearts must turn back to the days of Elizabeth—to the stirring times of Drake and Raleigh.

There is said to be no longer a field for that pluck and daring, or for that determination and persistency, which at one period made the name of the British famous throughout the world.

It would be idle, in this place, to inquire into the substance of these moanings and regrets, and it would be reasonable perhaps to allow that there may be some real or apparent element of truth in these lamentations over the man of the present.

Be this as it may, it will be agreeable to those who are most concerned in these forebodings to turn to the record contained in this volume, while those who view with some disgust the fashionable youth of the day, with his many effeminacies and affectations, will find in the pages which follow some wholesome relief to their distaste.

Dr Grenfell's narrative will take the reader away from the heated, unnatural and debilitating atmosphere of the modern city, from the innervated [*sic*] crowd, from the pampered, self-indulgent colonies of men and women who make up fashionable society, and will carry him to a lonely land where all conventionalities vanish, and where man is brought into contact with the

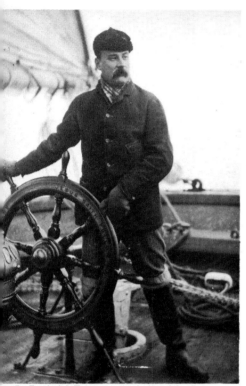

Dr Frederick Treves at the helm of the Deep Sea Mission's hospital vessel *Alice Fisher*

The Mission to Deep Sea Fishermen tended to the spiritual, social and medical needs of mainly British fishermen, initially in the North Sea and later further afield.

* Frederick Treves, Preface to Wilfred T. Grenfell, *Vikings of Today, or, Life and Medical Work among the Fishermen of Labrador* (London: Marshall Bros. 1895)

6

simplest elements of life and with the rudimentary problems of how to avoid starvation and ward off death from cold.

The present volume deals with a land of desolation, with a country hard, relentless, unsympathetic and cruel, where, among fogs and icebergs, a handful of determined men are trying to hold their own against hostile surroundings and to earn a living in defiance of dreary odds.

When the Mission to Deep Sea Fishermen resolved to send an expedition to Labrador, it was evident that the man to go with it was Grenfell. He was well known both at Oxford and in London as a hardy athlete; he was a skilled and able surgeon; he was profoundly interested in Mission work; and the sea had for him that magical attraction which a few centuries ago emptied nearly every little cove and fishing hamlet in Cornwall and Devon of its heartiest men, and carried them over the high seas to the ends of the earth.

Grenfell went, and the good work of the Mission was established on the Labrador. It was no little matter to bring into the hard and desperate life of the Labrador fishermen a touch of kindly and practical sympathy from the old country. It was no little matter to travel for many hundreds of miles along a grim, inhospitable coast, where buoys and beacons are unknown and where there is scarcely a bay or island which has not been the scene of some lonely disaster.

It will be seen from this book that the race of Vikings is not yet extinct, on the one hand, and that on the other the spirit of enterprise and daring is not yet lost to the English people, and that the modern rover of the sea differs from his predecessor in little save the motive of his expedition.

Those who know how to value the comforts of an English home, and who can appreciate the quiet content and the beauty of an English village, will be induced by this book to feel no little sympathy for those whose lives are cast among the dreary islands and deserted bays of Labrador.

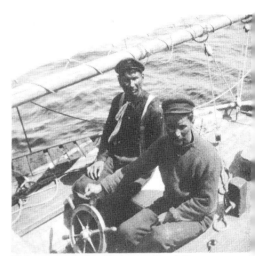

Fishermen at Indian Harbour—Grenfell's 'Vikings of today'

I AM ABOUT HIS BUSINESS*

Norman Duncan (1871-1916), born in Brantford, Ontario, graduated from the University of Toronto and in 1895 became a journalist in New York. In 1900, by arrangement with McClure's Magazine, *he came to Newfoundland to gather material for a series of sea tales. Duncan spent the better part of three summers in northern Newfoundland and one on the Labrador coast, travelling with Grenfell on the* Strathcona *in 1903. He quickly produced a series of articles and three books—*The Way of the Sea *(1903),* Doctor Luke of the Labrador *(1904) and* Dr Grenfell's Parish *(1905).*

Grenfell was already lecturing and fund-raising in Canada and the United States, but it was Duncan who, in the phrase of Grenfell biographer Ronald Rompkey, 'discovered' him for American readers. He presented Grenfell as a popular hero and contributed substantially to his success in print and on the lecture circuit.

Not many years ago, in the remoter parts of Newfoundland and on the long, bleak coast of Labrador, there were no doctors. The folk depended for healing upon traditional cures, upon old women who worked charms, upon remedies ingeniously devised to meet the need of the moment, upon deluded persons who prescribed medicines of the most curious description, upon a rough-and-ready surgery of their own ... Everywhere, indeed, there was need of a

---

* Norman Duncan, "Grenfell of the Medical Mission," *Harper's Magazine* 110 (1904): 28-37

Grenfell with young patient

physician of good heart and some skill to stop the waste of power and life. Death and pain were wanton on those coasts.

It must be said, however, that the Newfoundland government did provide a physician—of a sort. Every summer he was sent north with the mail-boat, which made not more than six trips, touching here and there at long intervals, and, of a hard season, failing altogether to reach the farthest ports. While the boat waited—an hour, or a half, as might be—the doctor went ashore to cure the sick, if he chanced to be in the humour; otherwise the folk brought the sick aboard, where they were painstakingly treated or not, as the doctor's humour went. The government seemed never to inquire too minutely into the qualifications and character of its appointee. The incumbent for many years—the folk thank God that he is dead—was an inefficient, ill-tempered, cruel man; if not the very man himself, he was of a kind with the Newfoundland physician who ran a flag of warning to his masthead when he set out to get very drunk....

While the poor 'liveyers' and Newfoundland fishermen thus depended upon the mail-boat doctor and their own strange inventions for relief, there was a well-born, Oxford-bred young Englishman of the name of Wilfred Grenfell walking the London hospitals. He was athletic, adventurous, dogged, unsentimental, merry, kind; moreover—and most happily—he was used to the sea, and he loved it. It chanced one night that he strayed into the Tabernacle in East London, where D.L. Moody, the American evangelist, was preaching. When he came out he had resolved to make his religion 'practical.' There was nothing violent in this—no fevered, ill-judged determination to martyr himself at all costs. It was a quiet resolve to make the best of his life—which he would have done at any rate, I think, for he was a young man of good breeding and the finest impulses. At once he cast about for "some way in which he could satisfy the aspirations of a young medical man, and combine with this a desire for adventure and definite Christian work."

I had never before met a missionary of that frank type. "Why," I exclaimed to him, off the coast of Labrador, not long ago, "you seem to *like* this sort of life!"

We were aboard the mission steamer, bound north under full steam and all sail. He had been in feverish haste to reach the northern harbours, where, as he knew, the sick were watching for his coming. The fair wind, the rush of the little steamer on her way, pleased him.

"Oh," said he, somewhat impatiently, "*I'm* not a martyr."

So he found what he sought. After applying certain revolutionary ideas to Sunday-school work in the London slums, in which a horizontal bar and a set of boxing-gloves for a time held equal place with the Bible and the hymn-book, he joined the staff of the Royal National Mission to Deep-sea Fishermen, and established the medical mission to the fishermen of the North Sea. When that work was organized—when the fight was gone out of it—he sought a harder task; he is of that type, then extraordinary but now familiar, which finds no delight where there is no difficulty. In the spring of 1892 he set sail from Great Yarmouth Harbour for Labrador in a ninety-ton schooner. Since then, in the face of hardship, peril, and prejudice, he has, with a light heart and strong purpose, healed the sick, preached the Word, clothed the naked, fed the starving, given shelter to them that had no roof, championed the wronged—in all, devotedly fought evil, poverty, oppression, and disease, for he is bitterly intolerant of those things.

"It's been jolly good fun," says he.

There is now a mission hospital at St. Anthony, near the extreme northeast point of the Newfoundland coast. There is another, well equipped and commodious at Battle Harbour—a rocky island lying out from the Labrador coast near the Strait of Belle Isle—which is open the year round; it is in charge of Dr

Cluny Macpherson, a courageous young physician, Newfoundland-born, who goes six hundred miles up the coast by dogteam in the dead of winter, finding shelter where he may, curing whom he can—everywhere seeking out those who need him, caring not a whit, it appears, for the peril and hardship of the long white road. There is a third at Indian Harbour, half-way up the coast, which is open through the fishing season. It is conducted with the care and precision of a London hospital—admirably kept, well-ordered, efficient. The physician in charge is Dr George H. Simpson—a wiry, keen, brave little Englishman, who goes about in an open boat, whatever the distance, whatever the weather; he is a man of splendid courage and sympathy: the fishing-folk love him for his kind heart and for the courage with which he responds to their every call.

"I wishes that poor man had one o' they launches," said a fisherman, as he watched the doctor put out in a punt when half a gale was blowing. "The Lord ought t' send un one."

There is also the little hospital steamer *Strathcona*, in which Dr Grenfell makes the round of all the coast, from the time of the break-up until the fall gales have driven the fishing-schooners home to harbour.

When Dr Grenfell first appeared on the coast, I am told, the folk thought him a madman of some benign description. He knew nothing of the reefs, the tides, the current, cared nothing, apparently, for the winds; he sailed with the confidence and reckless courage of a Labrador skipper. Fearing at times to trust his schooner in unknown waters, he went about in a whaleboat, and so hard did he drive her that he wore her out in a single season. She was capsized with all hands, once driven out to sea, many times nearly swamped, once blown on the rocks; never before was a boat put to such tasks on that coast, and at the end of it she was wrecked beyond repair. Next season he appeared with a little steam-launch, the *Princess May*—her beam was eight feet!—in which he not only journeyed from St. John's to Labrador, to the astonishment of the whole colony, but sailed the length of that bitter coast, passing into the Gulf and safely out again, and pushing to the very farthest settlements in the north. Late in the fall, upon the return journey to St. John's in stormy weather, she was reported lost, and many a skipper, I suppose, wondered that she had lived so long; but she weathered a gale that bothered the mail-boat, and triumphantly made St. John's, after as adventurous a voyage, no doubt, as ever a boat of her measure survived.

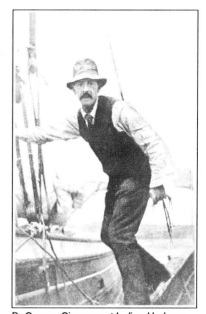

Dr George Simpson at Indian Harbour

A man of action, courage and conviction, he fit the Grenfell model.

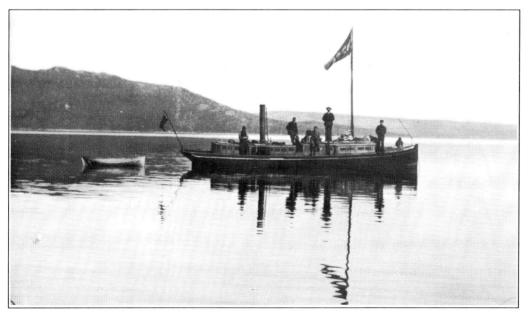

The steam launch *Princess May*, which journeyed the length of the eastern Newfoundland and Labrador coast in 1893

This particular voyage established Grenfell's reputation for daring but skilful seamanship. He is standing amidships.

"Sure," said a skipper, "I don't know how she done it. The Lord," he added, piously, "must kape an eye on that man."

There is a new proverb on the coast. The folk say, when a great wind blows, "This'll bring Grenfell!" Often it does. He is impatient of delay, fretted by inaction; a gale is the wind for him—a wind to take him swiftly towards the place ahead. Had he been a weakling he would long ago have died on the coast; had he been a coward, a multitude of terrors would long ago have driven him to a life ashore; had he been anything but a true man and tender, indeed, he would long ago have retreated under the suspicion and laughter of the folk. But he has outsailed the Labrador skippers—outdared them—done deeds of courage under their very eyes that they would shiver to contemplate—never in a foolhardy spirit; always with the object of kindly service. So he has the heart and willing hand of every honest man on the Labrador—and of none more than of the men of his crew, who take the chances with him; they are wholly devoted....

In the course of time the *Princess May* was wrecked or worn out. Then came the *Julia Sheridan* ... Many a gale she weathered, off 'the worst coast in the world'—often, indeed, in thick, wild weather, the doctor himself thought the little craft would go down ... Next came the *Sir Donald*—a stout ship, which in turn disappeared. The *Strathcona*, with a hospital amidships, is now doing duty; and she will continue to go up and down the coast, in and out of the inlets, until she in her turn finds the ice and the wind and the rocks too much for her.

" 'Tis bound t' come, soon or late," said a cautious friend of the mission. "He drives her too hard. He've a right t' do what he likes with his own life, I s'pose, but he've a call t' remember that the crew has folks t' home."

But the mission doctor is not inconsiderate; he is in a hurry—the coast is long, the season short, the need such as to wring a man's heart. Every new day holds an opportunity for doing a good deed—not if he dawdles in the harbours when a gale is abroad, but only if he passes swiftly from place to place, with a brave heart meeting the dangers as they come. He is the only doctor to visit the Labrador shore of the Gulf, the Straits shore of Newfoundland, the populous east coast of the northern peninsula of Newfoundland, the only doctor known to the Esquimaux and poor 'liveyers' of the northern coast of Labrador, the only doctor most of the 'liveyers' and green-fish catchers of the middle coast can reach, save the hospital physician at Indian Harbour. He has a round of three thousand miles to make. It is no wonder that he 'drives' the little steamer—even

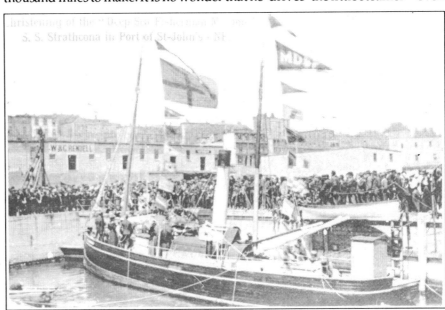

A Deep Sea Mission postcard showing the christening of the *Strathcona* in St. John's, 1900

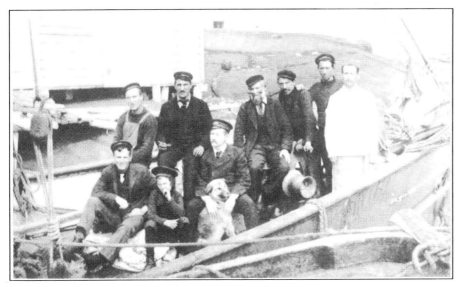

at full steam, with all sails spread (as I have known him to do), when the fog is thick and the sea is spread with great bergs.

"I'm in a hurry," he said, with an impatient sigh. "The season's late. We must get along."…

Fear of the sea is quite incomprehensible to this man…. Perhaps that is in part because he has a blessed lack of imagination, in part, perhaps because he has a body as sound as ever God gave to a man, and has used it as a man should; but it is chiefly because of his simple and splendid faith that he is an instrument in God's hands—God's to do with as He will, as he would say. His faith is exceptional, I am sure—childlike, steady, overmastering, and withal, if I may so characterize it, healthy. It takes something such as the faith he has to move a man to run a little steamer at full speed in the fog when there is ice on every hand. It is hardly credible, but quite true, and short of the truth; neither wind nor ice nor fog, nor all combined, can keep the *Strathcona* in harbour when there comes a call for help from beyond. The doctor clambers cheerfully out on the bowsprit and keeps both eyes open. "As the Lord wills," says he, "whether for wreck or service. I am about His business."

"What you going to be when you grow up?" I once asked a lad on the far north-east coast.

He looked at me in vast astonishment.

"What you going to *be*, what you going to *do*," I repeated, "when you grow up?"

Still he did not comprehend. "Eh?" he said.

"What you going to work at," said I, in desperation, "when you're a man?"

"Oh, zur," he answered, understanding at last, "I isn't clever enough t' be a parson!"

N. Duncan 1905

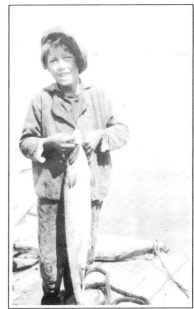

Duncan's fisherman in waiting

WE HAVE NO ORDAINED WORKERS*

By 1903, after eleven years of toiling, Grenfell had attracted the attention of American newspapers and Christian magazines. The Missionary Review of the World *published an article by Grenfell in which he emphasized the non-denominational aspect of his Mission's work.*

For the past eleven years we have been trying on the rocky coast of Labrador, to bring the living Christ as a transforming power into the lives of the twenty thousand fishermen who earn their livelihood there in the summer months. The Master has promised to make us 'fishers of men,' and He has proved His readiness to help us *catch* men if we are only ready to follow His bidding….

The governing body of our mission is a registered, limited liability, company called the 'Mission to Deep Sea Fishermen,' to which title our late beloved

* Wilfred T. Grenfell, "Among the Vikings of Labrador," *Missionary Review of the World* 16, no. 7, new series (1903): 481-2

During my early years on the coast a patient came to me with a hand practically blown to bits from a gun accident. He had been loading the little 'darling,' as he affectionately termed his ancient muzzle-loader, when it exploded. After weeks of hospitalization, trying to save one thumb and one finger so that he could pull on a line, it became necessary to graft skin on the newly made hand. My assistant at that time was a Scotchman, who donated good Scotch Presbyterian skin for the back of the hand, while I supplied English Church of England skin for the palm. The patient was an Irish Catholic—but the completed member did its work just as efficiently and perhaps more so, as an example of church unity.

W. Grenfell 1938

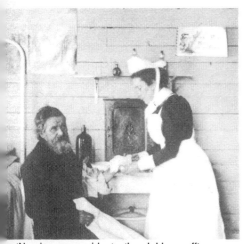

'Nursing gun accident—thumb blown off'

Queen added the title, 'Royal National,' in 1897, expressing the hope that it might do truly royal work in the service of the King of kings. The denomination of the work is best described by the boy who, when asked to what denomination his minister belonged, replied: "Well, I guess he ain't any special kind—just plain minister." We have no ordained workers. Our missionaries are our doctors, nurses, sailors, and fishermen.... It so happens that to-day our three Labrador doctors are respectively Episcopalian, Methodist, and Congregational, while the brother who left us last year and his wife, our nurse from Battle Harbour Hospital, were Presbyterians. What does it matter? We build no church, we have no settled congregation. We can not administer a different pill or plaster because our patients are Catholic, Protestant, or sceptic. There is no need to adjust a medicine to the idiosyncrasy of an Episcopalian or Salvationist. All we can hope to do is to draw the fishermen nearer to our Master, who, when He was on earth, loved fishermen so well.

AN UNQUALIFIED SUCCESS*

With Grenfell on the Strathcona *in 1903 was Dr Rufus Kingman, a surgeon from Boston who, at Grenfell's invitation but his own expense, took a month of his vacation to work with the Mission. So successful was the arrangement that Kingman became the first of scores of North American specialists who came north, bringing a calibre and range of medical and surgical services the envy of all other parts of Newfoundland. Through the years, these volunteers brought incalculable benefits to the Mission. Grenfell's following letter was written to the editor of* Among the Deep Sea Fishers.

Dear Mr Editor,

It is not every day that the fisherfolk on the Labrador have the opportunity of taking their ailments to an American specialist. Such, however, has been their luck this year, for Dr Kingman of Boston joined me on the 28th of July, and has been flying around visiting such cases as fell in his line, much to the advantage of many of them. I am beginning to think that we have solved a knotty point in our medical work. For it is a patent fact that in these days no one man can be as efficient in every line of medicine and surgery as a specialist who turns all his talents to one peculiar class of cases. Moreover, while this visit is good for our friends, it is equally good for us, affording us the very opportunities that we usually have to devote our vacations to seeking. I mean attaining some of the teaching direct from the great hospitals. Alas! This year I was only venturesome enough to arrange with one, for it was impossible to tell how such an experiment would turn out. It has proved such an unqualified success that I shall hope to repeat it without fail next year. Indeed, already one of the best known of Chicago surgeons has promised me part of his holiday next year.... We are now hoping next year to arrange with an eye specialist to visit us, and spend a month of his holiday going round in the *Strathcona*. This will add very materially to the boon our hospitals confer on the people, for not only will medical aid be placed within their reach, but that aid, as in the great centres of civilization, will be the best that can be obtained. This is the privilege of the poorest in all the great hospitals. At the same time the magnificent air of Labrador and its undoubted value as a health resort, specially adapted to people

* Wilfred T. Grenfell, "The Log of the S.S. *Strathcona*," *Among the Deep Sea Fishers* 1, no. 3 (1903): 6-8

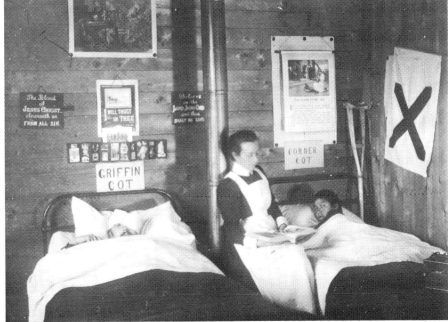

Interior of the Battle Harbour Hospital, a male ward

The religious sayings on the wall were typical of the Mission's hospitals. Subscribers and patrons provided funds for the upkeep of particular beds, which were then called after them.

who live in the heat and dust and noise of the modern American cities, will, we hope, become much more widely known. Not least to benefit has been our friend the surgeon, who goes back able to state that he can sleep well even after drinking tea, and that he can enjoy a pipe after meals without fear of semi-asphyxiation.

FAR TOO HEAVY A BURDEN*

Kingman's services to Grenfell extended beyond the medical, for he was among the first to suggest publicly the need of an American organization to support the Labrador work. This led to the founding in 1905 of the Grenfell Association of New York; in 1907 it became the Grenfell Association of America. Formed in 1907 also was the Grenfell Association of New England, with its headquarters in Boston.

In the following selection Kingman speaks to the enormity of the task Grenfell had set for himself, and conveys his immense, restless energy and dedication to the work in hand.

My two weeks spent with Dr Grenfell on the *Strathcona* impressed me most deeply, not only with the devotion, consecration and heroism of the man, but with the enormous and well-nigh overwhelming nature of the load of responsibility which he is carrying. He is strong, robust, seems scarcely to feel fatigue, and whether he is hungry or sleepy, or cold, or wet is alike immaterial and unnoticed if there is work to be done. But this ought not to be permitted. He is carrying far too heavy a burden, and unless something be done to lighten the responsibilities, the medical mind can only foresee a time when the breakdown must come. To preach the gospel, to care for the sick, to render all manner of surgical aid along a thousand miles of coast, to succour the starving and clothe the perishing, to direct the hospitals, to navigate the steamer, to devise and direct the various commercial agencies by which the people are taught and helped to help themselves, to administer the laws, and last, and worst of all, to listen to and sympathize with the endless tale of woe and suffering—how long, think you, can any one man do all this and do it properly and live?

It is well for us to sit in our comfortable homes while the winter storms pile the snow about our doors, or to make vacation trips in midsummer to the scene of these duties, but we owe a greater duty and service to this man and to his

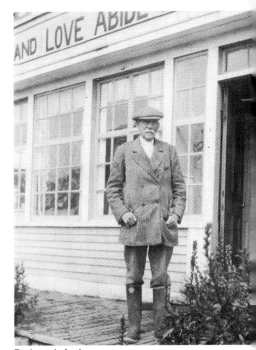

Dr Joseph Andrews

An eye, ear, nose and throat specialist from Santa Barbara, California, Andrews volunteered his services every summer for eighteen years.

* Rufus A. Kingman, "Personal Observations," *Among the Deep Sea Fishers* 1, no. 4 (1904): 5-6

associates … In my judgement some means must be found whereby a portion of this load of responsibility, and a large part of the worry and annoyance incident to the scrutiny and decision of points of minor detail should be removed from the present overburdened shoulders and be otherwise provided for. It is not for me to say how this is to be done. I simply record this as my earnest conviction, the outgrowth of close personal observation on the ground, and in this conviction I am sure those who were my fellow-travellers last summer will heartily coincide.

A SERMON WITH A CO-OPERATIVE STORE AS A TEXT*

Lyman Abbott was a Congregational minister in New York and the editor of Outlook *magazine when Grenfell first came to his attention in 1903. Sharing his commitment to social reform, Abbott actively promoted Grenfell's cause and became an influential ally. In Outlook's July 1903 issue, Abbott introduced the Labrador doctor and in the same issue presented Grenfell's own account of his life and accomplishments to date.*

In the following extract, Grenfell describes his initial, daring venture into co-operation at Red Bay, where in 1896 he established the first of his cash co-operative stores. Some of the stores survived but others failed: 'keeping the store for Christ' was no guarantee of sound management.

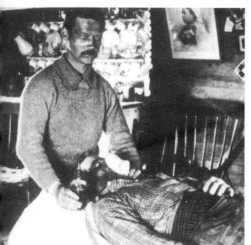

Grenfell administering an anaesthetic in preparation for home surgery

In the early days my great problem, and the cause of most of the disease and suffering in Labrador, was poverty; and that poverty was not, as in many places, the result of sin, as in indulgence-in-liquor cases, or of selfishness, but poverty resulting from helplessness. So, among the utterly scientific efforts to treat the ills of the Labrador and New-foundland coast, we had absolutely no alternative except to consider poverty as a disease to be remedied, as a condition calling for public health effort.

W. Grenfell 1930 (1)

Here other methods of commending our Gospel are also open to us, owing to the extraordinary poverty and isolation of the people. Lack of experience made us satisfied for the first three years to try and cope with the question of hunger and nakedness, by collecting and distributing warm clothing, and assisting the people in various ways to get food.

It was not until 1896 that, seeing the futility of giving financial help to men who had to pay from $7 to $8 for a barrel of flour worth $4, and $2.50 to $3 for a hogshead of salt which could be bought at St. John's for $1, we set to work to find a new sermon to preach on this subject. Many of our most piteous cases at hospital were the direct fruit of chronic semi-starvation. Thus our people fell victims to tuberculosis of glands and bones, owing only to the marasmus [a wasting away of the body] induced by insufficient food. This was more especially the case among children. A universal system of truck business prevailed: the 'catch' of tomorrow was mortgaged for the food of today. The people seldom or never saw cash. The inevitable results were poverty, thriftlessness, and eventually hopelessness. The contention of the trader was always that the men's poverty was because they did not catch enough to support themselves. The answer was that they got enough to support at least thirty traders.

We started a sermon with a co-operative store as a text. The people round it were all heavily in debt; most winters they received so much government relief to keep them from actual starvation that the place was known as 'The Sink.' The people were almost all illiterate and knew nothing about business, and the little store went through varying fortunes. They had very, very little money to put in, and even that they were afraid to put in under their own names, for fear the traders should find out and punish them. One trader wrote me denying our right to interfere with *his* people, as if those whom he had tried to lead me to think were only the recipients of his 'charity' existed solely for the benefit of his trade….

* Wilfred T. Grenfell, "Among the Deep-Sea Fishermen," *Outlook* 74 (1903): 695-701

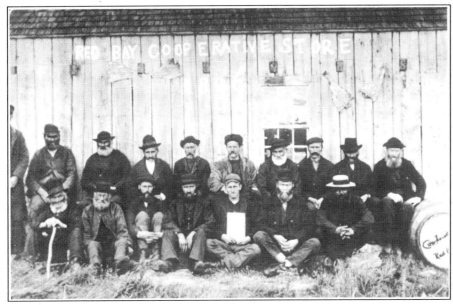

Grenfell's first producer and consumer co-operative at Red Bay, 1896, Grenfell seated mid-rear

Few of the co-operatives survived after the First World War, though in 1941 the store at Red Bay still carried on under the direction of W.Y. Pike.

Looking at the results of the sermon seven years afterwards, I find the people clothed, fed, independent, with a new little church building, and children far-and-away better clad and educated. The movement has spread; there are now five co-operative stores, with a schooner called the *Co-operator* which carries their products to and from the markets. The price of flour has been uniformly kept under $5 a barrel; the price of salt has been reduced nearly 50 per cent, and other things in proportion. We have had many troubles, owing to poor fisheries, to our own ignorance of methods of business, and to our isolation. But our storekeepers and crew are Christian men, well aware that the best Gospel they can preach is to keep the store for Christ.

Sir Wilfred Grenfell must be regarded as the father of co-operatives in Newfoundland.
J. Smallwood 1937

Co-operative distribution is one interpretation of the Christian religion.
W. Grenfell 1929

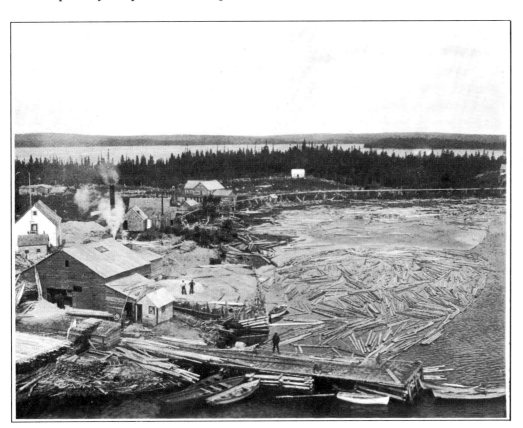

The sawmill at Roddickton in Canada Bay, northern Newfoundland

This was Grenfell's first attempt to provide off-season employment. Like his other industrial enterprises, he viewed it as a public health effort.

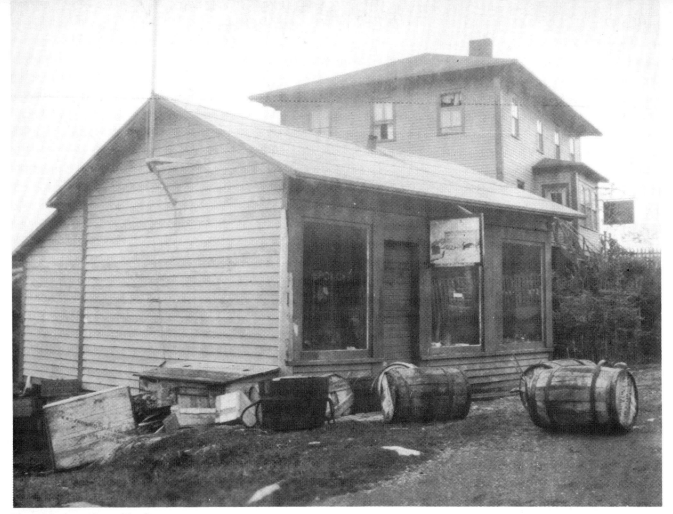

The original premises of the St. Anthony Spot Cash Co-operative Company

The sign, devised by Grenfell, shows huskies pulling a komatik laden with supplies to a settler's door. The inscription reads: 'Spot Cash is always the leader.' On the other side, a vessel named *Spot Cash* is seen bravely ploughing through towering waves and mountainous icebergs. It is inscribed, 'There's no sinking her.' Behind the store is St. Anthony's Inn, a Mission-run hostel for visitors.

OPPOSITION IN ST. JOHN'S

Grenfell's reputation as a benefactor was growing in the rest of North America, but in the city of St. John's he was losing ground. By 1905, opposition there had emerged publicly. Ranged against Grenfell, and willing to vent their grievances in the press, were forces resentful of outside interference in the affairs of the colony and hostile to anything that threatened vested interests. They included merchants, traders and ecclesiastics.

The Trade Review *spoke for commercial interests. For obvious reasons, they opposed Grenfell's co-operative ventures and distribution of used clothing and other goods. The* Evening Telegram, *which supported the governing party of Sir Robert Bond, adopted a more cautious approach. The anti-Bond* Daily News *opened its columns to Roman Catholic archbishop M.F. Howley, an ardent Newfoundland nationalist with an agenda of his own. Church leaders in general had been alienated by Grenfell's suggestion that they were neglecting their Labrador flock, as well as by his evangelism, his militant anti-sectarian stance and his advocacy of non-denominational schools. The* Royal Gazette *reflected the views of the Newfoundland governor, Sir William MacGregor, a Grenfell supporter.*

The following selections from the press over a three-week period in 1905, during Grenfell's fall visit to St. John's, reflect a variety of political, economic, religious and cultural views. They suggest the threat Grenfell posed to, if nothing else, local dignity and pride.

Trade Review 25 November 1905

This is about the time of year that a gentleman known in this country as Dr Grenfell begins to publish in some of the local papers what he calls his 'Log.' As the matter contained in the 'Log' is about as interesting as the back of a bill of lading, and as original as a police court summons, it is safe to say that not one man in a thousand reads it; but, if the writings of the doctor are not interesting, no one can deny that the doctor himself is an interesting man. He comes to us in the triple capacity of philanthropist, evangelist, and trader, his special sphere of action being the rugged coast of Labrador. What he has achieved in the first two capacities is problematical, but, there can be no doubt about it, he has made considerable money by his mission.

There are but few men sufficiently gifted to successfully point to the Heavenly Jerusalem with one hand and sell 'old clo'[thes]' with the other, but it appears that the doctor is one of the number. It is said that he can talk of the golden streets and dilate on the beauties of a $5 suit of clothes almost in one breath; that he can enlarge on the better life and buy a consignment of skin boots at the same time (at the lowest possible price), without ever turning a hair. That a man of such exceptional parts should make money on the Labrador coast is not to be wondered at, and we are not surprised to hear that he will soon retire from the mission with what the sinful and vulgar would call his 'whack of spondulics.' Of course, the doctor's principal object in going to Labrador was philanthropy, and if he has made money it is entirely against his will.

The doctor, like a number of other gentlemen who have visited us from time to time, discovered, a few years ago, that the Labrador fisherman was suffering untold hardships, and that nothing could make him so happy as the cast-off raiment of the benevolent Briton, especially if he were charged a good price for it. On looking over the ground, the doctor discovered that there were a number of Newfoundland traders trying to do business along the coast, and, ordinarily, it would be pretty hard to dislodge them; but, on deeper investigation, it was found that these foolish people were paying duty on *all* the goods they traded in, and the only way to down them [ie. put them down] would be to get goods in duty free, and be in a position to undersell these ordinary common people who had been in the business for so many years.

Accordingly the doctor applied to the Newfoundland government to be permitted to drum up all the old clothes he could get in Great Britain, alleging that he would sell them cheap for produce only; and at such low figures as would be of immense benefit to residents or transient fishermen on the coast. To enhance the offer, he promised to erect three hospitals on the coast, in which to treat sick or disabled fishermen. As an offset for his outlay on the hospitals, however, he asked a certain annual grant from the government, to go towards the support of these institutions. Premier Bond, who has always had a weakness for the stranger who drifts this way, favoured the proposal, though he was opposed by many of his Executive, and [he] closed with it, thus laying the foundation of Dr Grenfell's fortune. One result of the arrangement is that hard-working Newfoundland traders, who ought to have certain vested rights in the business, have been practically driven out of it....

The only figures of the doctor's doings that we could get, come to us in a roundabout manner, namely, through the registrar of births, marriages, and deaths. From these, we learn that the death rate on Labrador has increased by over a hundred per cent on the coast since the establishment of the doctor's hospitals. In the last enumeration, before the great philanthropist established his hospitals and imported his cast-off clothing, the Labrador death rate was 9 per thousand, while last year it rose to 20.52 per thousand. If we take the doctor's own valuation on the goods he got in duty free last year, it will be seen that, directly and indirectly, the premier (for he is mainly accountable) is paying Dr Grenfell nearly $3,000 a year to double the death rate on the Labrador coast....

We anticipate that a number of people will say: "Oh, but these hospitals have done a lot of good on the coast; Smith, Brown, Jones and Robinson, were cured in them last summer."... [S]upposing the hospitals are necessary, isn't it the duty of the Newfoundland government to build, equip, and own them themselves? Have we no shame in us as a people, that we must permit itinerant self-dubbed

The master mariner knows not the meaning of rest. He is a composite of Dr Livingstone, President Roosevelt and Evangelist Moody, and he is the highest ideal of the strenuous life... In the hearts of the people he is premier of The Labrador. If his election is not so recorded in St. John's, it is simply because the 'liveyers' have not had opportunity to exercise their franchise.

S. Briggs 1904
Managing director, Fleming H. Revell,
Grenfell's New York publishing house

Co-operative trade of any kind was looked upon with hostility by individual traders and suppliers, and complications serious to us and our work followed our early attempt to introduce cash co-operative stores—for we had to depend on public support for our other branches of work.

W. Grenfell 1929

philanthropists to exploit our alleged poverty and misery, and shake the hat for us all over the world? Must the name of Newfoundland and its dependency (Labrador) ever remain a synonym for poverty and misery, because some philanthropist (so called) wants to exploit their supposed condition, in order principally to make money?

Evening Telegram 27 November 1905

On Saturday night we interviewed Dr Grenfell in reference to the serious charges made against him.... Doctor Grenfell tells us he has no intention of retiring, and has not said so, and that he is but at the beginning of his life work on the Labrador; further, that he has made no money here, and that he is a poorer man now than when he came first.

... [T]he doctor said that old clothes are not sold, but are distributed to needy men, women and children. In case of the infirm no returns are exacted; in case of the able-bodied, labour is exacted but not money. The labour is rendered to the mission in nine-tenths of the cases, in the remaining tenth on public work, and never to any private or trading enterprise....

Further, the doctor informed us he has never got in dutiable goods duty-free for trading purposes. 'Tis true, he has initiated several co-operative enterprises, quite apart from his mission work, with a view to bettering the lot of the fishermen in the remote north. He has got the fishermen to put in money and he has put in money of his own, and borne himself the risk of the venture. Except in one instance ... in which he drew $10, he has never drawn any profits ... in one case, the only one which was unfortunate, he stood the whole loss himself and was out of pocket $1700.... The co-operative companies trade on precisely the same footing as to duty as any other trader....

As to the percentage of death rate on the Labrador, the figures quoted are absolutely unreliable as there is no compulsory registration of deaths, the floating population has never been enumerated, and it is impossible to make up any reliable percentage of death rate, either now or a decade ago.

Trade Review 2 December 1905

Soon after the *Trade Review* was published last Saturday, indignant denunciation began to pour in upon us by phone and letter ... and we now feel that we were not justified in making the statements we did against Dr Grenfell, or his work in connection with the Deep Sea Mission of Labrador.

Under these circumstances we feel that the straightforward and manly course for us to pursue is to recall our statements of last week, and we hereby do so most cordially.... Whatever doubts we may have possessed at the beginning of the week ... have been completely set at rest by the publication of the names of the men who stand behind the doctor in this city. Such names as Hon. E.R. Bowring, Hon. John Harvey, A.F. Goodridge, Esq., Sir R. Thorburn, Sir W.V. Whiteway, Judge Emerson, Hons. J.J. Rogerson, S. Blandford, J.S. Pitts, G. Knowling, J.B. Ayre, and C. Macpherson, Esq., would not stand for wrong doing in connection with the Mission, and we have therefore no hesitation in acquitting Doctor Grenfell of every charge preferred against him last week.

Daily News 5 December 1905
Mr Editor,

I will gladly avail of the offer which you make in all fairness to open your columns to a rational and unprejudiced discussion of the Deep Sea Mission question.

No one would for a moment question the good faith of all those engaged in or sympathizing with this work. At the same time may we not ask in all sincerity whether these philanthropic and charitably disposed people are not mistaken?

Just to show one instance of how bitterly the move to supply cheaper food was resented: one big firm withdrew its subscription from the hospital, removed the endowment plate from over a cot which it had provided for, and discontinued its support entirely (and we needed it badly) just because we had started a cash co-operative store.

W. Grenfell 1930 (1)

It is incredible that men and women content to leave England for a life in Labrador could be of a spirit willing to carry on for personal gain an illicit traffic in old clothes! Nor is it possible to argue that any section of the community—say the traders—can be really injured by that which affords the people such valuable essentials which they have not the purchasing power to obtain in any other way.

W. Grenfell 1905 (1)

Whether the Deep Sea Mission work is not only a mistaken charity as applied to Labrador but actually, a positive evil? … pauperizing and demoralizing the people …

[T]here can be no doubt but that it would ease the public mind very much if Dr Grenfell would abandon his trading concern and stick to his religious or missionary work. A very ancient authority tells us that no man can serve God and Mammon.… Dr Grenfell says he makes no money by the business, but in one venture alone lost $1,700. To the ordinary individual, it is difficult to conceive of a sane man entering into a business for the purpose of losing, or at least of not gaining.…

As to the mortality figures, Dr Grenfell says they are not reliable. Are the public to be satisfied with his word on this point? The figures are given in the official return of the registration of births, deaths, etc. Here they are:

Death Rate per 1000

Labrador	1901	1902	1903	1904
	9.35	8.88	18.74	20.52

… If not correct, why did the registrar give this enormous increase of mortality? Where did he get his figures from?

M.F. Howley

The higher mortality figures for 1903 and 1904 were attributed by Grenfell to epidemics of infectious disease among the Inuit to the north. Infectious diseases brought by white men took a heavy toll among Inuit people, for they had little or no immunity.

Royal Gazette **5 December 1905** (referring to Grenfell's lecture the previous day when, at a meeting chaired by Governor Sir William MacGregor, he spoke to a large body of supporters)

Of Dr Grenfell's lecture we can honestly say it was convincing. He spoke of the work of the Deep Sea Mission principally from the social and medical standpoint, and showed that on both sides it was working for the betterment and well-being of the people. Many photographs were shown of the sick and maimed, the halt and lame who by treatment in the coast hospitals had been relieved of suffering and made useful members of society. It does not lie in our mouths to say that the results cannot be commensurate with the outlay, because the population is scattered and cases demanding hospital treatment are few, for *we* pay but little towards the work. Moreover, when one considers what the relief from suffering is to each individual concerned, taken from torture and helplessness and lifted into a position to enjoy the blessings of life, criticisms must be silent and the words of approval must be spoken. We have no room in our hearts for such a question as 'To what purpose was this waste?' There is another objection rather feebly made that the medical treatment tends to pauperize the recipients; but putting aside the reply of Dr Grenfell that all his patients pay some little sum in acknowledgment, surely it is a mistake to assume that a free provision for the needy sick is an economic wrong, else were all the public hospitals and convalescent homes in the world to be condemned. Experience has, we think, proved to the hilt the usefulness all round of these splendid institutions whether in the town or country, and we cannot see that any peculiar conditions in the Labrador can lead to an opposite result.

Great though as, we believe, has been the benefit of the medical service of the Deep Sea Mission, in our view the social side of its work has a much wider usefulness, and a much greater significance. In the various attempts at co-operation made by Dr Grenfell, some of them successful and some unfortunately not, the doctor has started organizations which cannot but have a good effect upon the morale of our people. This will teach them to be thrifty, industrious, and self-reliant. It will add independence and a manly character to the people interested and fill them with a finer hopefulness, and finally enable them to turn their opportunities to the best advantage.

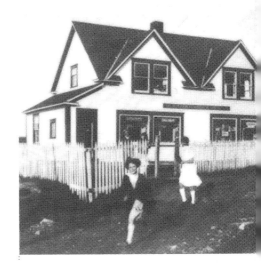

The successful Spot Cash store moved to larger quarters

A tea room for visitors is on the right.

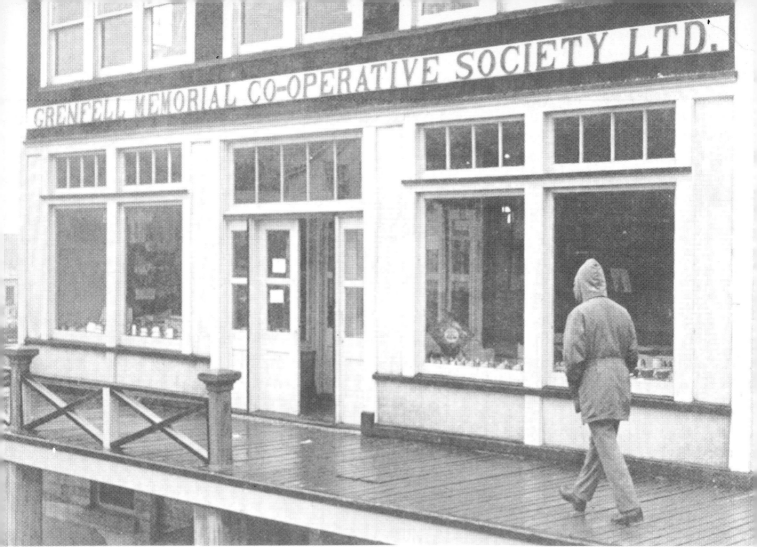

The Grenfell Memorial Co-operative Society
Limited in recent times

In 1940 the St. Anthony Spot Cash Co-
operative Company was reorganized
according to Rochdale principles and
renamed.

There is too the provision, through the kindness of an unknown donor
[Andrew Carnegie], of books and libraries for our isolated people by which Dr
Grenfell is helping splendidly in the education and uplifting of those who lie
within the scope of his work.... The people of Labrador and White Bay have
not many opportunities of obtaining books, and Dr Grenfell is doing them a
real service in bringing his libraries to their homes.

Such work as Dr Grenfell is doing on our desolate northern coast is the work
that the world now calls for.... [T]here never was a time in the history of the
world when greater importance was attached to all those social influences
which help men and women to live clean and happy lives. In the care of the
sick, the succour of the orphan, the feeding the hungry, the enlightenment of
the ignorant, and in the growth of the brotherhood of man the spirit of modern
Christianity finds its expression, and so far as we can understand the work of
the Deep Sea Mission on our coasts, it is all along these lines, and so can claim
the approval and support of everyone who has the welfare of those outposts of
civilization at heart.

Daily News **13 December 1905**
Mr Editor,
I said in my last letter that the means by which Dr Grenfell obtains financial
aid for his Mission is a degradation of the people of Newfoundland, and I am
surprised and pained that any person claiming to be a Newfoundlander or
whose children are Newfoundlanders, should tolerate, much less approve of
and abet, an enterprise supported by such means....

Dr Grenfell tells us that he collects abroad some $20,000 annually. This sum
he collects by means of lectures which he illustrates by lime-light views [magic

lantern slides]. These views are indeed taken from life, but that does not prevent them from being veritable and most offensive caricatures.... These pictures, taken from the very lowest and poorest of our people's homes, are highly coloured by an exaggerated verbal description, and the impression left upon the mind of the hearers is that such is the general and normal state of our people. Thus the poverty of a few (and very few) of our poorest settlements is exploited as a means of extracting alms from a charitably-minded audience.

Any one hearing Dr Grenfell's lectures and reading his publications must know that I am stating the truth.

In one of his articles, after graphically describing a hut on Labrador with "one room, a cracked stove, two wood bunks and a porch where the dogs sleep," he goes on to say "the mother and children took one bunk, four children in the other. Two children lay on the floor. All went to bed with their boots on." He winds up by saying "I think without any exception I was in the worst human habitation I had ever been in."...

But even if Dr Grenfell's most graphic descriptions are true, he must have but a slight knowledge of the poverty, wretchedness, filth, squalor and misery of the crowded populations of East London and the mining and manufacturing towns in England.... [Howley proceeds to quote from a variety of contemporary sources illustrating the state of the English poor.]

I do not make these said quotations by way of retaliation, but only to show how far Dr Grenfell is astray in his estimate of the poverty of Labrador.... If Dr Grenfell is overwhelmed with a spirit of humanity, of philanthropy, of Christian charity, could he not find ample field for his overflowing zeal and energy nearer home among these swarming millions of wretched sufferers [in England], instead of wasting his efforts among the few hundreds of hardy, healthy inhabitants on Labrador?

... I maintain then that this whole Grenfell business is a huge mistake and an indignity to us as a country and a government. There is nothing in the circumstances of Labrador that calls for extraneous help, or that our local government ought not to be able to cope with, by the use of their ordinary administrative machinery.... The Grenfell Mission is not needed on that shore ... it is not only useless but worse than useless. It is demoralizing, pauperizing, and degrading.

M.F. Howley

I regard the work that Dr Grenfell is doing in Labrador as one of the most simple, direct, and vital applications of the Gospel of Christ to human needs that modern times have seen.

H. Van Dyke, President
New York Grenfell Association
Quoted in Gosling 1910

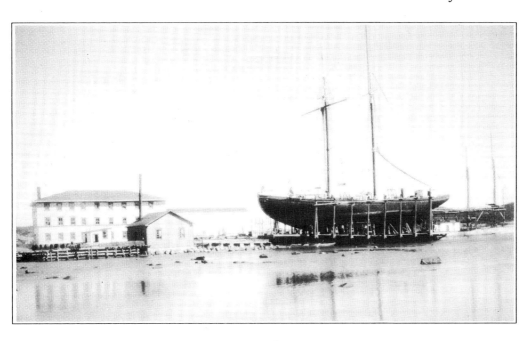

The Mission supply vessel *George B. Cluett* on the marine slip at St. Anthony, *c.* 1931

Another of the Mission's industrial projects, the dry dock was a valuable addition to the northern economy.

TWICE BLESSED INDEED*

William Gilbert Gosling (1863-1930), a director of the large and influential St. John's mercantile firm of Harvey and Company, was noted for his public spirit as well as for his sense of fair play. He was one of a relatively small number of St. John's businessmen actively committed to the proposition that the possession of wealth implied a corresponding responsibility for the welfare of others. His fine history of Labrador was published in 1910.

In a single month in the United States, in 1906, Grenfell raised twenty thousand dollars for his work, an extraordinary feat when one realizes that this was an English doctor with an upper-class accent asking Americans to support welfare work in a British colony.... Grenfell could size up an audience like a politician.

P. Berton 1978

I once attended a lecture given by [Grenfell] in a well-known church in New York. The building was crowded with a cosmopolitan gathering, representing many different nationalities and classes, all attracted by the fame of the lecturer and his philanthropic [*sic*] enterprises. "So shines a good deed in this naughty world." Grenfell's story was simply and unaffectedly told, with humorous and pathetic anecdotes interspersed, and although it was an old story to me, I listened again with deep interest—an interest unmistakably shared by all present, and practically demonstrated by the handsome collection which was taken up at the end of the lecture. I had previously thought how generous were the people of the United States in supporting a Mission which had really so little claim upon them; but now, after seeing and hearing, I came to the conclusion that they were getting good value for their money; it was a privilege to them to be allowed to help, and the lesson they received should be as valuable to them as the practical results to the people of Labrador. It was 'twice blessed' indeed....

There has been a somewhat natural feeling of shame, accompanied by resentment, that the fisher folk of Labrador and Newfoundland should be held up to the outside world as in need of charitable assistance. It has, however, been the comfortable and well fed who have assumed this attitude, and we have yet to learn that those in need have rejected the proffered assistance. It is so easy to be proud and independent when one's own 'withers are unwrung.'

The Grenfell personality has been, undoubtedly, the most valuable asset in the mighty business that his practical Christianity has become. Sheer bonniness has disarmed enemies who met him. His winning smile, his flashing sense of humour, his memory packed to the doors with a lifetime of episodes hazardous, funny, or heart-breaking, bring down the house year after year, and charm from hard-headed businessmen the needed river of gold to flow northward.

D. Peattie 1937

WE WORE IT OUT**

Grenfell was an effective fund raiser, if not a great speaker, possessing a fine sense of the dramatic, an innate talent for publicity and the knack of wringing tears as well as money from his listeners. On the lecture circuit, and in his many articles and books, he portrayed the local people as hardy, uncomplaining, fatalistic and worthy of help. Typical of his stories was this one, an old chestnut he had been trotting out for a minimum of five years (see Howley on p. 21).

It would appear that I possessed an insatiable love of lecturing. Nothing is further from the truth. Lecturing is without question the most uncongenial and least romantic task I have been called upon to do.

W. Grenfell 1932

The pitiable straits to which one or two bad seasons sometimes reduces these families, especially the more isolated ones, is the side of the picture that is perhaps most pathetic. I went one day up a bay, to visit a settler's family. It was dark when we arrived and hauled our boat up near the house. The father and one boy were away. The mother and seven others were home. The youngest was four months old. The house consisted of one large room, a central cracked stove, and a porch in which the inevitable dogs slept.

---

* W.G. Gosling, *Labrador: Its Discovery, Exploration, and Development* (London: Alston Rivers 1910)
** Wilfred T. Grenfell, *Down to the Sea: Yarns from the Labrador* (New York: Fleming H. Revell 1910)

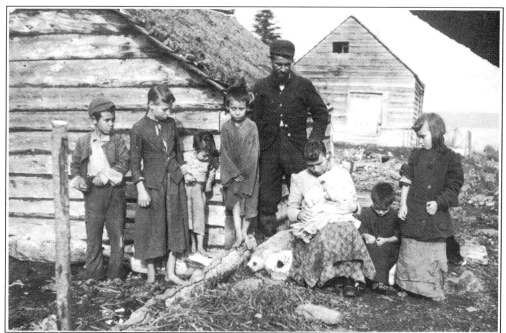

One of Grenfell's photographs, captioned 'The bread bag family. This is before I gave them the clothing for the wood.'

Our hostess remarked at once: "I am very sorry, sir, I cannot offer you any tea. We have had none in the house for over a month. Richard is away selling some seals." They had for their summer twelve quintals of fish at two dollars thirty a quintal, two bear skins, and six seals. The 'seven' were to all intents and purposes naked. Two threadbare cotton coverlets were the sole furnishings of the two beds. The semi-religious light of an exceedingly small lamp in some measure obscured the rest of the meagre surroundings. 'Soft loaf and water' had been their supper for many a day. Not even a drop of molasses was in the house. Two children slept with the mother, four on the other bed, two on the floor. Where the other two stowed away was a mystery. All turned in with even their remnants of boots on. We wrapped up in our blankets and slept on the floor.

"I don't see the blanket I sent you last fall," I ventured as we were stowing away. "Did you receive it?"

"Yes, sir. But five children sleeping under it soon wore it out."

THE LEND-A-HAND*

Grenfell's first winter on the coast, that of 1899–1900, was like subsequent winters spent at St. Anthony, filled with dogsled travels to visit the homes of remote liveyers. He became an experienced dog-team driver, capable of covering in a single season some 1,000 to 2,000 miles. Justifiably proud of his skill, he deemed northern winters "one long delight."

The 'lend-a-hand' is my komatik or dog-sleigh. We cut it ourselves from a stout old spruce—just where the stem joins the roots—so that the curved up 'horns' of the runners should carry the grain right on round the 'bend.' It is shod with enamel, sawn from the jaw-bone of an old sulphur-bottom whale which was killed off our harbour and towed in to be flensed of its blubber. Not a nail

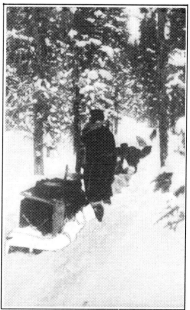

Grenfell and the Lend-a-Hand heading off through the woods

* Wilfred T. Grenfell, "Leaves from the Log of the Lend-a-Hand," *McClure's Magazine* 24, no. 6 (1905): 624-32

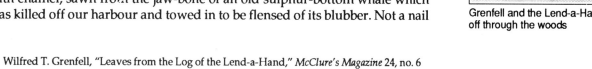

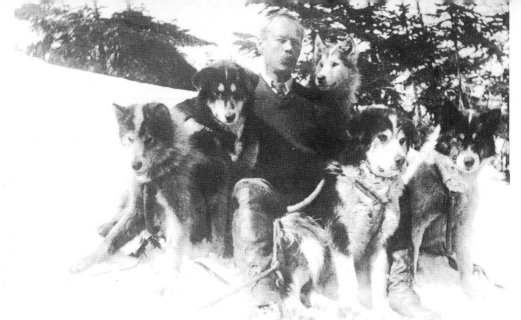

Grenfell and his dogs

is used to hold it together. Every piece is lashed to the next with stout thongs from the hide of an old harp-seal which one day pushed its inquisitive head out of a 'lake' in the Arctic ice a little too near the end of our rifle as we lay hidden behind a shelter of ice blocks.

Many a mile by night and by day this stout old friend has carried me. And many a hard knock it has endured, when, in glissading down icy hillsides, it has got beyond all control and ended by burying itself in the snow-drifts below, or by being brought up 'all standing' in the hummocky sea-ice; or, again, when missing the trail by night, we have launched ourselves into the air over some miniature precipice and so have even jumped over our own dogs, much to their surprise and ours.

IT WAS NO PLEASURE YACHT*

It is the fall of 1906. Grenfell has just moored the Strathcona *in St. John's for the winter and wonders aloud about inviting Governor Sir William MacGregor to inspect the vessel. His skipper advises against it, the* Strathcona *looks "too much as if she had been through a mill." Grenfell muses on.*

In truth there was no denying it, for she looked as if she had just come out of battle. The topmasts had been struck for the late gale, and the dainty rigging we sailed out with had been stripped off and stowed. Our ragged remnant of a flag fluttered now from an impromptu staff, which lashed into the large topgallant iron looked lost and forlorn. The masts were grimy with smoke, and weathered and salted with the sea spray. For the continuance of heavy easterly weather had given the men no chance to scrape down during the voyage home. As for her deck houses, the varnish, where any was left, had assumed the colour of skimmed milk from the continued driving sleet and spume. Up to two feet above the level of the rails most of it had been scraped off bodily by the heavy deck loads of pine wood, which we had been carrying out of the bays to the hospitals as our last contribution toward their winter comfort. The paint on her sides and bulwarks had paid such tribute to the sterns of countless fishing boats

When his steamer drops anchor all the inhabitants for miles about flock to her deck. Everyone has an ailment or trouble; all are listened to; something is done for each. I wouldn't be surprised if sometimes a healthy but complaining man gets a bread pill, but he departs satisfied.
G. Durgin 1908

* Wilfred T. Grenfell, "The Close of Open Water," *Among the Deep Sea Fishers* 4, no. 4 (1907): 8-11

alongside, that the once shiny black surface was mottled like a pane of frosted glass—while below the water line—well—even there we would like to go over her on dock ourselves before others saw her. For we had struck twice on a nasty day in the late fall when we tried to navigate a part of the Gulf of St. Lawrence on the way to the new Canadian hospital [at Harrington Harbour], a piece of coast that was new to all of us. She had, in fact, entered her last port like a man cut off without a moment's warning. Thus she certainly was not, as some would say, ready for inspection.

But as I stood on the wharf, running my eye over her familiar lines, to me endeared by so many happy days together, there was a sort of feeling that I would not have it otherwise. For she looked like a workman right from his field of labour. Her very toil-worn features spoke of things accomplished, and afforded some scant solace for the regrets that opportunities had gone by.

I could see again as I looked at her the thousands of miles of coast she had carried us along—the record of over a thousand folk that had sought and found help aboard her this summer—the score of poor souls for whom we could do nothing but carry them, sheltered in her snug cabin, to the larger hospitals where they could be better tended than by us at sea. I remembered visitors and helpers, whom she had faithfully carried, and who were now scattered where they could tell of the needs of our folks, and bring them better help in years to come. I remembered the ministers and travellers that had been lent a hand as they pushed their way up and down our coast—the women and children and aged persons that she had carried up the long bays to their winter home and to whom she had saved the suffering of the long exposure in small and open boats. One remembered the libraries she had distributed all along the bookless coast line, the children picked up and carried to the shelter of the orphanage, the casks of the food and drugs for men and dogs placed at known rendezvous along the line of water travel, making the long dog journeys possible. How often had her now boarded-up windows lighted up her cabin for a floating court of justice in lonely places where, even if the judgments arrived at had been rather equitable than legal, yet disputes had been ended, wrong doing punished, and the weak had been time and again helped to get right done them.

One remembered how she had been a terror to certain evil doers and more especially to those wretches, whose greed for sordid gain leads them to defy the laws of God and man, as they sell illicitly the poisonous drinks with which they lure brave-men-and-true to their ruin. On a truck on the wharf beside me,

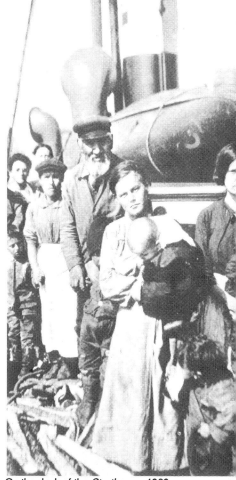

On the deck of the *Strathcona*, 1920

'We've come to see the doctor.'

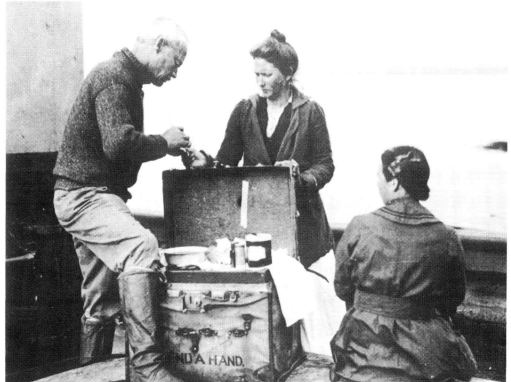

Treating a patient

Grenfell's medical chest also bears the inscription Lend a Hand.

25

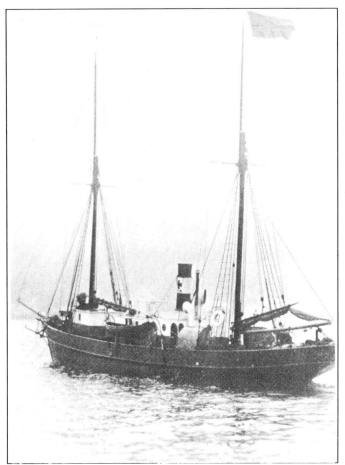

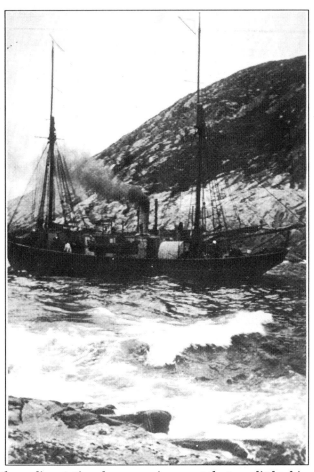

Left: *Strathcona*
Right: in rough seas

even now, on its way to the police station, lay a consignment that our little ship on one of her raiding expeditions had saved from doing the damage it was capable of. How like a confiscated bomb-shell it looked. One remembered pleasantly the comment of a fisherman friend on this, one of the most vital of her missionary efforts, at one specially troublesome settlement: "Bedad if the mission ship goes on like this long we won't be able to kape an ould bottle in the house to put a drop of ile in."

Again I could see her saving from destruction a helpless schooner abandoned by her crew and fast beating to pieces on a lee shore. I could see her cabin loaded with sacks of warm clothing for use in districts where dire poverty from failure in the fishing, or possible accident in their perilous work, had left defenceless women and children to face the coming cold of winter unprotected, and among those who had benefited in this way, were the crews of half a dozen unfortunate schooners, wrecked in the heavy equinoxtial [sic] gale of last September.

And beyond all the physical aid that had been rendered, one remembered the many sorrowful hearts to which she had carried messages of comfort and cheer. To some dying she had brought the joyful view of the realities of life beyond, and to some stricken hearts bereft of the hand they looked to for protection, she had brought with material help, the ray of hope which God permits the hand of a brother to carry as possibly its most precious burden.

The skipper who had come to the rail to insert a fender between the streak [sic, strake] of the wharf shores, noticed that I was still examining the ship, and he interrupted my reverie.

"Doesn't look exactly like a pleasure yacht, Doctor, does it?"

"Indeed she doesn't, skipper," and I almost added, "Thank God."

WHY I AM AGAINST ALCOHOL*

Grenfell was a strict prohibitionist from his days as a medical student when, working among the slums and docklands of East London, he saw firsthand the misery that alcohol could cause. One of the major functions of the Deep Sea Mission was to curtail the trade in liquor on the North Sea. Now, as a non-stipendiary magistrate, Grenfell was in a position to enforce an existing ban on the sale of liquor in northern Newfoundland and along the Labrador coast, where the temperance movement then in vogue had gained the upper hand. He did so with all the fervour of a true missionary, using such high-handed methods that he alienated many. In the following selection Grenfell suggests another facet of his complex character, an intolerance for the views of others.

Alcohol is not now allowed to be sold on any part of the coast on which we are working, but so surely as it comes and an illicit sales begins, one sees its evil results as quickly as if, instead of alcohol, it had been the germ of diphtheria or smallpox. Lying at anchor in Labrador harbours, women have come off to the ship after dark, secretly, for fear of being seen, to ask me for God's sake to try and prevent its being sold near them, as their sons and husbands were being debauched, and even their girls were in danger of worse than death.

I have seen it come among the Eskimos. It kills our natives as arsenic kill flies, and it robs them of everything that would differentiate them as human beings from the beasts around them....

I have seen ships lost through collision because the captain has been taking a 'little alcohol.' I have had to tell a woman that she was a widow, and that her children were fatherless, because her husband, gentle and loving and clean living, had been tempted to take 'a drop of alcohol' at sea, and had fallen over the side, drunk, and gone out into a drunkard's eternity. I have had to clothe children and feed them when reduced to starvation, because alcohol had robbed them of a natural protector and all the necessities of life....

Why do I not want alcohol as a beverage in a county where cold is extreme, exposure is constant, and physical conditions are full of hardship? Simply because I have seen men go down in the struggle for want of the natural strength which alcohol alone had robbed them of. The fishermen that I live among are my friends, and I love them as my brothers, and I do not think I am unnecessarily prejudiced or bigoted when I say that alcohol is inadvisable, after one has seen it robbing his best friends of strength, honour, reason, kindliness, love, money, and even life. I feel I have every right to say that it is inadvisable to have alcoholic drinks among sailors and fishermen.

Over twenty years' experience on the sea and on the snow in winter—and experience coming not on the top of the kind of life which would naturally fit one to meet these conditions, but rather after an upbringing in soft places—I have found that alcohol has been entirely unnecessary for myself.

There is no liquor sold in all this district, with the result that there is no crime.

W. Grenfell 1903 (2)

"Mr Grenfell is a good man, a very good man, but he has made brandy dear—dear beyond the reach of common men altogether—along the coast."

Louis Napoleon Partington
A Labrador trapper in the 1912 novel
Marriage *by H.G. Wells*

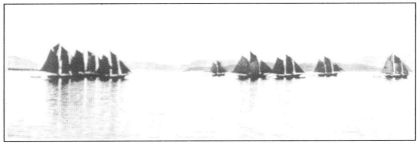

*   Wilfred T. Grenfell, "Why I am against Liquor," *Among the Deep Sea Fishers* 5, no. 1 (1907): 18-9

THE LADY DOCTOR OF MEDICINE*

So I offered my services to Dr Grenfell for a long summer season. He replied that he would gladly accept my offer, but he wanted to feel sure he could depend upon my promise to stay; he had been inconvenienced so many times by volunteers who failed even to show up. He also asked for my qualifications, that he might place me to the best advantage. When from my second letter he discovered I was a woman, he doubted if the fisherfolk would care to have a woman doctor. However, if I would call upon him at the *Outlook* office in New York we could discuss the matter. I did so at Christmas-time.

Dr Grenfell was a man of few word. "Would you be willing to go as a nurse?" he asked.

"No," I replied, "I must go as a doctor if at all."

A. Withington 1941

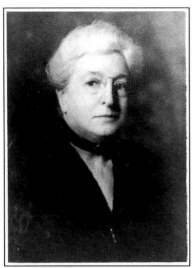
Alfreda Withington

Born in Germantown, Pennsylvania, Alfreda Withington in 1888 graduated from the Women's Medical College of the New York Infirmary, the pioneering medical school for women in the United States. For three years she studied and worked as a doctor in Europe and then set up practice in Pittsfield, Massachusetts. In 1907 she worked for Grenfell as a summer volunteer, paying her own expenses and bringing her own supplies. Withington spent most of that summer at Blanc Sablon. During the First World War she served overseas with the Red Cross. After the war she remained in France to pursue anti-tuberculosis work, and in 1921 she went to work in a remote area of the Kentucky Mountains. In his introduction to her autobiography, published shortly after his death, Grenfell claimed Withington was the first 'Lady Doctor of Medicine' he had ever met.

At Blanc Sablon one day a cry rang out, "The *Strathcona* is coming!" We all rushed to the staging to greet the little Mission hospital steamer, bringing Dr Grenfell from his headquarters in St. Anthony on the Newfoundland shore, his business manager, and a nurse bound for Harrington Hospital farther up the coast.

Hardly had Dr Grenfell touched foot to shore when he inquired, "Have you any ether? We have none." Fortunately I had ether and to spare.

He then asked me if I would go with him on the *Strathcona* some thirty miles westward to Bonne Espérance, an isolated part of the Canadian Labrador at which steamers rarely touched, and attend to the medical requirements there while he went on to Harrington; so having finished my rounds at the bunkhouses I quickly put together what might be needed for the trip and hurried on board.

Towards evening we found ourselves in a dense fog and lost among the shoals and icebergs. I remembered hearing that once upon a time, somewhere thereabouts, the intrepid *Strathcona* had gone over a shoal, up one side and down the other. Dr Grenfell said his captain knew every inch of the way, but what could one do with no bearings? We were wondering where we would anchor for the night when some fishermen sailing by told us that we were miles off our course. Just as we turned seaward again a whistle sounded, and creeping out of the fog came the midget steamer in which Dr Grenfell had formerly cruised the coast, the *Princess May*, now a fisheries launch belonging to Mr Whitely, owner of the Room at Bonne Espérance. She led us into the harbour, where I was presented to the Whitely family as one who had come to spend a week with them.

Early the next morning a man named Jimmy and a boy appeared in a small sailing-boat and asked for Dr Grenfell to go to Old Fort Island seven miles out at sea. But "that shockin' nice man" had already left, so I went in his place. Jimmy seemed to be in a tremendous hurry, and I supposed his anxiety was due to solicitude for the patient. But no, indeed! It was because an increasing wind was raising a high sea. I had grown accustomed to the ordinary upheavals of the ocean, but on this particular morning the huge seas that were running brought an involuntary gasp from me as we heaved this way and that.

… There was much speculation on the part of Jimmy's family as to who was coming; they had sent for Dr Grenfell and then had seen the *Strathcona* pass by. Who could the stranger with Jimmy be? Possibly that cousin from England who for many a year had promised them a visit.

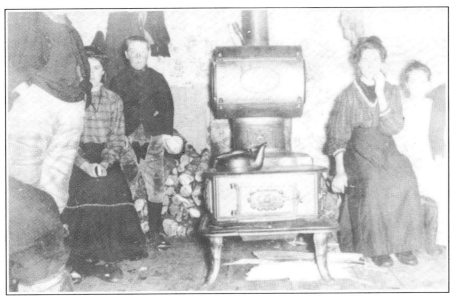

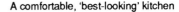

The patients were a mother with a slight pleurisy, whom I made more comfortable by strapping, and a boy who had a most exaggerated case of St. Vitus's dance. No one had ever seen anything like it, and the mother's heart was heavy. It was hard for them to believe that he could ever be made better, but later on came a letter stating that the last bottle of medicine had cured him, and "he doesn't twitch at all."

Dr Grenfell had told me whenever I found myself stranded to choose the best-looking house and tell the occupants I had come for a visit. The one I was in seemed comfortable, so after being invited to take off my hat and have a cup of tea, I suggested that I would like to stay until the wind changed. The mother had made me a dinner of bread, tea, and partridge berries, as they called the native cranberries, stewed in molasses; I ate it with zest except for the dust which sifted down through the rafters from someone's sweeping the room above. The storm had driven the men in from their fishing and the children from their chores; the whole household assembled. Even cousins from a house near by came over to have a look at me, and sat in a silent row watching me while I ate.

Then came the long afternoon with more time for intimate talk. Unconsciously the mother revealed her life, her unselfishness, and her hopes for her children. The father had had good luck the winter before with his traps, and they were planning to send their sons to Montreal for further schooling. "How I shall miss them!" she said sadly. "They are good boys. If only they don't get to drinking up there!" Her eagerness for their education was contagious, and by evening I too was ambitious for those boys.

Bedtime came with no diminution of the wind or rain. The loft had several compartments, one of which was for the men, another for the women. Mine was partitioned off with calico and had a feather bed in a box in the corner, all beautifully clean. On the floor were spread hooked mats, one of the handicrafts of Labrador. I once saw one with 'Don't Spit' woven in the centre, and wished its advice were more generally followed. Whenever I awoke I heard the howl of the gale and the roar of the sea, but the morning dawned fair. Although urged to remain, I felt that I must return to the mainland; but it was with a feeling of regret that I waved good-bye to the assembled family, including baby Alfreda who had been awaiting a name when I arrived....

Every morning [at Blanc Sablon] a row of men stood outside my surgery waiting to have wounds dressed.... Chatting with the men as I worked, to put

I had wondered what type of woman I should find on the Labrador. To my surprise I found her innately refined and forbearing. The wives and mothers had a hard time of it; their families were large, and they had everything to do, as well as helping with the fish. Their needles must have been in frequent use judging form the patches on the trousers—never were there so many or such variegated ones.
A. Withington 1941

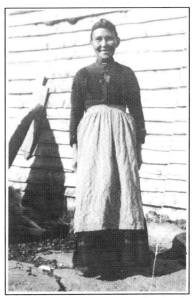

Granny Broomfield: innately refined and forebearing

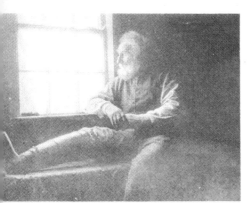

Withington's old man "who, with the initiative born of necessity, had made himself a wooden leg of barrel staves, as neat a piece of workmanship and as practical as any sent out by a metropolitan surgical supply store"

them at their ease, many a glimpse I caught of the steadfast patience of their natures, their meagre lives, their uncomplaining resignation to the inevitable. It would seem they had so little to be thankful for; they were so thankful for that little. This gratitude found expression in the names of their homes and settlements: Heart's Content, Heart's Desire, Heart's Delight, Heart's Ease—not empty words either, for barren and desolate and comfortless as they would seem to us, to the fishermen they were blessed havens of safety.

If a Labradorian left the coast, nostalgia often brought him back. There was a fascination for him in the rocks and the sea. His kindness to strangers and his cheerful brave response to the struggle for life were the qualities that impressed me most. If a net were carried away on a high sea, it had to be; if the food was scanty, if the salt for the preservation of the fish failed, these were facts to be accepted; if year after year children died of tuberculosis, it was simply so. "They went wonnerful quick," would be the comment, though grief was visible in their faces. Their ignorance as to the cause of tuberculosis prevented any way of escape from it; and their lives were adjusted to what seemed to them inevitable conditions. This resignation seemed born of the fact that nothing lay in their power, so far as they knew, to avert these evils.

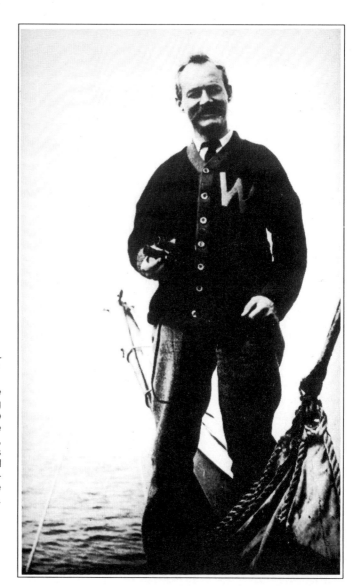

Grenfell at the bow in his Sunday best— the sporting look he so favoured

This photograph was probably taken in the summer of 1907. The following spring Grenfell set out by dogsled in response to an emergency call and, wearing only the football uniform he used as underclothing, nearly lost his life on the ice. The events surrounding his sheer struggle for survival and his equally daring rescue received international attention at the time, spreading his fame.

THE WHITE CURSE OF THE NORTH*

One of the Mission's more important roles was that of public health advocacy, and some of its greatest efforts were directed along these lines. The single largest cause of death in Newfoundland and Labrador, next to infant mortality, was pulmonary tuberculosis, with mortality rates far in excess of those in Great Britain, Canada or the United States. Grenfell pioneered both public health education and tuberculosis treatment in Newfoundland. He struggled to convince people that tuberculosis was infectious, not hereditary as they believed, and of the need to limit contact between infectious and other persons of the household. Recognizing that malnutrition was involved, he recommended good food, fresh air, sunshine and bed rest. In February 1908, following Grenfell's lead, a group of citizens in St. John's formed the Association for the Prevention of Consumption (APC) to combat tuberculosis and heighten awareness of public health issues throughout Newfoundland.

The following letters from Grenfell and Reverend J.T. Richards are addressed to the editor of Among the Deep Sea Fishers. *They suggest the nature of the Mission's anti-tuberculosis struggle.*

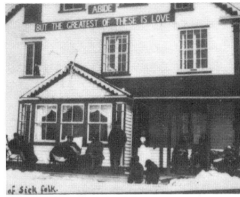

Tuberculosis patients in winter, St. Anthony Hospital, *c.* 1907

7 October 1905

Dear Mr Editor,

… The white curse of Labrador was again brought vividly to my mind here. A widow woman applied to me to get her the government widow's grant. I recognized her as a woman I had known further north some years ago, and asked after her husband. "He is dead," she said, "from consumption." "But where are your children?" "All dead of consumption," she said. "How many boys had you?" "Three," she replied. "How old were they, when they died?" "The oldest 17, the next 16, and the third 14." "And the girls, too? Surely they are not all dead of consumption." "All taken with coughing up blood," she said. "The eldest died when she was 18, the next at 16, and the youngest at nine." I remembered the tiny house, the fetid air, the windows that would not open, and the spitting on the floor, as I went back in memory to the visit I paid their house some eight or nine years ago. If anyone, Mr Editor, were to put in your paper that they had poured poison on the floor of a house until the father and all the six children had died from that poison, Newfoundland would rise in horror, and demand at any cost the extinction of such a scoundrel. And yet because it is only consumption that is doing this all over the country, no one appears to take any notice of it.

None of these had been able to read or write. What an awful tragedy from real life. Can anyone conceive that it would be right to say it was the will of God; their time had come. It was not anything of the kind. It was the culpable negligence of the rudimentary laws of health. Would that Newfoundland would establish a commission and spend some money on this great enemy of its people.

Wilfred T. Grenfell

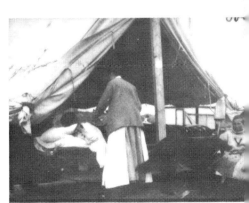

Open-air treatment for pulmonary tuberculosis

Outdoor shelters were erected at each of the Grenfell hospitals.

6 August 1906

Dear Mr Editor,

… We have been not a little amused of late by some of the comments on our endeavours to carry out open-air treatment for consumption. Alas! that this disease should flourish on so healthy a shore. The ignorance of man is largely

---

* Wilfred T. Grenfell, "The Log of the S.S. *Strathcona*," *Among the Deep Sea Fishers* 3, no. 4 (1906): 8-17; Wilfred T. Grenfell, "Dr Grenfell's Log," *Among the Deep Sea Fishers* 4, no. 3 (1906): 9-11; J.T. Richards, "Doings in the North," *Among the Deep Sea Fishers* 6, no. 2 (1908): 23-4

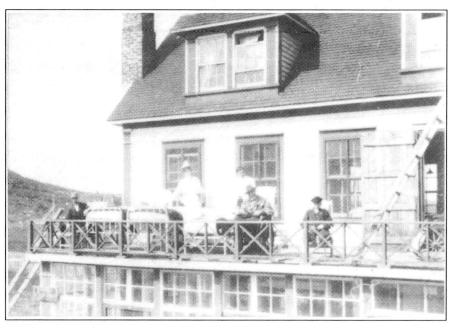

An enlarged St. Anthony Hospital, c. 1911

Glassed-enclosed sunporches below and second-story balconies above were for the benefit of tuberculosis patients, who accounted for a large percentage of admissions.

responsible for it, and our people have not yet learnt that while the sea may slay its thousands, this tiny bacillus is slaying its hundreds of thousands.

Returning to one place, where we had erected a canvas open-air shelter for the wife of one of the fishermen, we found her pale face now as brown as a berry, and that she was able to eat without effort just four times the quantity she could take only a fortnight before. She had only one trouble. The people were not accustomed to see a woman in bed on the side of their hill. The gauze that we use for dressings had served to keep off the mosquitoes; but nothing served to keep off the open-mouthed throng of youngsters, who were never tired of observing this strange phenomenon....

The scope of our work has largely increased of late years, owing to the number of volunteers who have come from Canada and the States at their own expense to help, actuated solely by a desire to do something. I am writing to you, Mr Editor, swinging at anchor among fifty schooners. A volunteer from Harvard, Mass., and a volunteer from Montreal are ashore building yet another open-air shelter for a lad with tuberculosis, and, incidentally, driving home the conditions necessary to give him a fighting chance for his life. The lad was lying in a half house six feet by twelve by six feet high, one closed window two feet by two, facing north. A large stove was burning, and the porch-door, which was only five feet six high, was closed. The patient was on a feather bed. The one idea was to keep him hot, out of draughts, and in semi-darkness!

Wilfred T. Grenfell

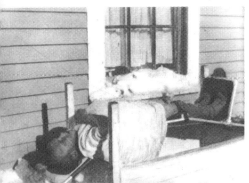

Post-operative bone-tubercular patient immobilized for healing

Orthopediac surgeons, summer volunteers from Canada and the United States, fused diseased bones with bone grafts, many involving children.

13 May 1908

Dear Mr Editor,

... It is cheering to note that our leading citizens and doctors at St. John's realizing that we are dying faster than we ought, have followed the example of our 'physician of the North' and are taking steps to teach our countrymen the rudiments of sanitation [by forming the APC].

Thank God for the great work of Dr Grenfell on this coast and on Labrador. For years we have had drilled into us by lectures, circulars and placards, the simple laws which, being observed, must certainly raise the standard of our health. The results are already, I believe, being felt. Windows are being flung open, or ought to be, by every home from White Bay to Port Saunders, and the pure breezes of heaven are invading consumptive nooks and corners and driving those demons of death to destruction; supplying in their place the pure health-giving atmosphere that God intends to inflate the lungs of man and carry a full supply of oxygen to his blood. Spittoons are becoming the order of the day, and now instead of the consumptive father, by that filthiest of habits, spitting the germs of consumption on to the floor, to be taken into the lungs in the next hour by the son or daughter whom, thus poisoning, he professes to love, we find the greatest care beginning to be exercised, for what father wants to be the murderer of his own child! What brother the murderer of his own sister! What husband would be the unwitting slayer of his own wife! If man by his carelessness lays death traps for his friends, God will not prevent those friends from walking into them, and we shall not be justified in attributing to heaven that which is due to man's folly.

J.T. Richards

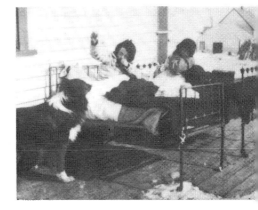
Young boys with tubercular joints

A CATECHISM OF SIMPLE RULES OF HEALTH*

Grenfell's first biographer, James Johnston, discusses in this selection another aspect of the Mission's public health program. Included in the Catechism *as well were sections on Washing, Spitting and Wounds.*

Besides his varied functions Dr Grenfell steadfastly discharges that of the hygiene and sanitary educator and reformer. Early in 1907 he compiled a *Catechism of Simple Rules of Health for Use in Newfoundland and Labrador Schools*, consisting of simple questions and answers. Scattering it broadcast he had the pleasure of finding the children in the schools well acquainted with its contents. Going also from house to house in one of the villages, he was encouraged to notice the reflex influence which it had exercised. He found windows open, doors wide open, dry floors, sunshine streaming in, and all the symptoms of the prophylactic measures having taken root.

As specimens of the *Catechism* we append three series of Questions and Answers.

THE AIR

Is fresh air good for me? I cannot live without it.
Is air ever bad? Yes, it gets very poisonous.
What makes it poisonous? Every time any one breathes he throws poison into the air.
What are these poisons like? Some are poisonous gases, some like tiny seeds.
Will they hurt me? Yes, they will kill me in time.
How can I avoid these poisons? By always keeping in fresh air.

THE SUNSHINE

Must I let in the sunshine? Yes—every bit I can let in.
Why must I let in the sunshine? Because nothing else cleans the room so well.
How does sunshine clean a room? It kills all the poison germs it falls upon.
Ought I to sit in the sunshine? Yes. I must always keep in it when I can.
Why must I do this? Because it will kill all the poison germs in my blood.

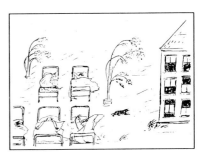
'Sick people need lots of fresh air'

This is one of Grenfell's many whimsical drawings with which he illustrated his books for the young.

* James Johnston, *Grenfell of Labrador* (London: S.W. Partridge 1908)

Must I open the window? Yes.
When must I open the window? All day and all night.
Will not the cold hurt me? Cold does not hurt anybody.
Why must I open the window? Because I cannot grow strong unless I do.
Will not the draught hurt me? I must try to avoid draughts as far as possible.
What good is it to open the window? It lets in the pure air to clean my blood.

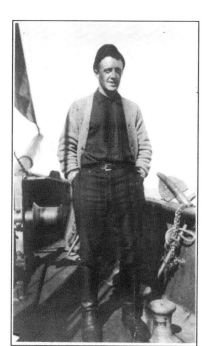

Dr John Mason Little on the deck of the *Strathcona*, 1907

The number of cases treated on board the *Strathcona* in the summer of 1907 exceeded 1,200. Besides these there were treated at each of the four hospitals maintained by the mission between 500 and 700 cases. There is a doctor at each of the hospitals, but operative work, unless urgent, is done when the *Strathcona* reaches them.

J. *Little 1908 (1)*

A WINTER'S WORK IN A SUBARCTIC CLIMATE*

John Mason Little (1875-1926) came from a wealthy Boston family. After graduating from Harvard Medical School in 1901, he studied for a further year in Vienna, completed a surgical residency at the Massachusetts General Hospital and then worked for five years as a surgical assistant to Dr Samuel Mixter, the noted Boston neurosurgeon. Hearing Grenfell lecture at this point in his career, and now a gifted surgeon in his own right, Little decided to volunteer. The summer of 1907 he spent with Grenfell on the Strathcona; *in October, he offered to stay the winter. He 'retired,' as he put it, to the St. Anthony Hospital and found himself at the centre of a busy hospital practice with adventure on the side.*

Little remained to enlarge the St. Anthony Hospital, and he established its reputation as a fine surgical facility. He left the Mission in 1917 to return to the Massachusetts General Hospital. Sadly he died at the age of only fifty-one, at the height of his medical career.

Unlike the rest of Grenfell's medical staff, Little was not an evangelical Christian. But he was an excellent doctor, he contributed to a number of professional journals, and he was a pioneer in the emerging field of deficiency diseases. His series of observations on beriberi in Newfoundland proved its association with a diet containing little fresh meat or vegetables. Little's following account of his medical work in the winter of 1907–1908 appeared in the Boston Medical and Surgical Journal *in the form of a letter to the editor. It was written in hopes of "reaching another circle of friends who might not through other channels become acquainted" with the Mission's work.*

I thought some account of the medical work up in this subarctic climate might interest your readers. As you can imagine, there are no automobiles here, but the work, though carried on in a different way is not unlike that at home. In the *Journal of the American Medical Association* of March 28, 1908, I published an account of the medical work done on the mission steamer, *Strathcona*, during the five months of open water last summer....

In the summer I had, with Dr Grenfell, travelled along the east Newfoundland coast as far south as White Bay; on the west coast as far as Flowers Cove; in the Strait of Belle Isle as far west as Harrington in Canadian Labrador; and on the Labrador coast as far north as Cape Chidley, Hudson Strait, and Killinek in Ungava Bay. Much of this ground had been covered not once but twice or even three times, and the operative work and supervision of four hospitals had been accomplished, so that in November, I found to my surprise over 1200 cases had been seen and treated outside the hospitals, 33 major operations performed, to say nothing of the numerous minor surgical procedures carried out with and without anaesthesia.

From this active professional life I expected to retire into the hibernation of a small hospital with, perhaps, two or three chronic cases, and the administra-

---

* John Mason Little, "A Winter's Work in a Subarctic Climate," *Boston Medical and Surgical Journal* 158, no. 26 (1908): 996-7

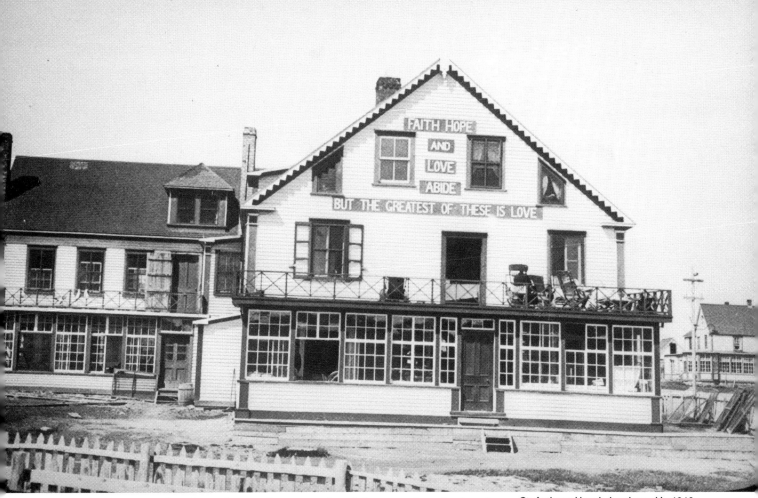

St. Anthony Hospital, enlarged in 1910, the Guest House visible on the right

tion of cathartics and tonics to the small community of about two hundred souls in which the hospital is situated. I had reasoned entirely wrongly. I knew nothing of the modes of travel in this snow and ice bound land, or of their efficacy. I realize now that in the very months in which I had supposed the people were most isolated, they are, on the contrary, the least so, and in fact, this is the time when they do most of their travelling. So now I am surprised in looking over the records for the last five months, November to March, that there have been 51 patients in the hospital on 27 of whom surgical operations have been performed, and that the out-patient record shows 1,012 new cases.

There are at present in hospital 12 cases.... [Little describes them as well as several tubercular bone and joint cases in the orphanage.]

I have said enough to show that from a clinical standpoint the material is interesting, but let it not be thought that this material reaches one who sits by the stove in the hospital and waits. Though the people are learning what can be done to relieve their sufferings, still by far the largest number of patients is found and persuaded to go to hospital by the doctor on his travels.

Up to the last of December, the water is open and patients come in vessels and open boats, and many from distances on the east coast, on the large mail steamer, which up till this time runs every two weeks from St. John's. After this time all travel is done on *komatiles* [*sic*] or sledges drawn by dogs. I have travelled nearly a thousand miles this winter and, given a good team of dogs that you know and proper conditions, I know of no sport to beat it. Also, I know of nothing so good for the temper when conditions are unfavourable and things go wrong. To show how conditions alter the aspect, I may say that one stretch of eight miles took from 8 in the morning until 3:30 that afternoon to travel and the same stretch was done in fifty minutes on the way back, five days later.

The hospital was even then considered superior to the General Hospital in St. John's, the only other hospital on the Island. Patients came on the government's coastal steamer and mail vessel from that far south.

In the last 5,000 cases seen in the out-patient department of the St. Anthony Hospital, the diagnosis of beriberi has been made 220 times. Beriberi is one of the deficiency diseases and develops whenever man is, for sufficient time, deprived of certain elements of his diet which have been called 'vitamins.'

J. Little 1914

35

Besides numerous short trips of from fifteen to fifty miles, I have taken four more extended trips, the first of twenty-three days, on which I got a splendid 36-point caribou and a doe, brought back three orphans, three patients for operation and one upon whom I had operated for acute osteomyelitis of the tibia. I saw 95 patients, did four operations, sent in [a] lunatic to the asylum [at St. John's], contracted for the building of a 70-ton schooner and straightened out the business of a lumber mill and general store, the manager having died during my presence in the vicinity—[all] this was before the mail boat had ceased to run on account of the ice.

My next trip was one of sixteen days, on which I saw 135 patients ...

Sometimes it is not all pleasure. A short while ago Dr Grenfell got on some bad ice and went through. He was alone. He managed to get [to] a small pan of ice with his dogs, but lost his sledge and everything on it. He was left on an open bay in which there was a heavy sea running. The ice was about a foot thick and about as large as a small room. He had on short running trousers, a light sweater vest, but no hat, coat or gloves. He was on this day and night during which time he was in the water three times. He drifted nineteen miles out to sea. He killed three dogs with his knife though bitten in the legs while doing so. He skinned the dogs and made a wind shield of their bodies, a coat of their skins, puttees of their harnesses and a flag-staff of their legs. His shirt he used as a flag. By an extremely lucky chance he was seen and rescued but his physical condition was rather pitiable when he finally reached the hospital, snow blind, hands and feet frost-bitten and looking twenty years older than before he left.

The winter is at last breaking up and we are looking forward to the life afloat on the *Strathcona*, with the new activities and interests that that provides both professionally and in other ways.

The Ice Pan Adventure of 1908 ... was typically Grenfellian. His impulsiveness, his incautiousness, his refusal to heed advice got him into trouble; his coolness and resourcefulness under pressure got him out. His sense of theatre and his courage turned the incident into an international act of heroism.
P. Berton 1978

Post-surgical patient heads home from hospital

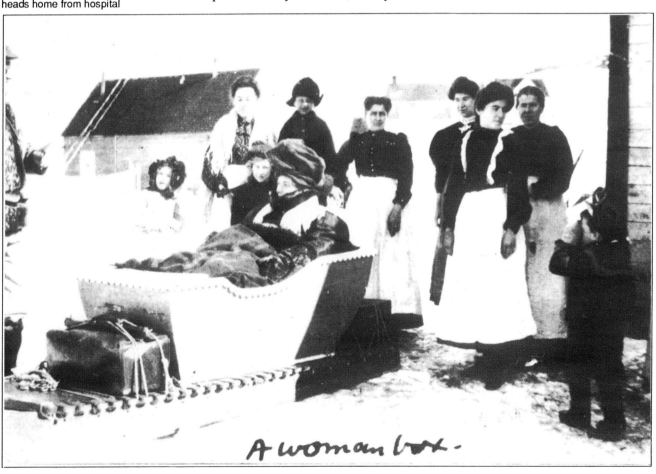

A woman box.

SPORTS DAY, 1908*

In 1900 Grenfell held a winter sports day at St. Anthony, initiating what was to become an annual event. The program included a shooting competition, a snowshoe race, a sack race, a komatik race and a greasy pole climb. Among the prizes to be won were barrels of flour, pork and beef, clothing and other goods. In a letter to the editor of Among the Deep Sea Fishers, *Reverend J.T. Richards described St. Anthony's 'winter sports' in 1908.*

The prophet of Labrador and northern Newfoundland, W. Grenfell, MD, CMG, having invited us to the St. Anthony sports, to take place on the 12th of March, the early part of this month saw us once more on the march thitherward. The most musical sound to the traveller in winter on this coast is the 'yappy yap, yap' of the dog team as they canter over the frozen snow, and on March 13th, one day late, we dashed down the incline into the commodious harbour of St. Anthony.

As we drove across to the house of Mr Boyd we saw the crowd assembled on the harbour in the vicinity of the hospital, and soon joined them. As we approached the scene of the sports the excitement of the onlookers apprised us of the fact that something very interesting was in process.

We had arrived just in time to see the closing tilts of the three last combatants in a bread bag fight. All the others had been put *hors de combat*, and soon the third last was put out of the fight by a very skilful manoeuvre on the part of Esau Hellier, who in turn was knocked out by John Pilgrim. The two last won the first and second prizes given by Dr Grenfell. It was then proposed by some mischievous onlooker that the doctors should do bread bag battle with the parsons. It was useless to refuse, and into the bags we were soon hustled. The only qualification for taking part in this unique combat is the pulling of a bread bag up over the body and tying it around the neck, thus rendering arms and legs useless. I soon found myself lying helpless on the snow, and was somewhat cheered on looking around to see several others in the same predicament—Dr Grenfell, Dr Little and the two Methodist parsons, Mr Wilson and Mr Brown. Only Father Tibeaux from Conche and Dr Stewart now held the field, and after a stubborn fight Dr Stewart succeeded in getting Father Tibeaux outside the line and was declared champion. Notwithstanding the bitter cold, the day passed merrily, and we felt thankful to Dr Grenfell for this much-needed diversion. What struck one most forcibly was the great patience shown by Dr Grenfell in amusing the boys. Whilst others were driven periodically into some abode to thaw and warm their almost frozen face and extremities, he never once left his post until due attention had been paid to all who wished to take part in the sports, by which time the shadows of evening were fast falling, and we were all glad to avail ourselves of the doctor's hospitality, which was most willingly and bountifully bestowed.

From the commencement of his work along the Labrador, Grenfell had never regarded his work as solely medical, but had always insisted that his concern was with the whole person, and his social, financial, religious and general health needs, his work, his recreation, and his place as a member of the community—and not only his, but hers; for the work of the orphanage, the school and the industrial centre was concerned as much with girls and women as with boys and men.

H. Willcox 1986
House surgeon
St. Anthony Hospital 1930-31

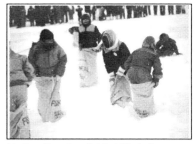

Modern flour bag fight at St. Anthony

This photograph taken by Dr William Mahood in 1991 shows the continuing tradition, though the bags are no longer tied around the neck.

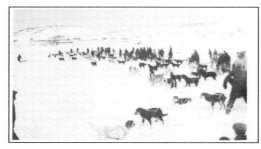

Komatik race, sports day, 1940

---

* J.T. Richards, "Doings in the North," *Among the Deep Sea Fishers* 6, no. 2 (1908): 23-4

THE DIGNITY OF LABOUR*

Edith Mayou, a former VON nurse from Ottawa, Ontario, served at Harrington Harbour on the Canadian Labrador. Harrington Hospital was opened in 1907, the Mission's fourth, and until 1916 was administered by Dr Mather Hare. He was a surgeon from Nova Scotia who had spent two years with the Canadian Methodist Mission in China West. Mayou, a regular contributor to Among the Deep Sea Fishers, *here discusses the Mission's clothing business and how it worked.*

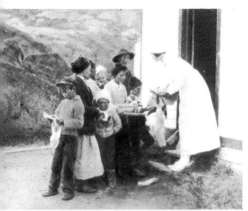

Exchanging handicrafts for clothing

New and used clothing were supplied by the Needlework Guild of America and friends of the Mission.

The splendid bales and barrels of new and second hand warm, well-made clothing, sent to the different mission hospitals have saved numberless men, women and children from perishing with cold, and falling victims to disease and death from exposure when insufficiently clad; and yet so eagerly is the clothing sought for, that the supply does not nearly equalize the demand. This clothing is not given away except to widows, orphans, and in cases of unavoidable sickness and poverty; but each article is considered as payment for work done, or articles brought, that the people may not be demoralized by pauperization.

Wages are paid partly in money, partly in clothing; the clothing is given as payment for carpentering, road making, land clearing, wood hauling and chopping, washing, sewing, cleaning, work of all kinds, and in exchange for fish, eggs, berries; in fact nothing, even if at the time apparently useless, is refused. A queer and miscellaneous collection there is some times on the deck of the *Strathcona* when she has stopped at one of the outports, and people have brought, to exchange for much prized clothing, a bowl of berries, barrels of capelin, whale meat or seal blubber for the dogs; winter food, wood for the engine, tree trunks for firewood or for building purposes, a squealing puppy, to be trained in the winter to draw a komatik with from seven to nine older dogs, some freshly caught fish, a partridge or wild duck, some rabbit skins, bottles of goat's milk, a stuffed bird or animal, skins for the skin boots worn in the winter, rag mats; from the Esquimaux, skin boots, and mats and baskets made of grass, and sometimes, a forlorn dirty little boy or girl soon to become a happy, clean, well cared for inmate of the orphanage at St. Anthony....

Dr Grenfell helps the people not by pauperizing and giving indiscriminate charity, but by showing them how to help themselves, teaching them the dignity of labour, that things must be earned to be possessed.

THE BISHOP'S TROUSERS**

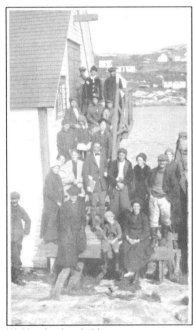

Waiting for the clothing store at Battle Harbour to open

Kate Austen, a Grenfell nurse in the late 1920s, told this story.

Sir Wilfred on his voyages along the coast is always giving away his clothes. If he sees a ragged, cold fisherman he gives him his coat, his sweater, anything. This he had never mentioned in his books, but it is a well-known fact. Usually he is not very far down north before he is suffering from exposure. And when his own clothes begin to run out, he starts giving away those of his crew and passengers. Anything that is lying around, Sir Wilfred picks up. "Here's a jacket," he'll say to a fisherman. "Keep you warm."

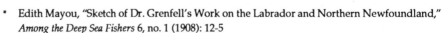

* Edith Mayou, "Sketch of Dr. Grenfell's Work on the Labrador and Northern Newfoundland," *Among the Deep Sea Fishers* 6, no. 1 (1908): 12-5
** Elliott Merrick, *Northern Nurse* (New York: Charles Scribner 1942) Reprinted by permission of the author, copyright, Elliott Merrick

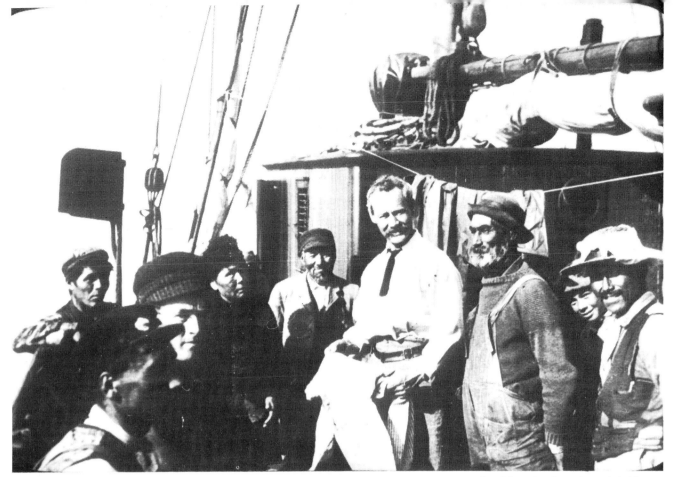

"Thank you, sir," says the fisherman.

"That's all right," says Sir Wilfred.

After a while his crew begins to get a bit naked too, for there are so many fishermen and they wear out clothes so fast.

Once many years ago Sir Wilfred took the bishop of Newfoundland north to give him a look at the Labrador. Right from the start the lop ran high, and *Strathcona*, narrow craft that she is, rolled like a barrel. The bishop was very seasick all the way up and across the Straits. Sir Wilfred was in fine fettle, and there was hardly a little fishing harbour anywhere that he didn't poke into. He soon had most of his own clothes given away as usual, and the bishop's sou'wester, and a few other odd articles had also disappeared. One day, it is said, the poor seasick bishop roused himself from his bunk just in time to see Sir Wilfred tiptoeing out of the cabin with some black broadcloth apparel slung over his arm. "My dear Sir Wilfred," said the bishop, "I would give you anything I possess, but how can I conduct a Sunday service without trousers?"

Grenfell sorting through used clothing on the deck of the *Strathcona*

He later admitted: "To tell you the honest truth, I hate rolling around on my hospital ship with the cabins clogged up with old clothes. I have slept on old clothes. I have spent hours sorting old clothes. I have gone through pack after pack looking for a pair of trousers for a man, and have spent an hour arguing with him that, as all I had was a lot of old ladies' jackets, one of those must be the thing he really wanted. I have seen the time when I could have taken a hammer and hit the postulant for help, however needy I knew him to be, because I was worn out physically with trying to find the right kind of garment among the debris of all that was left to me."

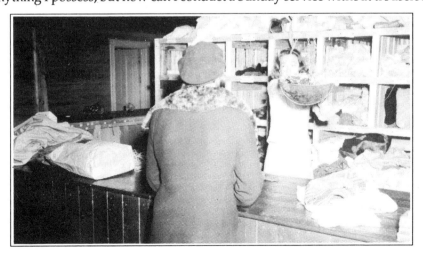

Clothing store at St. Anthony, *c.* 1940: sold by the pound

A SOUL-SATISFYING EXPERIENCE*

Francis Sayre (1885-1972) was born in South Bethlehem, Pennsylvania, the son of a wealthy American industrialist. While a student at Williams College he heard Grenfell lecture, and volunteered to work for him in the summer of 1908. He and fellow student Doug Palmer were assigned to the St. Anthony station. After his college graduation the following year, Sayre worked on the Strathcona *as Grenfell's secretary and general assistant, becoming his close friend. Afterwards he entered Harvard University Law School and married Jessie Wilson, daughter of President Woodrow Wilson, in a White House ceremony in 1913. For many years Sayre taught law at Harvard, and he held a variety of public positions, both at home and abroad. He did both with distinction. He remained one of Grenfell's warmest supporters to the end.*

In the following selection, Sayre conveys the effect Grenfell had on a young man in search of a useful career.

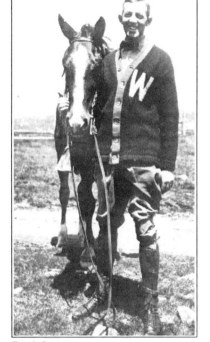

Frank Sayre

Frank Sayre was among the first of a species known as Wops, American college students who came north to 'do their bit' in response to Grenfell's call. Many of them, like Sayre, came from well-off families. 'Workers without pay' was the accepted origin of the acronym.

An hour later we entered Bonne [Espérance] harbour, passing close by the small eighty-ton steamer, the *Strathcona*, already anchored in the bay; and eagerly we jumped into the small boat and were rowed ashore. No sooner had we landed than we saw a knot of fishermen in animated conversation on one of the fishing stages over the water. In the centre of the group, joking and laughing, stood a man of moderate stature in rough sweater and seaboots, ruddy-complexioned, bareheaded, with rumpled hair and sandy mustache. At once I recognized Dr Grenfell. He caught sight of us and jumped forward to meet us.

"Well, Frank, so you're really here at last. I'm so glad. And Douglas Palmer, too. How jolly! You, Doug, are to take the mail boat south from Battle Harbour to our headquarters at St. Anthony. And for you, Frank, we have saved a bunk up forward on the *Strathcona*. Get your things off the *Home* and come right aboard. We'll be sailing at nine tonight."

Within half an hour the doctor and I were being rowed out to the *Strathcona*. Actually to board her and walk her crowded deck was like a dream come true. Here was the hospital ship which the intrepid doctor drove every summer, as long as open water lasted, through storm and fog and ice along the entire length of the Labrador to bring medical and other help to the isolated settlements along that desolate coast and to the fishing fleets sailing north from Newfoundland every spring in the search for cod.

I had read much about him; and so virile and winning a worker for Christ, I had wanted to know. During my junior year at Williams College he was raising money in the States on a lecture tour, and I had invited him to speak to our student body. He had come; and the day of his address I took him for an all-afternoon tramp through the woods and into the hills. It was plain that he loved the out-of-doors; and his enthusiasm for his work was so contagious that I longed to have some small part in it. No one I had ever met had impressed me so deeply. As a result of his talk to the college that evening we students set to work raising money for his mission, and it was then that I had promised to join him on the coast.

Now at last that June evening I stood on the deck of the *Strathcona* beside him, prepared to share in his work. No one would guess, seeing him as I saw him then, hatless, garbed in old clothes and seal-skin boots, that he was skipper of the ship, helmsman, physician, the King's magistrate, head of an international Mission, director of four hospitals, preacher of the Word and friend of all. I

* Francis Bowes Sayre, *Glad Adventure* (New York: Macmillan 1957). Reprinted by permission of Macmillan Publishing Company, copyright, Francis Bowes Sayre

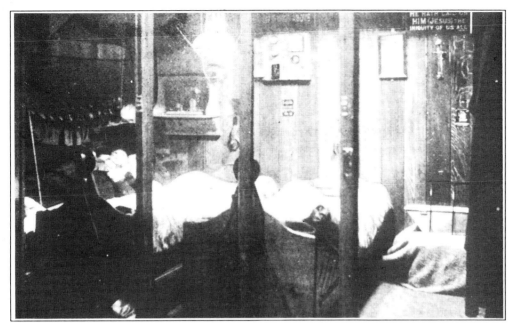

A splendid little hospital amidships

heard him call down to the engineer below; and shortly thereafter we were heaving up anchor and then threading our way through the fishing fleet where the men were still on deck cleaning cod by torchlight. Soon we were clear of the harbour, plunging through the open sea.

... All that [next] day we steamed west along the Canadian Labrador for Harrington, where was located one of the four Grenfell hospitals.

The *Strathcona* was admirably fitted for its purposes. Amidships below was a small hospital for carrying the seriously sick to one of the Grenfell hospitals; adjoining was the sickbay where lines of fishermen and 'liveyers' (i.e. 'live here') gathered for treatment whenever the little ship put into port or came to anchor. On the decks was all manner of cargo, being carried from place to place. Up forward were the wheelhouse and the chartroom. Here Dr Grenfell could generally be found, standing at the wheel or, when the ship lay to, sitting at work at his writing desk, or talking with fishermen who kept bringing to him their never-ending problems.

The first thing I saw on the wall as I entered the chartroom was the verse:

> So many gods, so many creeds
> So many paths that wind and wind,
> Just when the art of being kind
> Is all this sad world needs.

The *Strathcona* was the fascinating workshop of a man who at every turn was making his life count. "My own principle has always been where two paths are open to take the more venturesome," he once had said. He was emphatically a man of action. Furthermore he was consecrating his life to the joyful service of Jesus Christ. To him, his work and his religion were one....

Late in the afternoon we reached Harrington, where the simple white frame hospital with its limited ward was filled with patients. A Canadian doctor was in charge, with a resident nurse assisting him. Here we spent the night and the following day. I watched Dr Grenfell talking with the patients, always with a kindly sparkle in his eye, conferring with the doctor and nurse, settling problems, determining policies, going off to visit friends near by, ever alert and cheery and uplifting. He seemed, indeed, to win every one by his utter simplicity and selflessness, his sheer warmth and joy of heart. These people of the bleak north responded to it as to the sunshine.

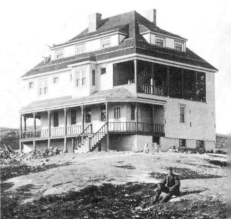

Harrington Hospital

Staffing, maintenance and equipment were the special responsibility of the Grenfell Labrador Medical Mission, the Canadian association headquartered in Ottawa. Grenfell is seated in front.

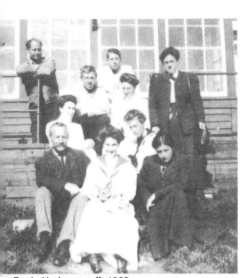

Battle Harbour staff, 1909

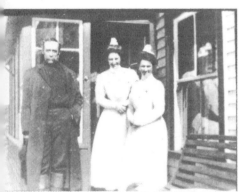

Arctic explorer Commander Robert E. Peary with Grenfell nurses, 1909

It was a crowded day, but time was pressing; and by late afternoon we were off again in the teeth of a gale, this time steaming back eastward for Red Bay, where patients were to be treated and a cooperative store tangle was waiting to be straightened out. From there, on along the Labrador coast to the important station of Battle Harbour, where another Grenfell hospital was located and various problems were waiting for decision. After a night at Battle Harbour, we headed south for St. Anthony in northern Newfoundland, passing now and again towering bergs of ice drifting southward in the Arctic current which washes the Labrador coast. Rocks can be charted, but icebergs cannot; and as we watched these mountains of ice and realized that eight-ninths of them were under water, we began to understand why Dr Grenfell, when the fog descended, would call the mate to take the wheel and would himself take his stand on the bowsprit of the *Strathcona*, straining his eyes for ice.

St. Anthony, the headquarters of the Grenfell Mission, was a fast-growing settlement. Here was the largest of the Grenfell hospitals, and also a Grenfell cooperative store and an orphanage housing some fifty [*sic*] children gathered in from various parts of the Labrador coast. Here were a bunkhouse for workers like myself and a little guest house for visitors. Mission boats lay to in the bay; and a stout wharf was piled high with lumber and building material. The Grenfell buildings formed the centre of a lively community.

A few days later Dr Grenfell departed on the *Strathcona* for his long summer trip down north.

The rest of that summer I was stationed at St. Anthony, working hard at a miscellany of jobs. I loaded and unloaded boats, shipped on a trip north as a schooner hand, went south to help dynamite a wreck, lent a hand at construction or in the hospital—even assisting at an operation or two—and one time played barber and clipped the hair off all the orphans, several heads being 'infested.' Doug Palmer was with me, and we tried to live by the doctor's creed: 'Wherever help is needed, try to give it.'…

That summer in Labrador had proved a soul-satisfying experience. In the months that followed during my senior year at Williams, Dr Grenfell and his work often filled my thoughts. Was Labrador the place where I could serve Christ best?

I completed my college work in three and a half years, and after a cowboy trip in Montana returned to Williams for graduation in June, 1909. Early in the year I had expressed the hope to the Williams trustees that they might confer upon Dr Grenfell an honorary degree; and to this they had gladly agreed. Hence I found Dr Grenfell attending my graduation to receive his honorary degree, and with him was his mother, recently arrived from England.

I had been chosen valedictorian, and at the conclusion of my address I remember my mother waving to me from the audience and sending up a little note of love and pride. Smiling and happy, Dr Grenfell sat near me on the stage. After receiving his degree he was asked to speak. As always he sounded the deeply Christian note in his uplifting impromptu address; and I think all the audience fell in love with him.

Following the graduation exercises, I again turned my face northward, bound for Labrador, this time to spend the summer on the *Strathcona* with Dr Grenfell, as his secretary and general assistant.

It was a summer of rare experience. Cruising northward from Battle Harbour along desolate rocky coasts and past drifting icebergs; avoiding many a sunken reef; often facing or riding out violent gales and storms; running up into Hamilton Inlet for a brief visit; touching at the Hudson's Bay post of Rigolet, to which the Montagnais Indians came from the interior with furs and deerskins to do their trading; on to Indian Harbour, where another Grenfell hospital was

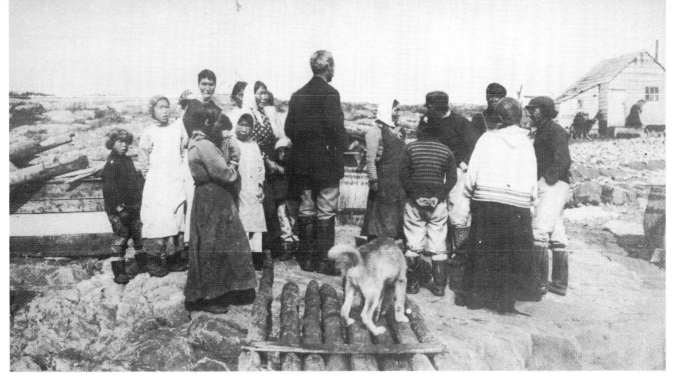

dispensing mercy in a very practical form; then on north to Eskimo country, stopping at Hopedale and Turnavik; coasting still farther north, past Nain, all the way to Okak near Cape Mugford, along a coast line of dark massive rock rising sheer out of the water for several thousand feet; rejoicing in the very substantial help we were able to bring to the needy in every little settlement. We kept in the very pink of physical condition, sometimes beginning the day and thoroughly awakening ourselves by throwing a rope over the ship's side and jumping into the icy water, with bergs floating near, and, needless to say, immediately climbing back on board. Of Dr Grenfell I was the constant companion, by his side in the chartroom, typing his letters or copying his manuscripts, helping when necessary in the dispensary, taking charge of the clothes box from which used clothing was dispensed, occasionally taking a turn on watch at the bow and straining my eyes to spot the low floating ice and the bergs. If ever we took a day off it would be to go ashore and climb the rocky coast, up into grassy hills above, and from the heights look over the magnificent wild northland panorama spread out before us, rocks and cliffs and endless sea. On Sundays we stopped in port and customarily held open-air services, often on the rocks overlooking the sea. Again and again I was reminded of the Gospel stories of Christ talking to fishermen and disciples gathered around Him on the shore.

In mid-August we had to turn and start the journey homeward. By September we reached Battle Harbour. To our surprise we found it filled with craft quite different from the customary fishing boats. We were greeted with exciting news: Peary, the explorer, had just unexpectedly made his appearance, returning from the North Pole aboard the *Roosevelt*, which we could see anchored off shore. Most exciting of all, after years of brave but unsuccessful attempts, he had at last actually reached the North Pole....

On November 18, 1909, Dr Grenfell was married. The story goes that, returning from England to New York, he met an unusually attractive American girl on the deck of the *Mauritania*, fell head over heels in love with her, and asked her to marry him. "Why you don't even know my name," she exclaimed.

"That makes no difference to me," he replied. "I want to change it."

The ceremony took place in Chicago, and I felt particularly honoured by being asked to be an usher and a member of the wedding party.

Almost exactly four years later he stood beside me as my best man in the East Room of the White House.

Grenfell visiting Inuit at the summer fishing station of Double Island

Mission doctors supplemented the medical services of the Moravian missionaries, making yearly or twice-yearly visits to the Inuit on the northern Labrador coast.

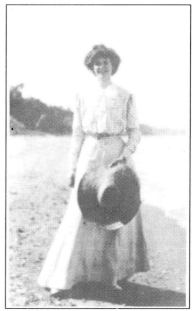

Anne MacClanahan Grenfell

Her Mission responsibilities rapidly became as onerous as his.

ONE OF THE GREAT MEN OF OUR ERA*

John T. (Pete) Rowland spent his boyhood sailing the shores of the eastern American seaboard. By 1907, when he entered Yale University, he was an accomplished small-boat sailor. The Grenfell Mission was at the time rapidly expanding its fleet of vessels, the majority of them provided by American philanthropists and university students; so Grenfell made use of his skills four summers in a row. In 1909 Rowland delivered the Pomiuk to Battle Harbour, and in 1910 he delivered the Yale. The following year he skippered the Daryl, which Grenfell had recently sold to the Hudson's Bay Company, from Harrington Harbour to the south side of Hudson Strait, crossing from there to Baffin Island. The year after, he brought the Mission's Floradel north.

The casualness with which Rowland in 1909 was taken on by Grenfell, the trust which was placed in him, was typical of how Grenfell operated. Many observers besides Rowland were struck by the serendipitous nature of it all.

More than anything else, I think, it was the doctor's ebullient high spirits and the warm kindliness which he radiated that drew me to him. In his efforts to better the lot of the fishermen he had made some powerful enemies, but they were all people who did not know him personally—and I have an idea that they avoided meeting him for fear of falling under his spell.

J. Rowland 1963

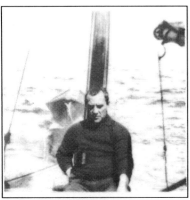

Dr Norman B. Stewart of Glasgow, shown here on the *Pomiuk*

Described by J.T. Richards as 'a big genial Scotchman,' Stewart spent over four years at St. Anthony, 1906–1911, moving to Indian Harbour each summer.

It seems almost as if Bob Carpenter and I had been preparing ourselves for a great adventure which stood closer than we knew. During the winter term Dr Wilfred T. Grenfell came to lecture in New Haven. We, of course, attended—and were astonished to see how few Yale students were there. For those to whom his name is no longer even a legend, Grenfell may be described as the Albert Schweitzer of his day....

In the course of the lecture at New Haven he described a hospital launch that had been donated to the Mission the previous year and taken down to Labrador by a crew of Harvard students. Then we sat electrified when he added, with a twinkle, that he would like to start a little Yale-Harvard competition of his own by having a Yale crew sail down a small schooner that was currently under construction.

Right after the lecture we went quickly and volunteered. The doctor looked at us keenly for a moment, then said: "Splendid! Miss White will make the arrangements. I'll see you at Battle Harbour in July."

That was it! Years later I inquired how he dared give such a job to a couple of college freshmen whom he had never before even seen. "I felt certain you would not offer if you did not know what you were about," he answered simply.

It would be flattering to think that Dr Grenfell saw competence and reliability blazoned upon our countenances. But that is not the answer. The fact was that he trusted everybody. Cynics may say that his type of service did not attract the sort of people who would be likely to let him down, but I think there was more to it than that. The doctor was a very inspiring leader ... generous in his judgments ...

Bob and I left the lecture walking on air. We were a little baffled over the identity of 'Miss White,' but not for long. She turned out to be the secretary of the New England Grenfell Association, which had charge of financial operations. A sweet little gray-haired lady, as meticulous over detail as the doctor was casual, she soon inundated us with correspondence. We spent a good part of the winter ironing out plans for the expedition ... [and eventually delivered the *Pomiuk* that summer.]

During the fall of 1909, Bob Carpenter and I founded a Grenfell Association at Yale. The immediate purpose was to raise funds for the building of a new and *perfect* hospital tender, in which we were unquestionably animated by our experience with the *Pomiuk* the preceding summer. Most of the money was

* John T. Rowland, *North to Adventure* (New York: Norton 1963)

raised during the Christmas vacation—from the student body, alumni, and friends.

The new vessel was designed by my good friend Charles D. Mower and built by Rice Brothers at East Boothbay, Maine. Both the designer and the builder donated their services. She was built for the actual cost of construction, without profit ... I consider the *Yale* the finest sea boat and one of the best sea-going sailers it has ever been my good fortune to command....

In the course of my four summers on the coast of Labrador I became intimately acquainted with one of the great men of our era. Given the opportunity, this was not a difficult thing to do, for, like all truly great men, Dr Grenfell possessed the quality of simplicity in a superlative degree. He spoke often of the tyranny of possessions, and whimsically poked fun at the 'unfortunate rich' who could never find time to do anything worthwhile. Himself he considered the luckiest of men because he was free; and this freedom he exercised joyfully, without fear or hindrance, in the service of the suffering and the oppressed.

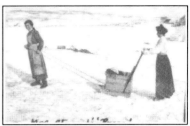
Mrs Stewart's pram

There was nothing sanctimonious about Grenfell, but he was a deeply religious man. Though a lay reader in the Church of England, he was no formalist; and his faith at times took odd and entertaining turns. Once while I was with him on the *Strathcona* ... an aged liveyer came aboard with a badly ulcerated tooth and a swelling the size of an orange distending one side of his face. The poor fellow must have been in great pain, so he was sadly disappointed when the doctor came up on deck for a breather between operations and told him he would have to wait. "Come back in the morning, Tom, and I'll pull it out for you then."

"Sure, Doctor," said old Tom, "she hurts me wonderful bad. Won't you just charm un, please, afore I goes ashore?"

The old fellow's earnestness was touching, but we who were watching could not suppress a smile. I half expected to hear the doctor rebuke his belief in witchcraft, which was then prevalent on the coast. Instead, he said calmly: "Why, yes, Tom. I'll lay a spell on it, if that's what you want."

Standing erect and bareheaded on the *Strathcona's* deck, Dr Grenfell intoned a Latin poem in a sonorous voice and made appropriate passes with his hands. When he had finished, the man looked up with grateful eyes. "Thank 'ee, Doctor! Thank 'ee, sor! Sure, she feels better already!"

He got in his skiff and pulled ashore, and the doctor went down to start another major operation.

Next morning I was on deck early to watch the *Strathcona* get under way. Out from shore came a skiff propelled lustily to catch us, and when it got alongside I scarcely recognized the rower as old Tom. He looked twenty years younger, his face was wreathed in smiles, and his cheeks were as flat as my

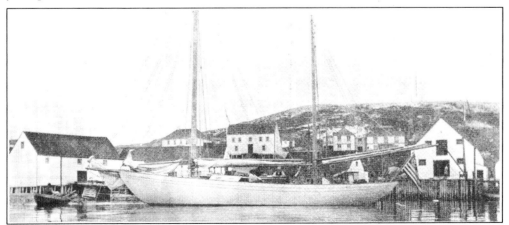

Yale at anchor in Battle Harbour

An auxilliary ketch, 45 feet long and a fine sea-going vessel, the *Yale* was eventually assigned to Dr Harry Paddon for use at Indian Harbour and North West River.

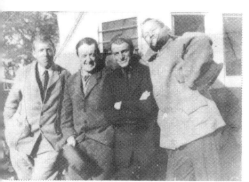

Doctors Grieve, Little, an unidentified man and Grenfell: 'a pixie-like sense of humour'

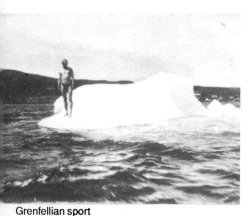

Grenfellian sport

Dr Arthur Wakefield takes a dip.

own. He held up a pair of prime silver fox pelts, worth a hundred dollars apiece, as a donation to the Mission.

"How's your tooth, Tom?" the doctor demanded.

"Sure, sor, she's sound as a dollar. Never gave me another mite of pain!"

"How in the world do you explain *that*?" I asked Grenfell later, as we were steaming out to sea.

"Medically I can't," he replied, "but there is no limit to the power of faith. Tom is a good man, and his faith must be in the power of good—call it what you will."

The doctor had at times a pixie-like sense of humour, and I think the picture of himself, a medical man and pillar of the church, solemnly reciting Ovid or Lucullus to 'cast a spell,' must have tickled his funny bone. But if the spell itself was a hoax, there could be no fraud about the deep sense of humanity that led him to commit it rather than dismiss the sufferer without giving him at least what he requested.

To a young man thirsting for adventure, Dr Grenfell's remarkable daring naturally made a great appeal. He told me that the little *Strathcona* had fifty-two dents in her bottom—one for every week in the year. When I asked how it was that Lloyd's kept up his insurance, with such a record, he replied: "Conscience! That is their contribution to the Mission."

This is not to imply that he was foolhardy—he was too good a sailor for that—but on a coast where fog and foul weather were the rule not much could be accomplished if one waited for a 'fair chance.'... The *Strath* was only 85 feet long, and so much room was taken up by her hospital equipment, which included a practical operating room, that not much was left for bunkers. On a long trip she often ran out of coal. At various strategic points where timber could be found, the native folk were encouraged to cut and stack cordwood of suitable length for burning under her boilers. During 'wooding parties,' when every available foot of deck space was piled high with fuel, the doctor himself set the example—and it took a strong man to match the pace he set. I have seen him do surgery all day, steam half the night, turn out at dawn to load cordwood, and then go on to another little port where the trap skiffs of the fishermen would be clustered thick about the *Strathcona*, bearing sick and wounded, the moment her anchor went down. Often I marvelled at his strength, when I had to drop down for a rest after only the physical labour....

One morning when we were anchored in American Tickle I crawled out of [my] snug berth to see a small iceberg—'calf' in the vernacular—drifting slowly past with the current. One side of this berg formed a gentle slope from its apex, some twenty feet high, to the base, where it projected as a shelf below the waterline.

"By Jove," said the Doctor, "a natural diving float! Who's for it?"

I stood shivering in my long underwear, and a couple of other young athletes showed no visible enthusiasm. The doctor threw off his bathrobe and pyjamas, sprang up on the rail, and dived overboard.... At this time Dr Grenfell must have been in his early forties. He had led a vigorous outdoor life ... With his clothes on, he was not especially impressive physically; but his body was well knit and strongly muscled, and he was quick as a cat....

The Magistrate — In addition to his regular duties, the doctor held the post of magistrate on the coast. Crimes were infrequent, but I played a small though essential part in bringing one culprit to trial. This man was a liveyer who dwelt at the head of Hamilton Inlet not far from the location occupied by the international airport of Goose Bay today. One of his neighbours charged him with making and selling an intoxicating liquor—spruce beer. It seemed rather silly, and I was inclined to admire the ingenuity of anyone who could make beer out

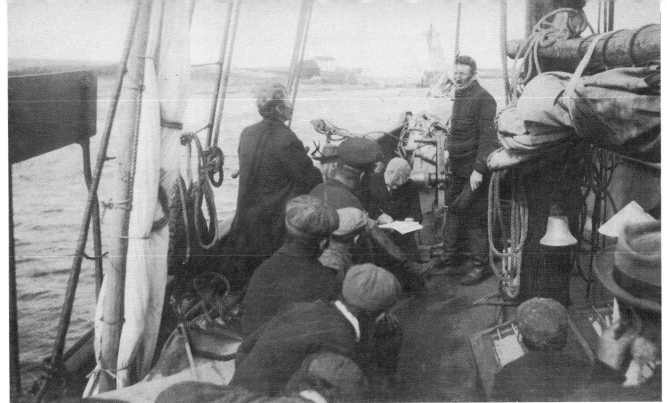

Trying a case on the deck of the *Strathcona*, 1908

Grenfell is barely visible in the centre wearing boots and a hat. His assistant is seated to his left.

of spruce gum, but the law had to take its course. Accordingly, Dr Grenfell made out a warrant for the poor fellow's arrest and sent me in one of the *Strathcona's* boats to bring him in.

The doctor first swore me in as deputy constable, in the course of which proceeding I had to take oath to serve faithfully 'His Majesty the King.' This caused him great amusement and might have been enough to throw the case out of court, had anyone been present to question its legality. I rowed a couple of miles to the man's dwelling and was somewhat nonplussed to be met at the landing stage by five stalwart young men, who were his sons. They inquired my business and marched on either side of me as I went up to the house. One, who moved in close behind me, made me wish for eyes in the back of my head; but I did my best to affect nonchalance. Within I discovered the object of my quest in the shape of a little old man with a wooden leg, sitting in front of the stove.

The stalwart sons ranged themselves along the wall, scowling and blocking exit by the door. I wondered if I was going to find it more difficult to get out than to get in. At any rate, there was nothing to be gained by timidity, so, after demanding of the old man whether he was the person named in the warrant and receiving an affirmative answer, I opened that impressive document and read "In the name of the King!" in a loud voice. This made a visible impression and did much to hearten me. No doubt that was part of its purpose. I read slowly and clearly while the old man listened with rapt attention. When I had finished he leaned forward and slapped his thigh. "Now, that's what I call proper!" he exclaimed.

There was no sign of resistance. Instead, he gave every indication of pleasure. He hobbled down to the shore, got into the boat, and appeared to enjoy his importance. I rowed back to the *Strathcona* and helped the prisoner on board. Somewhat to my relief, the five sons stayed behind.

On the *Strath's* forward deck an outdoor courtroom had been improvised. The complainants were there, and a number of other people from the settlement. There wasn't much to the trial because the defendant frankly admitted his guilt and in extenuation said only that he was too old to work and did not believe the spruce beer did anybody any harm. Dr Grenfell pointed out that the law had been broken and that he, as magistrate, had no choice but to impose

There being no regular magistrates for the north, we accepted also that most ungrateful task of unpaid and amateur dispensers of justice, to which we could bring only a sincere desire for equity without knowledge of precedent. It appeared to work satisfactorily, however, so long as no specialists of the sister profession of law were present to confuse issues, and intimidate our courts. Moreover, we were permitted to make our sentences *secundem artem*, remedial rather than retributive, and for lack of other entertainments our court trials were always exceedingly popular occasions.

W. Grenfell 1930 (2)

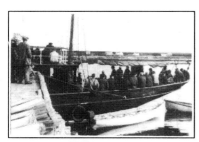

'For lack of other entertainments our court trials were always exceedingly popular occasions.'

This one took place on the deck of the *Strathcona II* in the early 1930s.

In my boyhood I used to collect postage stamps, butterflies, and birds' eggs. When we sailed to Labrador, however, a new chance presented itself, and I started to collect children.

W. Grenfell 1932

sentence. The fine was quite a heavy one, so that when he heard it the old man threw up his hands in despair. "I never had that much in all my born days!" he cried.

"Very well, then," said the doctor, "in lieu of money the court will take your wooden leg." He directed the bosun to unstrap it and lay it on the desk.

At this the old man crumpled. I have never seen anyone look so woebegone in all my life. It was unlikely that he could ever get another.

There was a long silence, during which I think even the complainants felt regret. Then the magistrate rose and picked up the wooden leg and stood turning it over in his hands. Suddenly he turned to the prisoner. "I am going to suspend your sentence," he said. "Do you understand what that means?"

"Do I get my leg back?"

"Your leg is no longer yours; it belongs to the court. But I will let you have it to use for as long as you behave yourself and do not break the law. If I have to take it away from you again you will never get it back." He laid the peg-leg on the old man's lap.

Despair turned to joy. I believe the old man would have kissed the doctor, had he been able to rise.

The bosun strapped his leg on again and then carried him over and set him on the rail, whence I helped him down into the boat. Then I rowed him home. Altogether I rowed eight miles that day in His Majesty's service. But it was worth it; and anyhow, what is a mere eight miles when you are tough and twenty—even in a pugnosed skiff!

The old man was pleased as Punch about the whole affair. And why not? His fame in Goose Bay would last as long as he lived, for had not the King sent a special messenger with a piece of writing to bid him to his court?

The five sons were happy too.

QUEER PROBLEMS*

"I had been summoned to a lonely headland, fifty miles from our hospital at Indian Harbour, to see a very sick family. Among the spruce trees in a small hut lived a Scotch salmon fisher, his wife and five little children. When we anchored off the promontory we were surprised to receive no signs of welcome. When we landed and entered the house we found the mother dead on the bed and the father lying on the floor dying [of influenza]. Next morning we improvised two coffins, contributed from the wardrobes of all hands enough black material for a 'seemly' funeral, and later, steaming up the bay to a sandy stretch of land, buried the two parents with all the ceremonies of the Church— and found ourselves left with five little mortals in black sitting on the grave mound. Thus we began what developed into our children's homes with the balance of the stock."

This was one Grenfell version—simple, direct, unadorned—of the beginning of the St. Anthony orphanage in 1905. Like many of what were undoubtedly Grenfell's real-life experiences, this one was later transformed into the pseudo-fictional moral tale, "The Joy of their Lord." It appeared in his fourth book, Off the Rocks: Stories of the Deep-Sea Fisherfolk of Labrador, *published in 1906. The following story is another example of this same process through which actual incidents were recast to serve the greater Grenfell purpose—publicity for the Mission. It opens as Grenfell and his mate Bill have set out from the* Strathcona *in a dory to find Tom Mitchell and his family, who were reportedly in trouble.*

* Wilfred T. Grenfell, "Queer Problems," *Down to the Sea: Yarns from the Labrador* (New York: Fleming H. Revell 1910)

"There's a smoke, Sir," said Bill at last, staring into a rather larger cove than usual. "Come on, Bill. If you can see nothing, I can't—where is it?"

Bill was right, however—there was a feeble smoke fighting its way up the side of a precipice face, but no sign of any residence could we see.

However, we landed, hauled up our boat, and went on a voyage of discovery, till at last we ran down a little fire-place in the open, by which sat a gaunt woman with a wizened baby on one arm, and stirring a sorry looking gruel in what appeared to be an old paint can with the other hand. "Good morning. Where's the tent?" I asked. "There she is," replied the woman, pointing with the gruel stick to a sorry roofing of matting and patches of canvas, which was stretched over some well-trodden mud against the cliff face. "Why do you cook in the open?" " 'Cos we hasn't got no stove." "Where's Tom?" He's away wid Johnnie trying to shoot a gull—here, Bill, run and fetch yer dad, and tell him Doctor wants 'un"–whereupon a half-naked urchin of about nine years promptly disappeared into the bushes. "What's the matter with the baby?" I asked. "Hungry," she replied. "I hasn't no milk to give him." She proceeded to show me the baby, which kept whimpering continually, like a little lamb bleating. "It's half-starved," I said. "What do you give it?" "Flour and berries," was her answer. "I chews the loaf first, or it ain't no good for him"—thus showing she had discovered a physiological truth.

A little girl of about five and a boy of about seven now emerged from behind the tent, where they had fled upon our arrival. Both were, to all intents and purposes stark naked, and yet as brown and fat as Rubens' cherubs. It was snowing a little, and the cold had overcome their shyness and driven them to seek the warmth of the fire. "I'm glad to see the other children are fat," I said. "They bees eaten' berries all the time," she replied. "What's t' good of t' gover'ment," she suddenly demanded. "Here is we all's starvin', and it's ne'er a crust they gives yer—there bees a sight o' pork and butter in t' company's store—but it's ne'er a sight of 'im us ever gets—what are them doin'? T' agent, he says he can't give Tom no mor'n dry flour—and folks can't live on dat." I was beginning to unfold to her the functions of a government, when a shuffling figure, with a very old, rusty, single-barrel, muzzle-loading gun, followed by two boys, appeared on the scene. He was somewhat shame-faced, I thought, carrying a dead sea-gull by one wing.

"You've had some luck, Tom," I remarked, inwardly referring to the fact that he had safely discharged the antique weapon without doing destruction at the wrong end. "It's only a kitty," he replied, "and I've been a-sittin' out on t' point all day." A 'kitty' is only a small gull, and Tom's tone of contempt was actuated entirely by the size of the victim. Tom's standard of values was graded solely by bulk, and involved no reflection whatever on the variegated assortment of flavours that these scavengers succeed in combining in one carcase.

"The gun isn't heavy enough to kill the big gulls, I suppose." "I hasn't much powder," he replied, "and ne'er a bit o' shot. I mostly puts a handful o' they round stones in her—t' hammer don't always set her off, neither. Her spring bees too old, I reckon," he said, playing with that extremely loosely attached appendage in a way that made me ask him to let me hold the weapon for a minute while I looked at it. Needless to say, I took good care to keep it in my hands till our business was through.

The truth is, Tom was reared on a truck system of trade, and had been all his life a dependent of others. He had never had the incentive to really look out for himself, for he had never been able to get clear of debt. This, and his Eskimo blood, left him bereft of all initiative, and so incapable, except when under orders from others, of earning a livelihood.

It is bad enough to put an orphan in an asylum here in America, but in Labrador we had none, and I used to bring these children to this country, and to Newfoundland and Canada, and some were sent to England, or wherever I happened to be going.

W. Grenfell 1907
Quoted in Johnston 1908

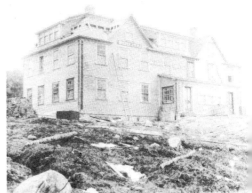

The St. Anthony children's home

Capable of accommodating about twenty children at the outset, the orphanage was soon enlarged. For ten years it was under the direction of Eleanor Storr, an English volunteer who left to become an army nurse during the First World War.

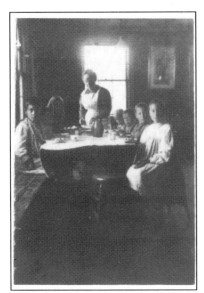
At the supper table: the children's home

Our little orphanage has assumed the somewhat unconventional role of a child incubator. For our newest arrivals have all got living parents, which is a good thing, but does not fulfil the functions of a living diet. We have, therefore, been assuming for periods of from one to four years the responsibility for the mental and physical development of several children, until circumstances shall alter sufficiently to make it reasonable to send them back to their own or other homes, where they will be adopted.

W. Grenfell 1908

"Tom," I said, "I want to help you—winter is coming on and you have nothing whatever to face it with. The only thing I can think of is for you to let me take charge of your two little boys, 'Billy' and 'Jimmy,' and the little girl. I'll feed them and clothe them, and send them to school till they can come back and help you along—and so long as they are with me I'll do my best to help you along also. They will certainly starve here during the winter—the snow is covering up the berries already, and you have nothing else." But poor Tom made no answer. He simple stood, his mouth wide open, and stared into space. "T' Doctor wants to take t' children," broke in the sharp-tongued wife. "Don't youse hear what un says? 'Tis the gover'ment that ought to feed 'em here, I says. I wouldn't let no children o' mine go, I wouldn't"—and she cuddled the wizened babe up closer, as if I had been about to pounce on that bag of bones and fly off with it like an eagle.

It took quite a long while to convince her that what a government 'ought to do' would not feed six children—especially as that government was so far away that we couldn't expect an answer before Christmas if we wrote to them. As for Tom, the intricacies of the problem had entirely failed to penetrate his dullard cranium, and yet, perplexed as he was, he showed the great wisdom of saying nothing.

"Why doesn't youse say something?" his irate spouse at last insisted. "Bees you a'goin' to let t' Doctor have youse childer?" but Tom only looked more and more puzzled, and merely reflected by taking off his hat and scratching his head.

Matters seemed to have come to a deadlock, when Tom, with a burst of eloquence suddenly ejaculated, "I suppose he knows." Backed by this moral support, I again advanced to the attack, and at length succeeded in extracting from Mrs Tom: "Well, youse can take Billy, I suppose, if you wants un."

During this prolonged debate my excellent mate had not ventured on a single word, though he was, in spite of his athletic dimensions, a most tender hearted father of many children. At this juncture, however, he cast propriety to the winds, and butted full into the debate by simply seizing the struggling Billy and putting him, kicking, under one arm, for he had in his mind the cheerful little children's home we had built near our southern hospital, and was familiar with the wonderful transformation that had been enacted there in other children that had been entrusted to us. But I had yet a hope of saving more of the children, and profiting by the evident resentment of Billy to be isolated from those he was familiar with, I pressed home on the mother how terribly lonely one child alone would be. I soon perceived that my logic was having its effect on her defences, and with fresh vigour proceeded to show her the advisability of sending a bunch together for company's sake. But I seemed somehow to make no headway till Tom, whose eyes had been glued to his struggling offspring, once more came to my rescue with his philosophy.

What it was impressed him so strongly, I can't yet say, but he broke in most opportunely once more with his "I says *he* knows what's for t' best," and then as promptly relapsed into the impregnable position of a deaf mute. I had already occupied much time—the snowstorm was all the while growing heavier, and white horses were capping the sea, to match the fast growing whiteness of the land. The *Strathcona*, which had followed us round the island, was evidently very uneasy, and already had blown her whistle several times to hurry us up. A final promise of a better gun for Tom, with a stock of powder and shot, of some spare old clothes for all the rest of the family, and of a note to the agent to give work, if the worst came to the worst, induced Mrs Tom to consent at last to my having 'Jimmy' as well as 'Billy.'

The subtlest argument I could advance seemed to make no impression on the enemy. I compared the tent with our fine house—I pointed to the mere semblance of a boat that was all they had to convey their family over a hundred miles in up to their winter station. I spoke of fine clothes, the schooling, etc., that we would give the baby girl if only she was allowed to come with us, and did my best to save her from the seeming starvation ahead of her. But all my blandishments fell on deaf ears—nothing I could say would tempt Tom to emerge again from his impenetrable silence, and I had at length to acknowledge discomfiture. My faithful mate, Bill, however, who had halted half way to the beach with his first prize, had no intention of risking the acquisition of a second, and long before I was through with the arrangements he was climbing into our dory with Billy under one arm and Jimmy under the other, their protesting lower extremities that stuck out behind notwithstanding.

We did not, however, fail to make good the rest of our bargain. The entire remnant of the family were conducted on board the *Strathcona*. They were fitted out with suitable clothing from the stock sent me by friends, and part of which is always in the strong box on the mission steamer's deck; besides which, some of my generous seamen contributed from their kits. A gun was loaned to Tom—his own old relic was overhauled and repaired by our engineer, to be given to John, the eldest boy, who was big enough to help with the hunt. Powder and shot were produced, tins of condensed milk were extracted from the ship's stock for the baby, our second axe was donated to their impoverished equipment, and indeed a heterogeneous collection, which included some needles and thread, soap, and other trifles in a couple of oil bags that had been sent us for sailors' use, all found their way into the Mitchell family's dilapidated houseboat. Before they left the paternal mate had Billy and Jimmy on shore in so well advanced a state of scrubbing and hair cutting, that Tom and his wife would have less difficulty in recognizing them when they shall return in the days to come. For this last impression of them, scrubbed and in clean clothes, formed a very marked contrast with that which they presented in their rags on the islands.

The boys soon got over a very, very short attack of homesickness, and neither of them was in the least affected by the tossing and the tumble of the sea.

Already Jimmy and Billy are numbered among the best scholars we have in our home. They are bright, affectionate, laughing boys—Billy a veritable Saxon, with his light hair and blue eyes. Jimmy takes after his mother, having the black hair and deep brown eyes of his Eskimo extraction. As they rush down to greet us now and 'purr' out their affection like pleased kittens, we shudder to think of what might have happened if we hadn't 'happened along' at the beginning of winter.

St. Anthony children headed to Sunday School

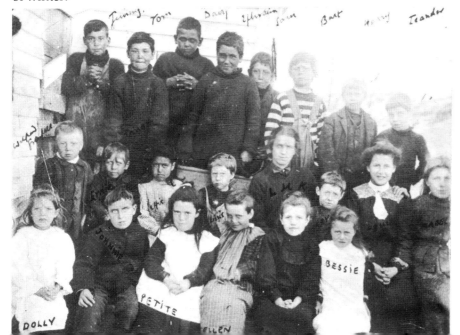

The Mission's children, *c.*1909

THE VERDICT*

Early in 1907 Grenfell purchased a small house near the St. Anthony Hospital to house himself and those of his staff not living in the hospital or in the orphanage. Known as the Guest House, by the winter of 1907-1908 it formed the centre of a lively little community. There was Dr John Little; craft instructor Jessie Luther; Cuthbert C. Lee, a wealthy Philadelphian youth sent by his father to work for Grenfell; and Lieutenant William Lindsay, a genial Irishman and Boer War veteran who was looking for something useful to do. There also was Ruth Keese, a schoolteacher from Ashburnham, Massachusetts, who had come to St. Anthony to start a kindergarten class. To her surprise, Keese had discovered when she arrived that though St. Anthony had a small school, it lacked a schoolteacher. Beginning with about a dozen students up to the age of fifteen years, she was teaching some seventy-five children within a year or two. Ruth Keese married Dr John Little in 1911 but continued to teach until they left for Boston in 1917. Ruth Little died in 1977.

The following story is not from Keese, but Grenfell. It appeared in Down North on the Labrador *(1911), another collection of his yarns where once again accuracy of detail is sacrificed to art. This is Grenfell at his best.*

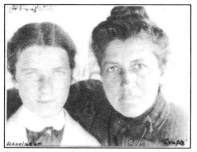

Schoolma'am Ruth Keese and craft instructor Jessie Luther

Christmas had come and gone, and even here 'away down north,' we were already discussing plans for the still distant season of open water. A flag raised one day on a high pole across the harbour heralded at breakfast that a dog mail had arrived that morning—and as we gathered round the log fire at night, each one was contributing for the general benefit titbits from the news received from our widely distributed homes.

It was our schoolma'am's turn to talk; she evidently had something on her mind. She was a poor dissembler of emotions. "A friend of mine who teaches a large kindergarten near home," she broke in, "has offered to come down for the summer, and help with the school. Do you think it would be any good telling her to come along?"

In a country like this, conundrums are our daily portion. But it was unusually unanimously, as if by instinct, that all hands plumped for a kindergarten, to be taught by a friend of our friend. After which, like so many children, we proceeded to discuss its possibility.

'Experimentum fiat' was the best verdict we could come to, even after prolonged discussion; and sure enough our first July boat deposited a trained kindergartner in our midst, with mysterious boxes of apparatus such as the sun had never shone on in our village before.

The question of installation was settled by clearing the diminutive schoolroom of all the impediments of rough board, forms and desks, that we had so laboriously collected and had previously been so highly prized. They were replaced by a few chalk lines on the floor, now resplendent from much soap and scrubbing. Some dainty little chairs occupied but little space, while in the corner stood the marvel of the shore—a real grand piano. It was no bantling, this piano—on the contrary, it had an added sanctity of years sufficient alone to commend it to our veneration.

Its size was appalling in its setting of our tiny school, while from the very first day the gorgeous polish of its mahogany case did for the ill-lit corners of the room what it has since been doing steadily for the far less penetrable corners of many small minds. It has been a veritable light to them that sit in darkness. How many of our little scholars stood open-mouthed and speechless, as, after

---

* Wilfred T. Grenfell, "The Regeneration of Johnnie Elworth," *Down North on the Labrador* (New York: Fleming H. Revell 1911)

bounding through the door with characteristic energy, its awful presence first dawned on their startled gaze. When at length they saw their beloved schoolma'am actually sit down and handle it with familiarity and force it to give forth sweet music, enthusiasm knew no bounds.

The grand piano had only one rival for many days, and that rival also had but just been unveiled. It was a large 'stuff' cow, that not only was as real as life, but the wise ones knew that if you 'slewed her head round' she would twist it back herself and give vent to a loud moo-oo as she did so. It was long the ample reward of the industrious to be permitted to slew that head.

And so the kindergarten got under way and our new helper could be seen surrounded morning and afternoon with an eager crowd of hitherto unappreciative youngsters, who in increasing numbers flocked to enjoy the marvel of modern kindergarten methods.

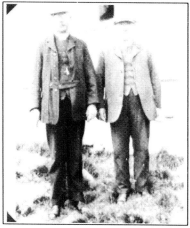
'Our oracles'

The hearts of all those who were interested in the children's welfare rose like sky rockets, and the gleam in many eyes betrayed that we were counting once again on leaving our southern, usually more favoured rivals, 'hull down' on the race for learning....

Among the pursuits that have received the irrevocable condemnation of the local leaders of religion, in spite of the concession of Solomon on this particular point, is dancing. It comes within the same category as dram-drinking, and must be unhesitatingly discountenanced. The laxity of foreigners on this particular article of the creed is proverbial. No wonder then that rumours were soon afloat that at the afternoon session of our kindergarten the 'thin edge of this wedge of sin' was being secretly inserted. Now if this scandal were permitted to spread it spelled nothing short of ruin for our most promising effort. It was obvious that this bull had to be taken by the horns, and that at once. There were two ministers who were our oracles on all such subjects at the time, in our harbour. I left in search of them without delay. It was agreed we should unexpectedly drop in at the very next afternoon session, and, if necessary, nip this poison plant while yet it was in the bud.

Three o'clock saw us, strengthened by the company of yet one more expert on vital matters of this kind, knocking at the kindergarten door. Our arrival, I must confess, seemed in no wise to disconcert the new teacher whose integrity was at stake. She certainly could not have realized the magnitude of the issues this solemn conclave foreboded. Politely but firmly we were ushered to the sole remaining wooden bench and told to perch ourselves well out of the way against the wall at the end of the room. Arrayed in a solemn row, and, there is no denying it, awed into silence by the atmosphere prevailing, we must have

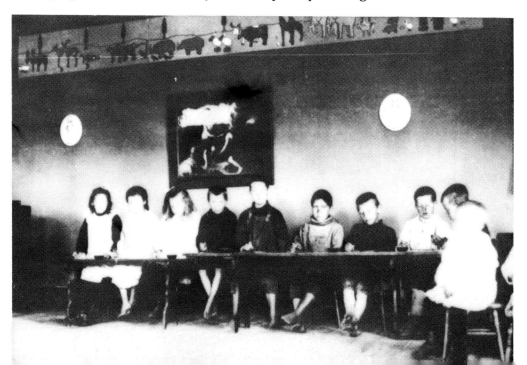
Ruth Keese's first class

appeared to an intelligent onlooker like a tenderfoot jury at a new quarter sessions. I confess to misgivings of conscience as I sat watching without a word the 'carryings on' we were shortly to pronounce on for good or evil. The first 'game' or two were irreproachable. The interrupted ball game was reenacted. Every child was sitting on the floor. No adverse comment was possible on this or on the second game, called 'Now we turn in, turn in,' 'Now we turn out, turn out.' For fortunately no one left the places allotted to them, though at the magic words 'I turn myself about' every one jumped round about. This game was certainly permissible.

But now the children are 'choosing partners,' and though, with the perversity of childhood, the boys had all chosen boys, and the girls girls to share the intricacies of the coming evolutions, I noted with trepidation that the suspicions of the vigilance committee were undoubtedly aroused. I could see it in their eyes, and, being unaware of what was to follow, I felt proportionally nervous. We were informed by the teacher that this performance would be a 'folk game,' and was known under the title 'Piggiewig and Piggiewee.' It was to be accompanied by singing.

There proved, to my intense relief, after all, no danger of our yet incurring theologic odium from this innovation on the road to the three R's. The children actually sat down part of the time, and the undoubted risks attaching to all forms of motor dissipation were then confined to rhythmic movements of the fingers. With a sigh of relief, I recognized we were still surviving the test.

Our teacher next successfully navigated us clear of any possible stricture through the game of 'All on the Train for Boston.' For, in spite of the motion, each player only held on to the shoulders of the one in front, and shuffled on after the engine along that apparently circuitous route. So that we could think of no form of dance (known to us in our unregenerate days of course) comprehensive enough to include this, as even a collateral. But we had scarcely begun to breathe freely when we were forewarned that the whole company would now 'join hands, and move round and round in a circle' to music. This was a very different matter. And now the whole committee realized that the supreme moment had arrived! With no little apprehension we saw boys and girls actually alternated, hands actually held in hand—and we noted that as all sang the undeniably secular script of 'Louby Loo,' many of the tiny feet positively left the floor as the circle went merrily round. We had seen sufficient. For we had now no doubt whatever that we had traced to their lair the very natural suspicions that had necessitated our visit. Without question there were those who would classify this proceeding 'as unbecoming to a wholly devoted religious person.'

With the most studied politeness we bade farewell to the prisoners at the bar, and adjourned to consider the whole problem at issue—*in camera*—on the nearest fishing stage.

The question now resolved itself into a very elementary one, viz., what should we do? It was no longer the kindergarten that was on trial, it was the committee. We, we, the irreproachable—we who were regarded as the patterns for the orthodox. It was *we* who were on trial. How were we to avoid becoming a stumbling-block to the feeble-kneed, and at the same time escape our own convictions that unregenerate scoffers might be justified in seeing a humorous side to our dilemma? I will not describe the vicissitudes of the session. There was nothing in Holy Writ to which 'Piggiewig and Piggiewee' was subversive, that was clear. Without any fear we decided that by no subtlety of construction could any known passage of even the most obscure portions of Scripture be construed into a ban on games restricted to the 'Piggiewig' class. By a natural process which gave us great relief and we hoped was not 'a falling back,' we

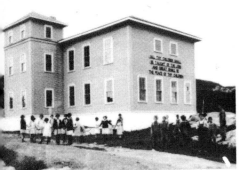
The Grenfell Mission's new school at St. Anthony

soon excluded also all but 'Louby Loo' from the 'questionable procedure group.'

An end has to come to all things. It was at length decided to put 'Louby Loo' to vote. On division we pretended to be seriously surprised that we were unanimously in favour of non-interference.

THE BIRTH OF THE 'INDUSTRIAL'*

In the spring of 1905 Grenfell was lecturing in Salem, Massachusetts, and went with his hostess to visit a small sanatorium at Marblehead catering to those suffering from 'nervous collapse.' The institution offered various forms of occupational therapy, a concept then in its infant stage, under the direction of Jessie Luther, a graduate of the Rhode Island School of Design and a teacher of arts and crafts. Grenfell was at the time looking for someone to teach weaving at St. Anthony, and was so full of ideas and fired with enthusiasm for the establishment of home industries that Luther in the summer of 1906 volunteered her services. She returned to St. Anthony in the fall of 1907, staying for one full year, and for a further year in 1909-1910. From then until 1914 she came to St. Anthony each summer. Through her craft and industrial development efforts, Jessie Luther contributed enormously to the Grenfell Mission.

Luther describes those early years.

The next summer, 1906, I was free and in early July started for St. Anthony. It was difficult in those days to get definite information as to the route, conditions of travel, etc., and Newfoundland seemed to everyone, myself included, very remote indeed....

We entered St. Anthony harbour in the afternoon ... There was then only a very small wharf, and the *Portia* dropped anchor offshore while everyone [was] landed in small boats—row boats, not the gasoline launches of today.

I had heard that a young doctor from Boston, Dr Soule, had gone down for the summer for out-patient work.... [He] had been there, I think, only two weeks. The only other staff members were Miss Storr from England, who had just arrived to open the new orphanage, then not entirely finished, and her friend, Miss Bailey from London, a trained nurse who had come over to help establish Miss Storr and who expected to return by the next boat.... The hospital ... was closed for the summer. Dr Grenfell was afloat on the *Strathcona* visiting the entire coast, and Nurse Williams, the only nurse at St. Anthony, had gone north to open the hospital at Indian Harbour, Labrador. Mr and Mrs Ashe were living at the hospital as caretakers, and Dr Soule slept there ... Miss Bailey decided to stay, and she and ... I lived with Miss Storr and the seven little orphans.

I found the looms and materials [donated by friends of the Mission] in the second story of a small building which was used downstairs as a carpentry shop.... While working on them I had many visitors, very shy and wondering what it was all about.... I soon found among odds and ends in the workshop a battered set of carving tools; and after putting them in order with the help of a grindstone, I found that several of the boys were interested in making use of them. So we started an evening carving class ... [which] consisted of Ted MacNeill [sic], John Newell and Archie Ashe, all honoured names in the Mission today....

That was a busy summer for us all ... one of the happiest summers I ever spent. Each of us was working about sixteen hours per day....

In the fall of 1908 Ted McNeill and Archie Ashe went to New York to take a technical course at the Pratt Institute. They were the first of many young people sent by the Mission to acquire technical and other specialized training in the United States, Canada and Great Britain.

* Jessie Luther, "In Retrospect," *Among the Deep Sea Fishers* 28, no. 3 (1930): 112-24

The women already made rugs of old clothing cut up into bits and drawn through the meshes of burlap or 'bun' as it is called locally; and the rude adjustable frame on which they are made is found in nearly every home. They also know how to spin, but the yarn is used to knit jerseys, stockings, caps and mittens and no one had ever woven the yarn or had ever seen a hand loom.

J. Luther 1907

Scarcely a day passed without visitors in the loom-room; some asking all sorts of questions; some coming in shyly, simply to gaze at the unfamiliar objects. Visitors from neighbouring hamlets were always brought to see the new work.

J. Luther 1907

We saw Dr Grenfell only once during the summer when he came in on the *Strathcona* and spent a day and a night. He came into the orphanage wrapped in a long cape, carrying a ship's lantern and, for the only time during my long acquaintance with him, wearing a beard. We had only time to show him what we were doing and talk things over, and he was off again.

It was obviously impossible to establish such a major industry as weaving on a permanent basis under such conditions and in so short a time.... So the following September [1907] saw me again on the way.

During the year much had improved. A small house formerly used by a trader had been added to the Mission buildings ... It was called the Guest House and was barely ready for occupancy when I arrived. Four members of the staff [Little, Keese, Lindsay and Lee] were already there.... A doctor and a nurse were installed at the hospital, and Miss Storr was still at the orphanage.

In the loom room ... the work went well, the girls came more regularly and we really felt that something was being accomplished. The whole work began to take form....

That first winter, 1907-1908, was an eventful one. It was the year of the epidemic of influenza ... the coming of the reindeer ... the year when Dr Grenfell so nearly lost his life on the ice ...

At the end of that long happy winter of 1907-1908, the early boat brought changes. A man from New York came to install an electric lighting plant of inestimable value to the Mission. The first wops made their appearance, unloaded coal and made themselves generally useful.... I first met Minnie Pike, who came to learn to weave and afterwards returned to her home at Red Bay to establish a new weaving centre.

After a year with my hospital work at home, I was granted another year of absence and in the fall of 1909 returned to St. Anthony. Again there were changes. The personnel of the staff was enlarged. The Guest House was filled to overflowing. Dr Stewart at the hospital had married and a little house had been built for him ...

I think it was during my third summer that I first went down the Labrador as far north as Indian Harbour in an attempt to direct the native embroidery on deerskin.... [After that] I took a short trip down the Labrador coast each summer, having learned the names of, and in many cases having met, those in each community doing the best work.... [From the Hudson's Bay Company] I bought skins and other materials, left them with the people for their winter work, and the following year sent word to the workers by the mail boat before that on which I expected to arrive, and they came to meet me with their product, were paid for their work and received more material for another year. Those living near centres like Indian Harbour or Battle Harbour sent their product there and were often paid in clothing which they usually preferred to cash....

[Another] of the native Labrador products that we found saleable were baskets made from native grass. These in form and texture were aboriginal and not influenced by the industrial department ...

I think it was in 1912 that Dr Andrews from Santa Barbara came to St. Anthony. It was the first time an oculist had ever visited us, and the news quickly spread in the mysterious way of remote localities that 'the eye doctor' was on the field. Those who had been blind for years came by the mail boat with happy hopes, only in many cases to meet disappointment. One of these cases was a young man who had lost one eye by an accident and whose other eye was badly affected. He was growing hopelessly blind and could barely distinguish light from dark. The mail boat stopped only once in two weeks and this man, unhappy with disappointment after being examined, wandered about while waiting to return home and found his way to the industrial school.

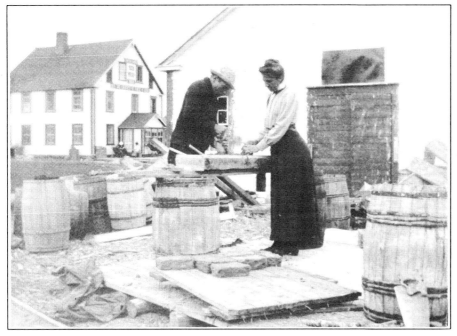

We had a little material for reed baskets and in the hope of giving the poor fellow something to fill the long hours of waiting I taught him basketry, a craft, of course, often taught the blind, but to him it was an absolutely new experience. He was interested at once and grew so proficient that when the mail boat came he took with him enough material to make several baskets and for some time afterwards he was supplied with material each year ...

While this blind man was working on his baskets two crippled boys, patients at the hospital, joined the class, and the three used to sit at work quite happily on the sunny porch. It was really our first occupational therapy attempt at St. Anthony ...

During the early period of my Mission work, I saw many native mats; the floors of nearly every house were covered with them, and many were brought in to sell for clothing or cash. There were some beautifully made mats in St. Anthony, some with interesting native designs ... but the traders had begun to offer pieces of burlap stamped with ugly designs in glaring and inharmonious colours with 'pound packages' of bright colours for patterns, and as a result many were well done but very ugly and unsaleable as a product.

We accepted many because those who made them were in sore need, but we did not know what to do with them. It seemed reasonable to suppose that mats of good workmanship, of colouring that would not clash with average household furnishings and with designs of local significance, might find a ready market; and I began to offer such designs, usually with a plain centre and border of seals, walruses, deer, rabbits, komatiks and dogs, etc., treated conventionally. Most of the material, some woollen and some outing flannel, was dyed in the loom room ... our object being to obtain colours that would be durable. These mats, with the patterns marked on them, or with the stencil to mark them themselves, were given out to the people in their homes ... After a while Dr Grenfell began to make designs himself in the nature of interesting pictures—bears on ice, ducks flying over trees, komatik and dogs on the snow, a lone owl, etc....

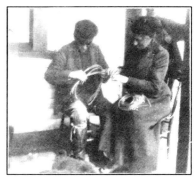

Basket making: 'blind leading the blind'

In the weaving and in all the other work I tried to set high standards and to make the workers understand that a permanent and profitable industry depended upon themselves, that we had a reputation to live up to and a lowering of standards would react on themselves. This was the principle of our

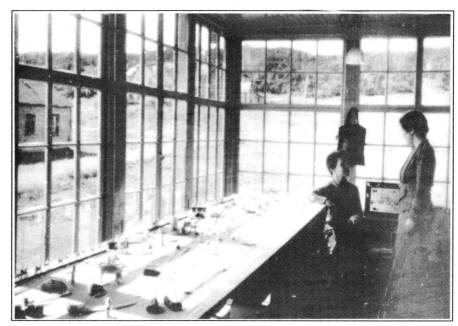

Industrial goods on display at Grenfell House, the Grenfells' St. Anthony home

An early view of St. Anthony

On the left is the orphanage. In the centre, left to right, are the guest house, hospital and industrial centre. The Mission had acquired a large tract of land, cleared it, drained it and created a settlement.

work, but there were exceptions when in cases of extreme poverty poor work was accepted because the immediate need was so great and what the people brought in was all they had to offer for money or clothing.

The summer of 1914 was my last on the coast. It was no longer possible to give the time to volunteer service, and, after a futile attempt to direct the industry from a distance, it was passed on to other hands during the winter of 1916. I knew it would go on. Lady Grenfell with great interest was extending the hooked mat industry over a large area. Mrs Wakefield was independently supervising spinning and knitting on the lower Labrador; new weaving centres were in operation.

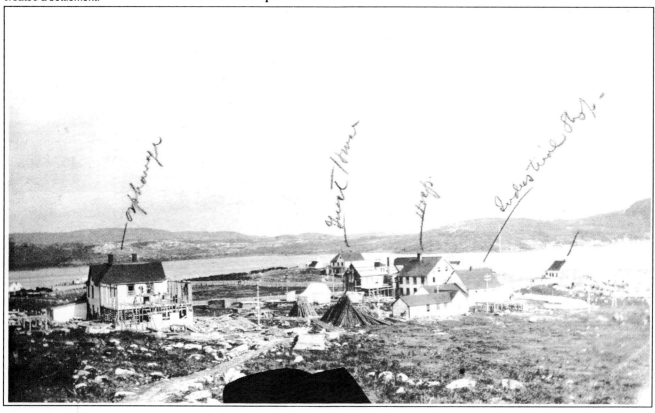

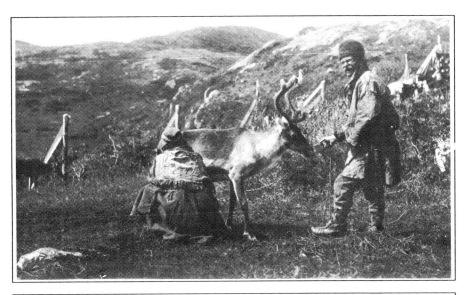

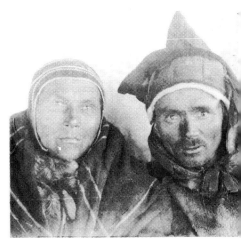

REINDEER TRIALS

The reindeer fiasco was one of Grenfell's more bizarre experiments. Convinced that reindeer could provide milk, meat and skins, replace the vicious and unpredictable sled dog for winter transport/travel and support collateral industries in leather, cheese manufacture and the like, he raised the necessary $15,000 to import three hundred domesticated reindeer from Lapland in 1908. They were accompanied by three Lapp families to act as herders. A visionary, daring and probably foolhardy scheme, dogged by misadventure from the start, the original herd had tripled in number by 1913. The experiment failed ultimately: the Lapps went home, the Newfoundland government was reluctant to see game laws enforced, and poachers killed off much of the herd.

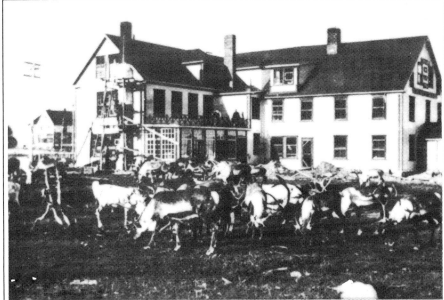

Counterclockwise from the top:
Lapp herders
Milking the herd
Grazing by the St. Anthony Hospital
Harnessing up

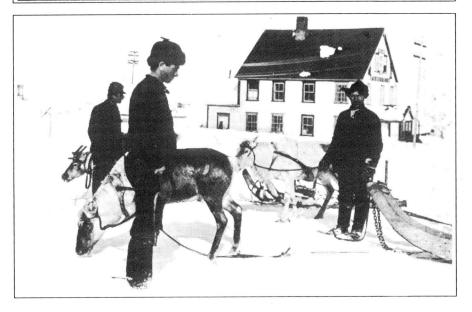

MORE THAN A WIFE*

Dr Arthur W. Wakefield, a former member of the Royal Army Medical Corps and a Boer War veteran, took charge of the St. Anthony Hospital in the summer of 1908. Working for two or more years at St. Anthony and on the Labrador coast, he then paid a visit to the Younger family of Montreal, whose head was a director of the Imperial Tobacco Company. When Wakefield returned to the coast, he brought Younger's eldest daughter, Marjorie, as his bride. A modern languages degree acquired from McGill University hardly prepared her for events ahead. The Wakefields spent time at St. Anthony, Forteau, Mud Lake and Battle Harbour, where Marjorie Wakefield was involved in industrial work. After the First World War the Wakefields left the Mission for good and eventually settled in Keswick, England. Marjorie Wakefield died in 1976.

The following was contributed by her son.

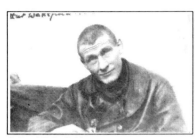

Arthur Wakefield

At her first introduction to the operating room, when she was required to hold a man's leg for amputation, she related how she was grateful for the supporting wall behind her back.... Dr Wakefield's bride, the honeymoon scarcely over, became 'dogsbody' to everyone. After helping at operations she would sterilize instruments, scrub the table and floor and, every fortnight when the mail boat arrived, she coped with the doctor's sack of letters in the 23 hours before the boat returned to civilization.

With her husband and an Eskimo driver—trained by Dr Wakefield to act as anaesthetist—she travelled hundreds of miles by dog team to attend patients. She is reported to have been the first white woman to have set eyes on Churchill Falls (then called Grand Falls). When babies arrived in the doctor's absence she delivered them; when teeth had to be extracted because no one was qualified to fill them she took a three months' practical dentistry course in Montreal and added this to her other duties. Dentures presented no problem. The patient obtained them by mail order, merely stating whether a male or a female, and whether upper or lower sets were required. "There was plenty of adventure," she used to say. "I've been lost in the snow, dumped out of a canoe into an icy river, half strangled by a dental patient during an extraction, and my first child was born on the Labrador coast while my husband was away."

In 1914 Dr Wakefield sailed for France with the forces. Mrs Wakefield remained in Labrador to make arrangements for the patients and staff at the hospital before returning to Montreal for the birth of her second child. But the need for medical help in Labrador was so great that in 1916 she spent another summer on the coast doing first aid and dentistry work after leaving her children in charge of a nurse in Montreal. After the war Dr Wakefield found himself too restless to settle in any one place and for a few years the family, now with three children, crossed and re-crossed the Atlantic some nine times.

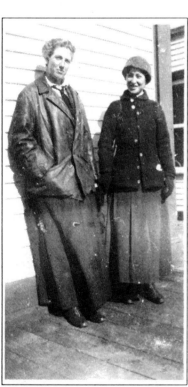

Nurse Williams and Marjorie Wakefield
at Battle Harbour

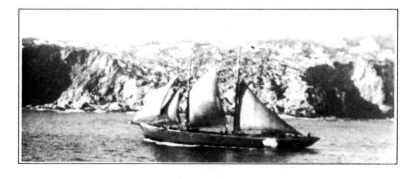

* R.W. Wakefield, "Mrs A.W. Wakefield," *Among the Deep Sea Fishers* 74, no. 1 (1977): 16-7

BATTLE HARBOUR*

George W. Corner (1889-1981) was born in Baltimore and entered Johns Hopkins Medical School in 1909. In search of summer experience after their third year of medical training, he and fellow medical student Grover Powers offered their services to the Grenfell Mission. At Battle Harbour they worked as medical and surgical assistants to Dr John Grieve. They also worked as pharmacists, boatmen, house painters, ditch-diggers and general labourers. At the end of the summer the Battle Harbour hospital was semi-closed, the summer staff scattered, and Grieve readied his dog team for winter rounds. Corner returned to Baltimore for his final year of medical studies, acquired his MD and returned to Battle Harbour for one more summer, this time working with Dr Arthur Wakefield. He went on to become an exceptionally productive medical scholar, publishing 240 papers and fifteen books, including his 1958 autobiography, Anatomist at Large.

Corner here provides a good description of how medicine in a Grenfell hospital actually worked. He indicates as well the medical conditions most frequently seen.

Battle Harbour Hospital is situated at a strategic point that was selected with much foresight. It stands on a little island at the southeastern apex of the coast, just where the gulf enters the sea…. Every one of the fishing vessels passing to the Labrador for the summer, or southbound for Newfoundland in the fall, must course within sight of [it] … Beside the local residents and the schooner men, the parish of the hospital is increased by the fact that Battle Harbour is the terminal port for three of the mail steamers which visit the Labrador, and a port of call for two others, making altogether nine stops each fortnight from June 15 to December.

Admissions to the hospital are in various ways. The young men of the staff often sleep half clad, with boots by the bedside, in expectation of a midnight blast announcing the arrival of a steamer. A patient may be dragged in on a sailcloth stretcher by his despondent schoonermates. A woman was brought twenty miles in the open Atlantic, lying helpless on her back in the bottom of a rowboat in a chilling, heavy rain. The mission steamer *Strathcona* brings a few patients from the remote unvisited harbours, but the mailships are the bearers of the majority of those seeking medical attention, either as they come of their own accord, or are sent by the government physician who travels on one of the ships.

The hospital building has grown from a small house … until the establishment is now a simple but neat hospital of 20 beds. There are wards for men and women, respectively; an inside room of three beds suitable for ether recovery, for ophthalmic cases, and the like; two verandas for open-air patients; a small operating room; a tiny place for infected dressings and miscellaneous examinations, and a room, now overcrowded by being used as drug room, dispensary, and clinical laboratory.

The building also contains a large and convenient kitchen and pantry, a sitting room for patients, and a hall about 20 x 30 feet, which served last summer by turns as a dormitory, unpacking room, lecture hall, dental operating room, loom room, and chapel. The staff makes the best of a few rather small sleeping rooms, with a small dining room and sitting room. Besides the hospital, the mission group also contains two store houses, a wharf, and a small laundry … The fleet at Battle Harbour contains a small auxiliary schooner, a launch, a barge, and a skiff for harbour use….

Patients arriving at the St. Anthony Hospital

The majority came on the government's coastal steamer and mail vessel to be embarked by rowboat. Eventually the Mission constructed a large wharf at St. Anthony which accommodated large vessels.

* G.W. Corner, "Hospital Work of the Labrador Mission," *Modern Hospital* 3 (1914): 72-8

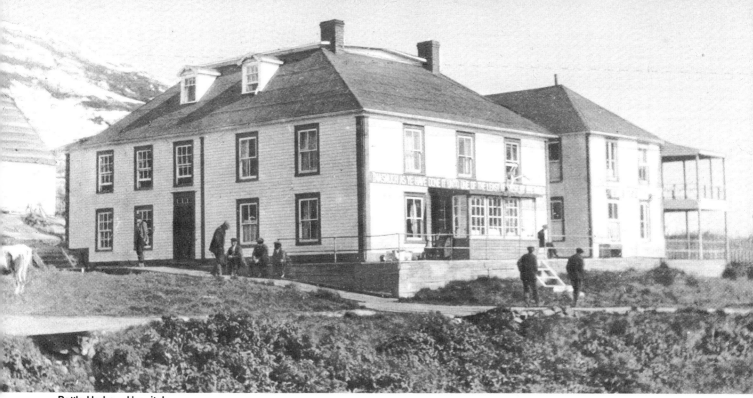
Battle Harbour Hospital

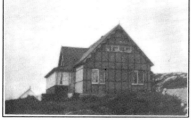
The doctor's house at Battle Harbour

Staff — About the middle of June the little town begins to rouse from its winter quiet. The doctor has returned from his dog-sledge trip in March, and since the first of May has been cooped up on the island by the weakness of the ice, which prevents all travel to and from the seaward isles. But with the first steamer which pokes her nose through the remains of the ice-pack come the summer helpers who are to take their part in the season's work. The most important of these newcomers is naturally the head nurse, who is either a volunteer, qualified by several seasons' experience with the mission for the peculiar difficulties of her position, or, as was the case last year, one of the very few paid nurses of the staff—that is to say, she receives a stipend called a salary by courtesy....

Some summers there is a regular housekeeper; otherwise the head nurse has this duty also. The housekeeper has the task of training six or seven Labrador girls in the service of kitchen and wards.... The kitchen, therefore, becomes a training school, for the girls are brought to the mission not only for the good of the work, but in the knowledge that when they return to their homes they will be missionaries in turn, taking to remote villages new ideas of cooking, household management, and hygiene.

The housekeeper must feed forty people, the sick and the well, on a diet every article of which, except fresh fish and berries, has to come in tin can or barrel by vessel. She must concoct a milk-and-egg diet, when ordered, from tinned milk and egg-powder; and she has to feed invalids who are deeply suspicious of custards, broths, and such unfamiliar things, and who complain if they are not given salt pork and sinkers.

Of late years the increasing work of the hospital has required three other nurses, and these are volunteers, who have only their expenses paid. They have come, in different seasons, from a number of the English training schools, from Massachusetts General, St. Luke's, Presbyterian (New York), from Johns Hopkins, the Sick Children's Hospital of Toronto, Sibley in Washington, and many others. The physician in charge has for assistants a recent graduate and one or two medical students, who pay their own travelling expenses in return for the instructive summer's experience. Usually three or four college students volunteer for the summer's work about the boats and in the general work of the station.

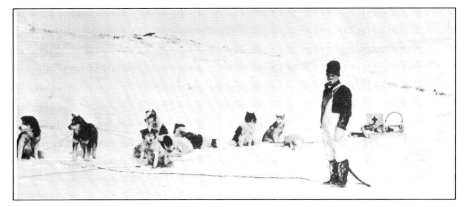
Dr Grieve's dogs

Medical conditions and patients — The medical work, of course, does not differ greatly from that of a small village hospital and dispensary in the United States, and yet there are special conditions which add immensely to the burdens, and, one might add, to the interest of the situation. First, the widespread occurrence and disastrous results of tuberculosis. In the absence of statistics it has been estimated that one death in three in Newfoundland and Labrador is caused by this disease, besides those in which an intercurrent infection carries off a tuberculous patient. The blame for this condition can fortunately be definitely traced. Spitting is the national sport of the fishermen, both indoors and out; and, when practised by an infected man, in a tight, overheated, one-room shack, among a family of underfed children, the result may be imagined. A lad was admitted to Battle, and died the next day, whose sputum showed at least five hundred tubercle bacilli in every field of the sample taken for study. He had been lying for seven months in a room also occupied by six brothers and sisters, and had never in his life been told that it is wrong to spit on the floor.... Of course, the problem is tangled up with the questions of food and housing, as it is everywhere, but on the whole things seem hopeful. The Labrador or New-foundland fisherman who has tuberculosis is much better off, if he can get good advice and will follow it, than the inhabitants of East Side tenements or the alley-dwelling negroes of our southern cities.

Strangely enough, another serious disease of this northern country is one that everyone thinks of as distinctly tropical—namely, beri-beri, or endemic peripheral neuritis. About 12 percent of admissions at Battle Harbour are cases of this disease. In etiology the northern cases agree with the experience of tropical physicians, who attribute the disease to a diet formed chiefly of polished rice, the husks, which are discarded in the process of polishing, containing a substance necessary to prevent neuritic degeneration. In the north the winter diet consists largely, sometimes entirely, of tea and bleached white flour. This diet lacks the same substance which is wanting in polished rice, and which seems to be present in the rice and wheat husks, in fresh meat, and in many vegetables....

In the spring of 1913 an epidemic of pneumonia invaded many harbours, with an unusual number of fatalities. The other common respiratory ailments are frequent, notably enlarged tonsils and adenoids. Scurvy, of course, and all the forms of diseases due to malnutrition are ever occurring. The vexing and yet hopeful side of this matter is that in most cases the faulty diet is not due to forced starvation but to ignorance of the people as to how to lay our their resources for proper food. Accidental lesions and wound infections send many of the fishermen to the mission dispensaries, violent pyogenic [pus producing] infections of cuts caused by fishing tackle are frequently seen.

Inflammations of the conjunctiva and other parts of the ocular apparatus give occasion for much ophthalmic practice. Pterygia [corneal abnormalities]

Remembering how difficult it had been in the Battle Harbour operation room to administer ether for tonsil operations with the old-fashioned ether-mask always in the surgeon's way, I built during the winter my own version of an apparatus for administering ether vapour by pharyngeal tube, recently introduced at the Johns Hopkins Hospital, and by special permission tested it on ten dogs in Harvey Cushing's experimental surgery laboratory. For this I received undeserved praise for inventiveness when the device was successfully used at Battle Harbour the next summer.

G. Corner 1958

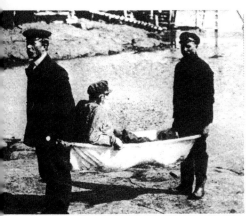

Labrador ambulance

During the previous winter and again after my second journey to the north, I was so eager to help the Grenfell Mission that I had a set of lantern slides made from my own negatives and gave lectures before any church and school groups that would have me.

G. Corner 1958

are very common, as is to be expected from the weather conditions. Skin diseases, especially eczemas, cause much suffering among the fishermen aboard schooners, where it is next to impossible to keep clean. Scabies is prevalent, and pediculosis is the bane of the nursing staff—it is found in every ward patient. The mission doctors do no obstetrical work, except when called in complicated cases; not from unwillingness, but because of the enforced slowness of travel, and because the patients favour local help, and will not send for the physician. Native treatment, needless to say, is of the most ignorant old-wife type; the late results of obstetric neglect are common and serious.

The venereal diseases are practically unknown at Battle Harbour—*O fortunati nimium*—in six hundred dispensary patients there were four cases; none of them were acquired in Labrador. A package of salvarsan lies unopened on the shelf. Yet the prevalence of arteriosclerotic lesions is distressing, a fact to be blamed on the constant exposure and dreadfully hard work of the fishermen. A man told me that the nets belonging to his crew were set in a place three miles away from his schooner. He and his mates had pulled their heavy boat the six miles three times a day, in gale and calm, all summer long. Let the reader try a few minutes at a fifteen-foot sweep, in a heavy sea, and he will appreciate what hard labour really is.

Those of us who go to the Labrador fresh from metropolitan hospitals are surprised and not a little instructed to learn how much can be done with the small equipment of a mission station. A critical visitor to Battle Harbour will find neat histories of every case, recording complete blood counts, gastric analyses, and even in a few instance pathological reports, made on the basis of free-hand-razor-blade sections. Autopsies are made in a little shed which serves between times as a dynamite store house. St. Anthony Hospital rejoices in a microtome and a bacteriological incubator.

At Battle the house officer finds time to make the routine physical examinations in spite of numerous other duties, being, as the mission magazine says, 'house surgeon, house painter, and stevedore.' It is no unusual thing for the staff to be called from 'public hygiene' work, in the shape of drain digging, to undertake major operating. The little operating room, which the British members of the household insist on calling the 'theatre,' sees the same moments of excitement, is filled with the same spirit of mutual dependence and mutual confidence that are known in marble amphitheatres at home.

The fisher-folk of northern Newfoundland and of Labrador, viewed as hospital patients, are admirable in some ways, highly annoying in others. The deeply pious nature of the people takes outward effect in a spirit of listless dependence on Providence, so that necessary treatment is postponed, or operations declined, in spite of every argument and threat. A man brought in with a fractured hip proved to have had chronic gastritis for eight years, with vomiting after each meal for the past two years. The patient said that he had never bothered to see a doctor, and, moreover, that as he had stood his ailment so long, he would rather continue vomiting that be put on a milk diet. A woman 62 years of age appeared at the dispensary suffering with an ovarian cyst, which after removal weighed twenty-eight pounds. She and her family greatly feared the operation, but finally gave permission. During her convalescence her husband came to visit her, and on leaving remarked to Dr Wakefield, "Well, Doctor, so ye've come through with this terrible thing. Who'd a thought it? But, then, all things is possible with the Lord. And now, Doctor, since ye've done so well by me wife, I just think I'll let ye test me eyes." Yet, when the occasion demands, the Labrador can show its examples of bravery.

Tradition and superstition are held with tenacity, oftentimes blocking the efforts which are being made to teach the prevention of common ailments. I have already referred to the prejudice against dark [wholewheat] flour; this seems to have arisen in days when darkness meant dirt. Another tradition is that of the danger of fresh air in the house. Hospital patients think it a crime to let the cold air on them, even when protected by five or six blankets. To make a tubercular patient sleep out-of-doors is the refinement of torture. Still, twenty years' preaching of these reforms is not without result, and whole wheat flour, the open window, and even that amazing novelty, the tooth brush, are beginning to invade the villages of Labrador.

Alas, alas, the patent medicine faker finds among these simple people an easy field for his trade. One audacious firm even sent a case of its cure-all liniment as a contribution to the mission. The people are invariably surprised if told that medicines are not necessary or are inadvisable for their complaints, and leave unsatisfied if not given pills and potions. Large doses of bitter drugs are preferred, and will be faithfully taken with much satisfaction on the part of the patient.

It is always amusing to see with what naive surprise certain things are regarded which are very familiar to us; for instance, the clinical thermometer, which is thought by many to be a kind of medicine. The bath tub is the greatest novelty. Battle Harbour possesses three of these, the only ones in Labrador, if I am not mistaken. "Doctor," said one of the patients, "has I got to strip off me clo'es and git into that thing? You folks is shockin' hard on us pore sailors." Of course the art of bathing has to be taught and its performance supervised. How often would you bathe if in winter you had to melt every drop of the water from snow, and in summer the water about your schooner was at a temperature of 38 or 40 Fahrenheit?

My possession of an MD diploma and a certificate to practise won me greater responsibilities [the second summer]. Before I left in the autumn Dr Grenfell offered me charge of the winter station at the village of Pilley's Island, where I would have commanded my own tiny hospital, staffed by a trained nurse and a sledge-driver with his team of eight Newfoundland huskies. Surely no young physician ever faced two such contrasting opportunities, under leaders of such different eminence as Grenfell in his ice-bound mission and Mall [Francis Payne Mall, the renowned professor of pathology at Johns Hopkins] at the metropolis of medical science; but with only passing regrets I returned to Baltimore and to anatomy.

G. Corner 1958

WE'VE HAULED THE WOMAN ABOARD*

Born in 1876 in Lynchburg, Virginia, into a well-off family, Rosalie Slaughter Morton left the promise of an easy life in the south to enter the Women's Medical College of Pennsylvania in 1893. During vacations, she worked in the slums. After graduation she did three years of post-graduate work in Europe—Berlin, Vienna, Paris, London... In Russia she was befriended by Tolstoy; in Scandinavia, by Ibsen. In India, she studied bubonic plague under the noted bacteriologist, Haffkine, and then worked in Manila. Returning to the United States, Morton pursued a career as a surgeon in Washington and New York, held major hospital appointments, and was in the forefront of the American public health movement. During the First World War she served with the Red Cross on the Salonika front, organizing and conducting field hospital units. After the war she founded the American Women's Hospitals and the Serbian Education Committee.

In New York before the war, Morton had met Grenfell several times. In 1915 she learned from Emma Dorset, the New York secretary of the recently formed International Grenfell Association, that because of the war he was unable to secure his usual complement of volunteer doctors to supplement his salaried staff that summer. Although Morton was at the time considering war work for herself, she decided to work for Grenfell first. En route to Labrador she stopped in St. John's, where she stayed at the Mission's fine new King George the Fifth Institute.

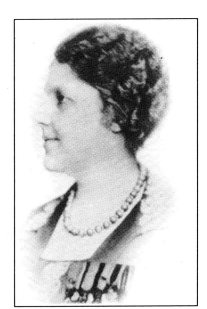

Rosalie Slaughter Morton

When we crossed the straits between Newfoundland and Labrador, we passed from the temperate to the subarctic zone. On our way up the coast our

---

*   Rosalie Slaughter Morton, *A Woman Surgeon: The Life and Work of Rosalie Slaughter Morton* (New York: Frederick A. Stokes 1937).

At St. John's, Newfoundland, Mr Sheard, the tall, genial business manager for the Grenfell Association, proudly showed us the comfortable Seamen's Institute. It was a dream come true for both Mission and men. The chapel was also used for illustrated lectures; there were rooms for pool, billiards, reading and writing; gymnasium, restaurant, shower baths, bowling alleys and even a swimming pool.

R. Morton 1937

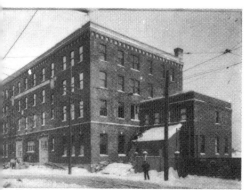

The King George the Fifth, or Seamen's, Institute

A four-storied red brick building on Water Street East, St. John's, the Institute was opened in 1912 at a cost of $175,000, all raised by Grenfell. The International Grenfell Association (IGA) had its main business office here. In the 1920s management of the Institute was taken over by the YM-YWCA.

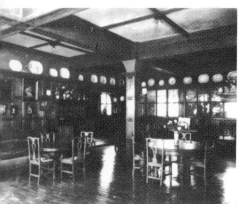

The Institute's temperance bar

little steamship was surrounded, whenever she anchored, by fishermen who had rowed out from their small harbours ... The men rarely asked anything about the war or for any news of the outside world. Their one persistent inquiry was "How's fish?"

On the Labrador coast things date by fishing events, such as 'the summer that the run was the poorest,' or 'the year of the good catch.' We found that there was much anxiety regarding the discontinuance, by command of the Admiralty, of the wireless station. It had been installed to keep the fishermen informed as to the condition of the ice and the locations of plentiful fish. This year they had to depend on passing steamers for information. They were obviously worried, asking, "Where are the fish? Why do they not come? They are late!" ...

Dr and Mrs John Grieve, three nurses and several of the 'Wops,' as the college lads dub themselves, met us [at Battle Harbour]. Dr Grieve, a Scotchman, had been in charge of this station for nine years. He heartily welcomed me as a coworker ... and put me in charge of his hospital and neighbourhood practice, for he was anxious to organize a cooperative store.

The cases were many and varied....

Dr Grenfell had sent me several messages of welcome although I had not seen him. He was in St. Anthony, Newfoundland, the chief Mission station of the chain, busy with hospital work. One day to my delight we heard that he would soon arrive on his small hospital boat, the S.S. *Strathcona*, in which during the summer he made trips to the settlements along the coast. He invited me to join and assist him. At every port people crowded the deck with all sorts of injuries, many of which in Labrador were regarded as minor, which in the States would have been major. The skiffs of patients were tied around the rail of our ship so that from a distance we must have looked like a hen with an oddly shaped brood of chickens. We remained in one harbour only so long as we were needed, then hoisted sail and Dr Grenfell steered for the next. At each place we put off a large box of books which were eagerly read by the villagers and sent on to another town. We also left clothing and food. Twenty first-aid boxes were entrusted to each village.

One evening at dusk we ran up on the rocks. The doctor said that he usually did this two or three times a season. Not a boat or habitation was in sight in the evening calm. But gradually people with hawsers, cables, poles, boat-hooks and other implements appeared on the cliffs above us. They soon cleared us, and we continued on our way....

Our medical cruise on the *Strathcona* ended at St. Anthony, for Dr Grenfell wished me to see the hospital there. On our way we stopped at Forteau on the Strait of Belle Island [sic], Nurse Bailey's station. She had just returned from making her 1,184th visit to 592 out patients in less than a year. She also had fourteen sick people for whom she was caring in her own cottage. As we neared her harbour, there appeared on the shore the first growing vegetables that had gladdened my eyes for many months....

As we neared our destination, the large St. Anthony Hospital with its wide porches for convalescing patients and the sunrooms below represented the most tangible of blessings—restored health....

The adaptability of all the doctors was such that one day, when an orthopaedic specialist who was visiting Dr Grenfell did some bone surgery, the rest of us rolled and prepared the plaster bandages because the nurses' hands were full with their regular work. During my stay in St. Anthony I had the privilege of assisting Dr Little. The release of a club foot from its shortened tendons; the restoration of the mind of a boy by relieving the pressure of a piece of bone on his brain, which had resulted from a severe fall and a crushed skull;

a tumour of the bladder; the removal of a kidney stone which had given agonizing hours to a man; and many others were especially interesting in view of the fact that before Dr Grenfell began his mission only such relief was available as a blacksmith could give....

The arrival of a ship in a Labrador harbour is something like the coming of Judgment day—every one knows that it will come but no one knows when. As the time approached when I had to depart [Battle Harbour] or be ice-bound for the winter, my packed steamer trunk and duffle bag were taken to our little wharf. Perhaps the steamer would dock in a day or two, more likely in ten. I was due back in New York to take up my hospital and private practice.

As I wished to be busy until the last day, however, I responded to the request of a villager who asked me to call. She confided that for ten years she had, without mentioning it, carried a very uncomfortable abdominal tumour. She had been waiting for a woman surgeon. She also confessed that she had waited to see how my patients 'got along.' Now her mind was made up. Would I operate? Yes, if she would come immediately to the hospital. Without hesitation, she gathered together a few things and we walked to the hospital.

The next morning, the operating room set, the patient drifting into etherized unconsciousness, assistants in place and everything ready to make the incision, the low toot of a steamer sounded. The nurses and I exchanged glances. We knew that meant that the boat would come and go within an hour. Should I let my patient out of ether, to face years of discomfort and perhaps a degeneration of the growth? I had a promise to keep. I proceeded with the operation. The ship's whistle sounded again, louder and nearer. Some one knocked on the door and asked what I was going to do. Dr Grieve insisted that it might be impossible for me to leave for eight months if I did not go at once. He added that it was just like that woman who had needed an operation for ten years to insist on having it done during the last ten minutes of my stay.

I am not Scotch, but I have just as much determination as Dr Grieve. Twenty busy minutes passed; there was another rap on the door. Some one had hurried up the hill. A breathless voice assured me that the captain had said I was not to hurry. He would hold the boat until I was ready to go. I nearly dropped an instrument. When I finished the operation and ran down the cliff to the wharf, the captain greeted me.

To my amazement, none of the passengers was annoyed. I told the people leaning over the rail, and calling to me as if we were old friends, that I thought they were very generous not to object to the delay. The captain escorting me up the gangplank, said quietly, "You are here to help our people. Why wouldn't we wait for you?"

But he took the edge off the elegance of this expression of gratitude by calling to the crew, "Cast off! We've hauled the woman aboard!"

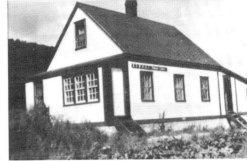

The nursing station at Forteau, Dennison Cottage

The first of the Mission's nursing stations, it was opened in 1908.

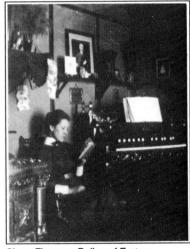

Sister Florence Bailey of Forteau

Her district included eighteen to twenty settlements stretching along sixty miles of coast. Bailey was with the Mission for eighteen years.

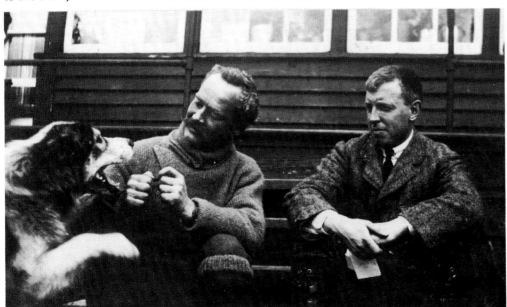

Grenfell and Dr John Grieve at Battle Harbour

A FORCED OPINION*

P.K. Devine (1859-1950) was born at King's Cove, Bonavista Bay, and taught school at Harbour Grace. In 1891 he joined the staff of the St. John's Evening Telegram; in 1911 he became clerk of the Newfoundland House of Assembly; from 1912 to 1918 he was editor of the Trade Review. He is best remembered as a collector of Newfoundland folklore.

Devine's following commentary appeared in the Trade Review in 1915, suggesting that the value of the Mission's medical work continued to be questioned in St. John's. It suggests also that differences between local commercial interests and the Mission were far from resolved.

In considering those early days of the Labrador fishery, there is no thought that challenges one's faculty of enquiry with greater force than the almost total immunity from sickness amongst the fishermen. The great contrast that has in this respect arisen in the past 25 years is, no doubt, the cause of this. Before there were so many visiting doctors, hospitals, and medicine dispensaries on the coast, there were very few cases of illness amongst the fishermen. It would be such a rare thing to have a man die on the Labrador, or to have a sick fisherman brought home before the voyage was over, that the whole coast would be talking about it for months afterwards. There is the fact, make what you like of it. Old men of 80 and 90 still living, will verify the truth of it. The most frequent cases of incapacity amongst the men would be when one of the crew would have a 'bad hand' caused by driving a hook in it, or cutting it with a splitting knife.

Since Dr Grenfell and his assistants have been going to Labrador, the cases of illness of different kinds—many never heard of before—have multiplied every season. I am not going to take the stand of saying that Dr Grenfell is not doing good work because I don't know that he is, or that he is not. But, if there was less sickness before he went there, and cases of illness began to take on a sudden increase when he began to go there, an opinion is forced upon one, whether he likes to accept it or not.

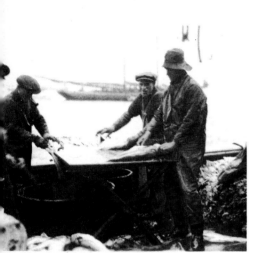

Cleaning fish aboard a schooner

BUT THE MUD HAD BEEN SLUNG**

In 1917, mercantile interests in St. John's petitioned the government asking that the Mission's duty-free privileges be abolished. The Mission was unfairly competing in the marketplace, the merchants claimed, because of advantages gained through customs concessions. Money squeezed from American philanthropists was giving it a further competitive edge. The Mission as a result had become 'a menace to all other mercantile concerns on the coast.' In response, the government of Newfoundland appointed a commissioner, Magistrate R.T. Squarey, to investigate the Mission's business dealings. In the process of his investigation, other issues emerged.

Magistrate Squarey heard evidence in St. John's, Harbour Grace and Carbonear before he and his entourage travelled on—via Strathcona—to visit Mission stations at St. Anthony, Battle Harbour, Cape St. Charles, Forteau and Pilley's Island. After examining sixty witnesses, Squarey found he was unable to find any connection between the Mission and the co-operative stores. The inquiry, but not the tensions, ended there.

It is to the sectarian issue raised during the inquiry that Grenfell speaks here.

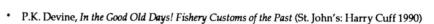

* P.K. Devine, *In the Good Old Days! Fishery Customs of the Past* (St. John's: Harry Cuff 1990)
** Wilfred T. Grenfell, "Medicine in the Sub-arctic: The Mary Scott Newbold Lecture. Lecture 22," *Transactions and Studies of the College of Physicians of Philadelphia* 52 (1930): 73-95

The starting of the cooperative cash stores ... brought us more serious opposition, and we woke one day to learn that at the request of many merchants, all of whose names were recorded, a commission was to be sent down by the government to investigate our irregular incursions into commerce. The list of accusations, however, were not confined to cooperative stores. Every department of the work was under attack, and even (we being Protestants) our doctors were accused of sectarian discrimination. This was made possible by intense sectarian fears, arising from the fact that all the educational grants in the country are divided 'per caput' amongst the leaders of the varying sects and creeds.... The commission sat at our headquarters at St. Anthony ... [and heard evidence from] the medical officer in charge ... Perhaps not unnaturally, the procedure on that occasion is fixed in my memory with unusual distinctness, for I subsequently printed 20,000 copies of the whole findings, for free distribution.

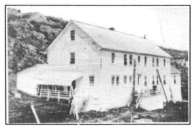

The Pilley's Island Hospital in Notre Dame Bay, the Mission's hospital furthest south

Established in 1911 in a hotel formerly owned by a mining company, its first medical officers were two young Americans, Harrison Webster and Hugh Greeley.

"Are you a doctor of medicine?"
"Yes."
"What is your name?"
"Louis Fallon."
"Your university?"
"Pennsylvania."
"Are you in full charge of this station?"
"Yes."
"Do you discriminate in your treatment of patients?"
"No."
"Do you give a Roman Catholic the same treatment as a Protestant?"
"Yes."
"What is your salary?"
"I am a volunteer, without salary."
"How long have you been here?"
"Six years."
"What is your religious affiliation?"
"I am a Roman Catholic!"

The reports were criticized as the best publicity that this work could possibly have received. But the mud had been slung.

PATCHES DIDN'T CONCERN HIM A BIT*

Florence Grant was born early this century at Blanc Sablon, where her father, Edwin G. Grant, was manager of a large fishing establishment. Her summers were spent at Blanc Sablon living in the 'Big House,' her winters at Trinity. Around 1933 she married Captain Percival Barbour, sometimes skipper of the IGA's Maraval. *Florence Barbour speaks from the perspective of an outport Newfoundlander who knew the Grenfell Mission well.*

Of all the guests at the Big House I think I am safe in saying that Dr Grenfell came more often than anyone. He came in the *Strathcona* and so he did not need accommodations. He loved to have a meal with us and many times told mother she was the best cook he ever came across. Father knew Dr Grenfell when he first came to the country in 1892. We all knew him from our earliest childhood days, and we were always so pleased to see him.

---

* Florence Grant Barbour, *Memories of Life on the Labrador and in Newfoundland* (New York: Carlton Press 1973).

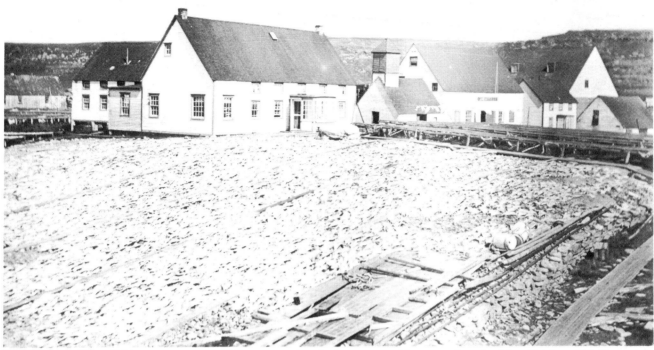

The 'Big House,' Blanc Sablon

The Big House was part of an extensive complex of salt fish processing and storage facilities owned by Job Brothers of St. John's.

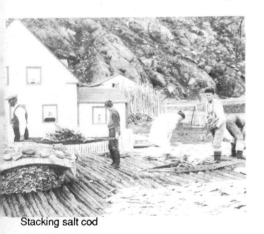

Stacking salt cod

Many a patch or button my mother sewed on for him. Patches didn't concern him a bit. He was known up and down the coast simply as the 'Doc.' He had a very pleasing manner, lots of personality, and was warm-hearted and humble. His chief concern was the sick. Yet he was very fond of joking and pulling the leg at times. On one occasion he had with him a Dr Andrews of California, the best [eye, ear,] nose and throat specialist on the Pacific Coast. At dinner one day he made an attempt to pull Dr Andrews's leg. Dr Andrews told him that he had seen a very large lobster that morning on the bottom over the stage head.

"Was it red?" asked Dr Grenfell.

Dr Andrews, with a glower, said "No, green."

For the convenience of Dr Grenfell and others, attached to the back of the house was a room we called the surgery. There were drawers full of clean linen for bandages, and about all the nostrums then in circulation, such as iodine, liniments, salves, antiflo-jistine, Radway's Ready Relief, castor oil, and epsom salts. The two latter remedies were supposed to be the panacea for all ills....

It was in the surgery that my father helped Dr Grenfell saw the bone of a man's gangrenous leg in order to save his life. My father was a very tender-hearted man; he told Doc he did not think he could do the job. However, Doc had such a persuasive way with father, that the next thing father knew he was helping to save the man's life. I heard my father tell the story and say he felt faint many times at the smell of ether, but Doc kept saying, "You're doing fine, Ned. Keep up the good work." At last it was over.

It was this same room where I had part of my tonsils removed, under a local anaesthetic and by the feeble light of a small kerosene oil lamp. Dr Grenfell had arrived that night with a Dr Little, who was a surgeon. He told mother it was the one chance to do the job. Some years before Sam [my brother] had one of his tonsils removed; when he saw the blood, he refused to have the second one touched. Sam bet me fifty cents that I would not go through with it. Fifty cents was a lot of money to a ten year old in those days. When I looked up, after the first tonsil was removed, I saw Sam's face peeping through the window at me. But I had one up on my brother because what he did not know was, that both doctors had promised me fifty cents if I stayed still and behaved myself. You bet, I stayed still and behaved! Who wouldn't for three fifty-cent pieces? All I could think about was all the material I was going to be able to buy for dolls' clothes once I got back to Trinity.

Once during the summer Doc would take part of a day to go up the river for some trout. He never went in a boat. He took a couple of sandwiches in his pocket and loved to walk up on the Canadian side of the river to the falls. He always brought back a dozen of the largest speckled beauties. On his return, we had a nice hot meal ready, to which he would do full justice.

One evening he was later than usual getting back. Mother became anxious when it became dark, so father sent Sam and his chum Alfred Wilson, who worked in the office, to look for the doctor. With a lantern, they found him fast asleep on the mossy bank and covered with sand flies. What a mess he was! However, he did not seem a bit concerned about himself, although it was difficult for him to see, since both eyes were swollen with fly bites. He was full of apologies to mother and father for causing them so much anxiety. Mother bathed his eyes with vinegar and water. After he had eaten his supper, he refused a bed for the night, lay down on the old couch, and was soon fast asleep. We knew better than to disturb him when we went to bed. He was up and away before the crack of dawn....

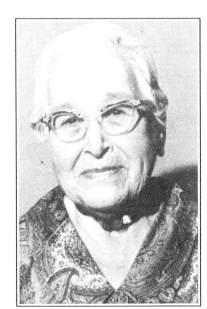

Grenfell conducting a service at Battle Harbour

We were all glad when the Doc arrived at Blanc Sablon to stand behind the table with the red plush cloth [in the fish store and conduct the service]. He was a man of medium stature, but with a big, big heart; he was clad in ordinary clothes, which sometimes had been patched by my mother the night before. He needed no robes to give him a saintly look and a dignified appearance. It was all there in the weather-worn face of the miniature St. Peter—the love of God, the divine gift for the healing of the sick and the saving of men's souls. Sometimes he read prayers from the Church of England *Book of Common Prayers*, but more often he prayed straight from the heart and faith that was within, prayers which I wish could have been recorded. He spoke as one inspired by God, and I have no doubt he was. When he preached, he spoke of the love of God, the forgiveness of sins, and the salvation of souls; in other words, he preached Christianity. When the benediction was said, we went back to the house fortified for another week's work, or for whatever life would bring our way. I am sure Dr Grenfell had a lasting influence for good not only on our lives, but on the lives of quite a number of people.

THERE WAS NO OTHER WAY OUT*

Dr Wilfred Grenfell dominated the early years of the Mission, which was so closely associated with his name. As the Mission matured, however, others became involved who would have an equal, if not greater, impact on the areas they served. Though Grenfell during the late teens, twenties and early thirties continued to lionize the Mission in the public mind, the Mission's business took him away from the coast for long periods of time. Day-to-day business was actually conducted by a handful of dedicated staff members who worked quietly and efficiently behind the scenes, in many cases shunning the recognition and honours that Grenfell sought. Dr Harry L. Paddon was one of these.

In the summer of 1912 Dr Paddon came from England to work for the Mission at Indian Harbour. That winter he and Dr Arthur Wakefield established a winter clinic at Mud Lake, at the extreme end of Hamilton Inlet, to serve trappers in the vicinity. Soon Paddon married Mina Gilchrist, a Grenfell nurse from New Brunswick. In 1915 the Paddons moved their winter base from

Elizabeth Goudie

* Elizabeth Goudie, *Woman of Labrador*, David Zimmerly, ed. and intro. (Agincourt, Ontario: Book Society of Canada 1983)

My father, Harry L. Paddon, came from middle-class English stock. As a boy, he had heard Grenfell lecture about Labrador—an experience he would never forget—and had announced to his family that he, too, wanted to work as a doctor in Labrador. After a good primary education, he attended Repton, an English public school, then went on to Oxford to study the classics … In due course, he departed for St. Thomas's Hospital, London, where he received a sound medical training.

W. Paddon 1989

Father's first two years were busy and marked by odd occurrences. Of two winter volunteers who worked as outdoor and general helpers, one managed to blow off most of his leg with a shotgun, and the second— an alcoholic sent by the ever trusting Wilfred Grenfell in the pious hope that the north and a bout of Christian service would make a man of him—contrived to drink virtually any liquid that would not freeze, in hopes that it might contain alcohol. In some cases it did—as in the cases of vanilla extract, surgical spirit, cough syrup, etc. and in others such as benzene, tincture of iodine, shoe polish and metal polish it did not. The reform process had to be cut short before the candidate demolished the last of his glomeruli and his hepatic cytostructure.

W. Paddon 1971

Mud Lake to North West River, a nearby fur trading centre. They built a hospital and raised four sons, including W. Anthony (Tony) and Harold G. Thereafter the Paddons spent their summers at Indian Harbour and winters at North West River.

The author of the following selection, Elizabeth Blake Goudie (1902-1982), knew the Paddon family well. She was born at Mud Lake of Inuit, Indian, English and French ancestry, and attended school there for three years. Her family eventually moved to Sebaskachu, a tiny settlement about eighteen miles away; in 1917, she went to work for the Paddons as a hospital aide. Married in 1920 to Labrador trapper Jim Goudie, she had eight children. During World War II the Goudies moved to Happy Valley-Goose Bay, where Elizabeth Goudie produced her autobiographical Woman of Labrador, *published in 1973. In 1975 Memorial University awarded her an honorary degree.*

Dr [Harry] Paddon was always busy. On his sick rounds he would also be preparing his songs for his yearly fair and concert. He was a good singer and a good actor. He always had one big sale about the twentieth of April. Everybody would gather in from around the Groswater Bay and join in the Grenfell Mission Spring Fair. The money was raised to help keep the Mission at work. The ladies would make handwork and the men would make pieces of furniture which would be put up for auction. Sometimes they would raise 700 dollars. Once they made 5,000 dollars. This was something the people looked forward to every year.

Dr Paddon always took time to think of the children at Christmas. I remember the first time I saw Santa. I was thirteen years old at the time. Dr Paddon sent gifts to our home, eighteen miles from North West River, and had the old gentlemen put up a Christmas tree. He sent word around to my mother a week ahead and then brought Santa on his dog team all dressed up in his red suit. This was one of the things Dr Paddon did apart from his medical work.

When he came to visit he would often tell us a little about city life. Although we listened we didn't pay much attention because we knew nothing about it. He always ended up saying, "I am glad to be in Labrador and to be among the people. I love it here and all the beauty of its land, the mountains and all its trees and rivers." He would chat away in this manner and we enjoyed him very much. He was always a welcome guest in our home and I guess in all our homes because he was our only doctor at that time to travel the coast and look after our ills.

When he would leave us he always shook our hands and said to us, "Now children, eat all the meat and fish and red berries you can if you want to build strong bodies." This would be when he was leaving for his [winter] trip on the coast south. Then when he came back a month or six weeks later he would tell mother and father about the poor people and their problems and I sat and listened. He would say that the homes were so cold and they hadn't enough bedding and the food situation was very poor. There was little nourishment for the children and they were poorly dressed and I could see by the look on his face that he was very concerned about these problems. My mother and father were concerned too because their uncles, aunts and cousins were tied in with the situation, and they were saddened because Dr Paddon couldn't take enough supplies for himself and the people. He had to travel as light as he could. The weather was cold and fierce to travel in, thirty and forty below zero most of the time, but I learned more and more that he was really concerned about the people and I always believed he loved them very much.

His wife also was a wonderful helper to him and she was a good nurse …

In 1917 I went to work for the Grenfell Mission in Indian Harbour and was paid four dollars a month and ten dollars worth of used clothing in the summer. This was what the Mission gave their girls at that time. I served as an aide on the women's ward.

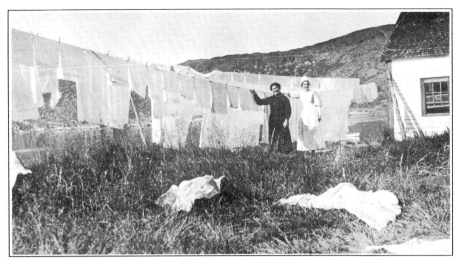

Indian Harbour, 1915: laundry work at the end of the season

We were out of bed at five in the morning and on our feet until seven in the evening. We got one afternoon off a week and we were let off to go to church on Sunday....

Mrs Paddon's children were small then. She had a nursemaid for them. The doctor and his wife had a little bungalow on the hill back of the hospital. The girls on staff that summer were the nursemaid Rachel Flowers and her helper Annie Baikie; the cook Kitty Montague; the parlour maid Beatris Flowers; and Jarmel McLean and I were the aides. The men's staff included Uncle Fred Blake, the two kitchen boys Austin Montague and John Montague; the crew on the *Yale* were Judson Blake and Tom Elson. Either Dr Paddon or Fred Blake went in the bay each trip the *Yale* made. Dr Paddon went every trip if there were sick calls to make. He had two student doctors the summer I was there plus two nurses and his wife. There were fresh-air shacks on both wards that summer and they were always full of TB patients. One aide and one nurse were on duty all day. Dr Paddon was a minister every Sunday as well as a doctor every day. Every man and women in Labrador in those days who was able to work at all had to be a jack-of-all trades. There was no other way out.

Two years before I came out here, Dr Grenfell wrote me an epistle of some four lines telling me that "all knowledge is useful out here. Learn all you can of house-building, plumbing, agriculture, stock-farming, etc., etc." How many times this summer have I wished I were a certified engineer!

H.L. Paddon 1915
In McGrath, comp. 1978

DAD WAS HOME*

Harold G. Paddon was born at North West River in 1915, the second of four sons born to Mina and Harry Paddon. In 1926 he and his older brother, Tony, went to a boarding school in New England. Harold graduated from an American forestry school in 1937, cruised timber in Labrador, and turned later to trapping. In 1950 he opened a sawmill near the American military base at Goose Bay, moving to British Columbia around 1956. Here, Harold Paddon captures the spirit of winter in Labrador through a child's eyes.

Winters, in those early days, were probably the happiest times of all for us. We had 'buttoned-up' for nearly eight months of isolation from a less friendly world. All preparations had been made to do entirely on our own, and now we could get on with the business of living and there would be no annoying disturbances such as visiting dignitaries or unwelcome news from outside. The men had faded into the back-country to earn a living for their families while

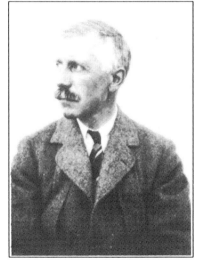

Harry L. Paddon, c. 1930

* Harold G. Paddon, *Green Woods and Blue Waters: Memories of Labrador* (St. John's Breakwater 1989). Reprinted by permission of Breakwater Books, copyright Harold G. Paddon.

For our family, Indian Harbour was a summer adventure; North West River was home.

W. Paddon 1971

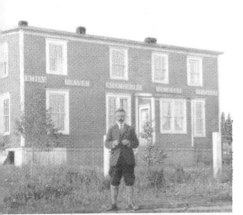

The Emily Beaver Chamberlin Memorial Hospital at North West River, Dr Harry Paddon in front

the women, and those children big enough to get around, became absorbed in the business of bringing food from the woods and water to the table. It was in winter, too, that there was some time for social gatherings. The women got together in the long evenings to sew for the annual fair that would raise a little money for church and hospital, or to prepare for the big celebrations of Christmas and New Year, when some of the men would be home again for a brief stay before returning to the woods for the spring hunt.

Christmas at North West River was an occasion to remember in those days of simplicity and neighbourliness. For several weeks we would prepare for the Christmas concert. Dad would write a play, a slapstick comedy with a thread of story. His bubbling sense of humour, and deft touch with the ludicrous, combined to produce the food for rib-cracking laughter that was so appreciated in a life accustomed to solitude. Everyone would pitch in; nurses, Hudson's Bay clerks, Dad, anyone else who was inclined, and learn a part. A couple of days before Christmas people from outlying hamlets would begin to arrive, and would move into the first household they came to that was not already bursting at the seams. The men brought choice bits of fish and game, the women took charge of the kitchens and the youngsters were sent to the woods for trees and brush. Later they were put to making wreaths and decorating the buildings, while the women cooked and baked and the men got their fur-trading and shopping out of the way.

The real fun began on Christmas Eve, shortly after dark, with the village Christmas tree. Someone, usually Dad, would don a Santa costume and arrive at the old community hall with a galloping team of huskies. A glib line of patter, aided by an intimate knowledge of the life of every child present, went with the gift that every child received. The last two or three presents on the tree were always good-natured jibes at some of the adults present and brought gales of laughter....

After the Christmas tree, everyone retired to the big social room in the old hospital for a tremendous supper and much good talk. The boys and young men washed the dishes and swept up afterwards while the older folk went on ahead to ready the hall for the play and concert. About nine o'clock, when suppers had settled, the play got under way. For perhaps an hour the gales of mirth carried far on the frosty night. Later, the whole group sang a few folk songs and carols. Then the youngest, and a few of the oldest, went home to rest while everybody else settled down to dance the graceful figures of the old square dances to the strains of harmonica and violin.

Christmas morning at the hospital was very much our morning. It belonged to the children and, though they enjoyed it as much as we did, it must have seemed to our parents that sleep had not yet been invented. Crazy with excitement, we'd be out of bed hours before daylight. Dad would get up and build a huge fire in the open fireplace while Mother busied herself with the coffee pot on the kitchen stove. We'd all sit by the fire while Dad took the packages from the tree and read out the names on the labels, and passed them to one of us to carry to the recipient. We boys might get a box of .22 cartridges, a roll of snare wire, and an axe or pocket knife, and always a book or two. Equipment to keep us going in the outdoor activities we cared about with good, carefully selected books to be read and reread when the weather kept us indoors. We got a far greater thrill and far more lasting pleasure out of these things than today's youngsters get from the wide assortment of more sophisticated gifts.

We ate our Christmas morning breakfast by candle-light, with cups and plates balanced on our knees or on the floor among the welter of treasures and wrappings. It was a family gathering on which no one intruded, though with

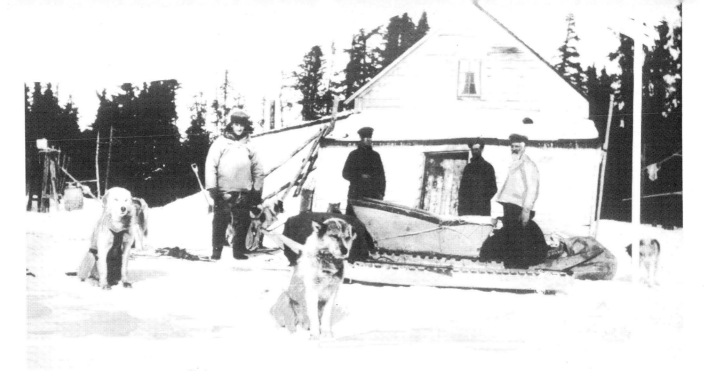

Mid-day rest

the coming of full daylight people began dropping in with a word of greeting, to sit over a cup of coffee and take their leave again until the Christmas morning church service.

Once Christmas was over, we began to eye a little gloomily Dad's preparations for his long trip, for we knew that after he left we would neither see nor hear of him till spring. We had great confidence in his wiry toughness and his ability to get anywhere at any time. Besides, on these trips he was accompanied by Jim, the best teamster in the business. Silent, taciturn Jim who could, I'll swear, communicate with dogs in their own language.

Dad's position as the only doctor on the coast from Battle Harbour to Hebron kept him away from home a great deal. In the summer he made his medical patrols by small boat, and in winter he could cover his territory only by dogteam. Leaving North West River in early January, he would travel south to Cartwright, then north along the coast to Nain. From Nain, unless there was a call for him to go on to Hebron, he would turn south again to Cartwright, then back in the bay to North West River. It wasn't the twelve hundred miles between these points that put the distance and the months into his long trip, it was the side jaunts; twenty miles off track to see two families here, forty miles up that bay to see another family or two. The more isolated the little groups he visited, the more of his time they needed, even though they might all be well. Many lived so far out of the way that nearly the only news and mail they received in a winter was what he brought them. Even though there was no sickness in the home he had to stay a night to relate all the news from along the way and give them a chance to read and reply to any mail he might have brought them.

Many a family without neighbours had been having a hard winter, and many a child's eyes glistened at the little delicacies he brought them from his 'grub box.' Dad was a great traveller and, when the going was hard, could snowshoe forty miles and more in a day to break trail ahead of his dogs. It was lonely at home when he was gone, and what it was like for Mother I can only guess. I am sure that had she not been so busy with the nursing and housekeeping at our little hospital, even Mother would have found it hard to take. As it was, she loved those early Labrador years as much as did the rest of us.

The spring would be well-advanced before Dad returned from this long trip. Leaned right down and iron hard, he nearly always came the last seventy miles from Valley's Bight in a single day, frequently walking the whole distance

One blustery drifting day he attempted to harness what appeared to be a stray husky dog trotting behind his komatik. The animal politely declined to join the team and finally walked away in frigid dignity to the horror of my father's driver, who was frantically shouting against the wind that it was an Arctic wolf and not a husky dog. On rejoining the team my father was advised never to harness any stray dog over three or four feet in height.

W. Paddon 1971

ahead of the dogs to break a trail. Nearly always he arrived well after dark, without warning. We would know nothing of his arrival until we heard the team pull up at the door. He would come in, snapping the icicles from his mustache and wiping the frost from his eyebrows, and would snatch us all into a squirming armful and laugh. Two minutes with us and out he'd go again into the dark to help unlash and unharness, while Mother hurried about getting a hot and hearty supper for him and Jim. As a family, the best times for us were between the close of navigation at the end of October until the saltwater ice got firm at the end of December, and again during the spring breakup from early May to early June, for during those times Dad, except for short trips to nearby settlements, was home.

PATIENTS ARE SO HARD TO KILL*

Dr Harry Paddon never left Labrador, except on furlough, when he would study and upgrade, lecture and raise money. In 1936 he addressed the Medical and Physical Society of St. Thomas Hospital in London. In order to illustrate the nature of his practice, he told this story. Paddon and a small group of Labrador men were at work enlarging the hospital at Indian Harbour in the spring of 1914, when these events took place. The young American in question was a Mission volunteer (see margin note, p. 72).

In the sphere of general surgery a small, scattered population does not afford enough practice to maintain any degree of dexterity, and assistance and equipment are often defective. A single illustration ... I was marooned on a small island, on the coast, early one spring before navigation opened, with a dozen local workmen who were extending accommodation at the cottage hospital. The [medical] equipment was almost all at the winter base. A young American, who had spent the winter on the coast, was included in the party. In a sally after some ducks a shot-gun went off accidentally, passing through the side of a small boat, and then entering the right leg of the American. On examination, numerous pellets were felt embedded in skin and fascia. A small marginal fracture of patella could be palpated; and synovial fluid, from an acquired synovitis, was leaking from a small lacerated wound where a few pellets had converged. With no nurse, anaesthetist or assistant, and the patient's natural reluctance to lose a limb unnecessarily, the only course was to clean up, splint and await developments, despite a strong suspicion that the joint was invaded. After forty-eight hours, with rising pulse and temperature, a modified drainage operation was done. Some septic-looking blood-clot was found, but no foreign body could be found in the joint, and no lesion of the cartilage detected. Drainage and frequent boric lavage reduced pulse and temperature to normal in two days, though pus was present. On the sixth evening the temperature rose to 102°, and the following day to 104°. There was no doubt of osteo-myelitis, or of the need for amputation under most unfavourable conditions. The choice of weapons for bone section was between a carpenter's cross-cut saw, an axe, and a phalangeal saw; and the one tourniquet which was to be found had the rubber rotted by frost (which was one reason for shifting nearly all equipment to winter quarters). The most intelligent of the Eskimo half-breeds was coached in the elements of anaesthesia; another was coached, without much optimism, as assistant; and a night was largely spent in sterilizing, and trying to put some

* Harold L. Paddon, "Labrador Today: A Lecture to the Medical and Physical Society," *St. Thomas Hospital Gazette* 35 (1936): 283-7

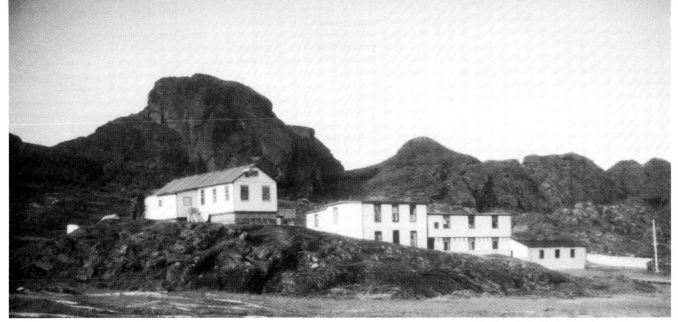

The hospital at Indian Harbour, the Paddon home at left

Note on the cliffs behind the profile of an Indian gazing at the sky, giving the harbour its name.

ideas of asepsis into the 'dirty-nurse.' The operation, which was neither brief nor bloodless, began; but soon the anaesthetist succeeded in over-dosing the patient with chloroform (it was too cold for ether). Artificial respiration had to be done, at a complete sacrifice of any remnants of asepsis, and the operation completed with all possible 'speed.' Infection was expected, and duly manifested itself, but free drainage arrested the process and saved the flaps. The patient ultimately survived to enjoy an effective artificial leg, and a useful career. Needless to say, these experiences are not related as triumphs for the operator, but with devout thankfulness that, when a man does his best, patients are so hard to kill.

While such considerations should not, of course, influence the efforts to achieve recovery, it certainly does 'rub it in' if failure to cure a patient renders the doctor liable not only to read the burial service, but also to dig the grave, as may easily happen where man-power is short.

FROM THE JOURNAL OF THE "LABRADOR PARSON"*

The Anglican minister Henry Gordon (1887-1971) was born in England and in 1909 graduated from Keble College, Oxford. Sent in 1915 as missionary to Cartwright, his parish extended from Batteau to Cape Harrison, including Sandwich Bay and Hamilton Inlet. Though Gordon had no official connection with the Grenfell Mission, he worked closely with it. Returning to England in 1925, he served in various English parishes until his retirement in 1952.

Gordon admired greatly Dr Harry Paddon. In order to care for the forty or more children in Sandwich Bay orphaned by the epidemic of Spanish flu in 1918–1919, he founded the Labrador Public School with Paddon's help. Gordon respected Grenfell, while observing him closely. The following extracts from his journal cover events in the summers of 1916, 1917 and 1919.

We spent our first night at Snack Cove, on Huntingdon Island. There I met a most interesting and charming personality—Miss Ethel Muir, a doctor of Ethics of Painesville University, Ohio. How she had got down to the coast and landed up in such an out of the way spot as this could be explained in a single word—Grenfell! With that inconsequence, which was both the admiration and

---

*   Henry Gordon *The Labrador Parson: Journal of the Reverend Henry Gordon, 1915-1925* (St. John's: Provincial Archives of Newfoundland and Labrador 1972)

Ethel Muir, PhD, was responsible for organizing the IGA's summer school program, a program whereby scores of young Americans from universities and colleges in the eastern States volunteered to teach the basics of reading, writing and arithmetic to a handful of children in remote villages. In addition, they did child welfare work. Dr Muir taught for about thirty summers in places like Snack Cove, Eddy's Cove and Brig Bay, and finally built a combined school/summer home at Black Duck Cove.

George Williams, an American manufacturer of shaving soaps and other sundries, came annually to Labrador to fish salmon.

despair of his friends, he had lured this gifted lady to come north with him for the purpose of organizing a system of summer schools for the children of the coast. He had then proceeded to land her at one of the fishing stations and left her to get about as best she could till he picked her up again on his way out. It had been part of the arrangement that he was to let me know, so that I could assist her in her investigations. Needless to say, he forgot to do this. To add to her troubles (which she took in a most sporting spirit) her personal luggage had gone astray. She was under the impression that it had been consigned to my care at Cartwright. Then the awful thought dawned upon me that I had given it away to some of our needy cases—under the impression that it was part of a consignment of clothing that had been sent to me for charitable distribution.

Before leaving next day, I fixed up for her to be run into Cartwright where she was to await the arrival of *Strathcona*—Grenfell's hospital steamer. I secretly rejoiced at the ticking-off the doctor had in store for him.

We met consistently strong head-winds all our way south to Batteau and, with no protection from the showers of spray that *Good Hope* bestowed upon us, we were in a perpetual condition of saturation. We spent the first night of our return journey with the Grenfell medical unit on Spotted Islands. This particular station is entirely the care of Yale [*sic*, Columbia] University, who supply the personnel and finance the expense of the station and the little motor-launch *P and S*. The present team of medical students consisted of three lively young sparks named Adams, Barnes and Smith. As things in the health line were very slack just at present, they were very keen to take a trip to the next Grenfell station at Indian Harbour. It appeared that one of the nurses there was having a birthday and they thought it a good idea to join in the celebrations. As they didn't know the way, and I did, I was persuaded to accompany them as pilot....

It had been my intention to get away as soon as possible on my main summer trip, to the north, but a succession of visitors delayed us for more than a week.

The first to arrive was Mr George Williams in his lovely *Jeanette*. He put into Cartwright for a night on his way up the bay to catch salmon in the Eagle River. I received a very pressing invitation to accompany him for a few days, but had reluctantly to decline.

Jeanette had scarcely sailed when two very business-like gun-boats came in. They had come north to investigate reports of German submarines having been seen off the coast. I am afraid that I didn't put much faith in the report, nor, apparently, did the gun-boat people, for they went up the bay and were later seen having some good sport with the salmon.

Then last, but very far from least, came S.S. *Strathcona* with Dr Grenfell on board. It so happened that a party of us were on the end of the [Hudson's Bay] Company's wharf preparatory to a dip in the water, when the steamer appeared from round the Harbour Point. Even before she had her anchor down, Grenfell was poised on her bulwarks in bathing kit, bellowing out "Wait for me." He then dived overboard and as we had also taken off, we greeted one another in salt water. This was my first meeting with Grenfell since I had last seen him at Parkgate in 1914. He had been down on the coast the previous summer, but we had missed one another.

There followed three very enjoyable if rather strenuous days during which time I was a guest on board *Strathcona*—if the word 'guest' can be applied to anyone who lodges with the doctor. He was one of those people who don't seem to need more than three or four hours sleep and worked both himself and his associates at full pressure. It was the same when he took time off for recreation, which he did for part of one of the days he was here. This took the form of a fishing picnic up Muddy Bay Brook. By the time we had rowed a heavy ship's

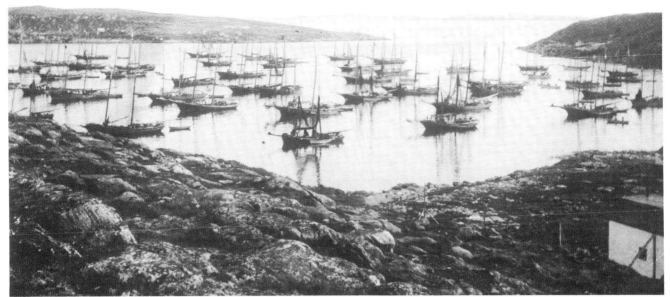

Newfoundland fishing schooners anchored at Indian Harbour

boat the five miles there and back, with some tough scrambling up the side of the brook, we were pretty tired—but not Grenfell. All the same I welcomed this opportunity of such close association with such a fascinating personality. It was little wonder that he was so universally loved by the people of the coast....

[Later that season our paths crossed at Indian Harbour.] Grenfell rowed out to inform me that I was invited, with himself, to have dinner on board *Jeanette*. Protests that I hadn't any decent clothes to wear and that what I had were dirty and creased, were of no avail. I had to go. *Jeanette's* saloon was beautifully decorated, and with a couple of white-coated stewards in attendance, I felt very out of place, but not for very long. Grenfell saw to that. A couple of millionaires (for Mr Williams had a guest with him) and all the frills of a six-course dinner didn't perturb him. He had us all in fits of laughter with one humorous story after another, and then, when the meal came to an end, he quietly said "That was a grand meal! Now lets have a few prayers and thank the good Lord for giving us such a happy time." And there was something really lovely to see the way that everybody, stewards, cook, deck-hands and all at the table joined in a hymn and knelt while some prayers were said. I doubt if anyone but a Grenfell could have brought this off....

1917 — We left Cartwright on July 19th in the same lovely weather that had been such a feature of this summer. It was a good week before we came into Indian Harbour, which was, as usual, well crowded with fishing schooners. Since last summer an additional wing had been built on to the Grenfell hospital, but even with this Dr Paddon and his staff were barely able to cope with the flood of patients. Profiting from past experience, I had brought along my most respectable suit, but even in this I felt very scruffy among the spotless white of the hospital personnel. But compared with certain persons who were due to arrive at any minute I was eminently respectable. These were of a species known as WOPS.... Four had been allocated to Indian Harbour, and they arrived on *Sagona* during the second day of my visit. Under the impression that they were coming into the wilds, they had adopted what they felt was [*sic*] the appropriate attributes. I shall never forget the scene that attended their arrival. There, on the hospital platform stood the doctor in his white linen coat, with Mrs Paddon (who acted as matron) and her three nurses in their starched blue and white. And up the gangway came four—well, I can only think of the word 'tramps': bearded, and in little better than rags. One could almost feel the force of the shock that struck the poor chaps as they realized the position, and I was glad that my sense of humour got the better of me and started a burst of laughter

This [1917] was my first meeting with Mrs Grenfell, and it didn't take long to come to the conclusion that she was the ideal mate for the dynamic doctor. The fact that he was not in his usual mad rush, and announced his intention to stay put for three days, was abundant evidence of her restraining influence. During their visit, I took up my quarters on board *Strathcona*, where such peace and order prevailed, that I hardly recognized her.

H. Gordon 1972

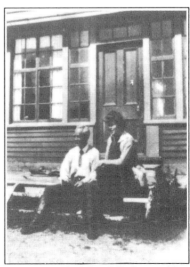

Anne and Wilfred Grenfell: she was his closest advisor

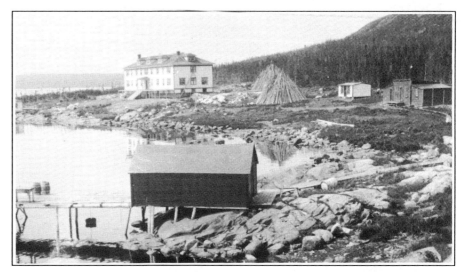

Boarding school at Muddy Bay

The Labrador Public School was a combined orphanage and boarding school at Muddy Bay, four miles from Cartwright. Henry Gordon and Harry Paddon between them raised $25,000 for its construction; with the help of a local committee, Gordon ran it. Grenfell, a vigorous opponent of church-run schools and in favour of centralized schooling at St. Anthony, was reluctant about the project from the start. But in 1922 he informed Gordon, "with his usual frankness and delightful inconsistency," that he had been converted to the idea of a regional school for Labrador. The IGA thereafter ran the facility.

I have always felt that Harry Paddon did more for the people of Labrador, and of southern Labrador especially, than the famous head of the mission, Sir Wilfred Grenfell. Blessed with great humour and a love of man and Christ, Dr Paddon went about his work with quiet efficiency.... He was quiet, competent, utterly dedicated and rather given to understatement, especially in reference to his own work.
F. Peacock 1986
Moravian missionary in Labrador

in which everyone joined, and so unfroze the icy atmosphere. Our doughty four were hardly recognizable by evening-time, after a shave and a change of attire....

1919 — One of my main objects of my northern trip was to see that all the emergency burial places that had had to be made during the 'flu, were safely fenced round. In answer to our appeal, the government [of Newfoundland] had shipped down on *Sagona* a large consignment of strong wire-netting, and made us a sufficient grant to cover the necessary expenses of erection. As I went on my rounds, I made measurements of the grounds, and arranged for the local men to prepare stakes, and have them in place as soon as possible.

Apart from this, the trip went off as usual until we arrived towards the end, at Indian Harbour, on August 20th. Here we met Dr Grenfell in his *Strathcona*, and nothing could ever be usual or normal when he was around. His energy was as unbounded as ever, and he was full of new ideas and schemes. He did, however, settle down for a long and serious discussion with Dr Paddon and myself about the future welfare of the [orphaned] children. I felt that he was not in favour of our project of a local school, but he was too large-hearted a man to do anything to damp our enthusiasm, and he wished us all success.

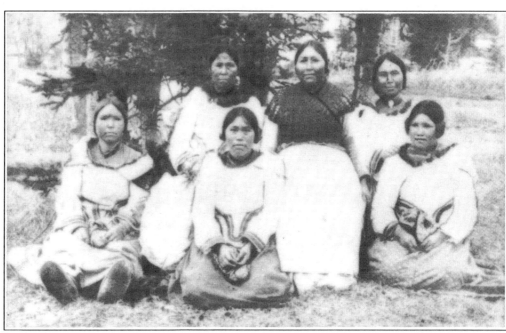

Inuit women

The Spanish flu epidemic of 1918–1919 killed an estimated 21 million people worldwide. In Newfoundland it killed 972; in Labrador it killed 410, nearly a tenth of the population. Hardest hit were the Inuit owing to their poor immunity: in a matter of weeks 353 Inuit, more than a third of the population, died.

To the Colonial Secretary from
Dr Wilfred Grenfell, 22 August 1919*

The following is the text of a letter from Grenfell to the Newfoundland colonial secretary concerning the aftermath of the Spanish flu epidemic. It has not previously been published. The 'unimpeachable authority' in Holy Orders referred to is Rev. Henry Gordon of Cartwright, who from October to December, 1918, had dealt personally with the epidemic in the Sandwich Bay area where nearly a quarter of the population had died. In January, Gordon had written the Newfoundland government requesting help for the survivors, not the dead. The government, with no further communication, had dispatched a doctor, an undertaker, a policeman (to maintain order) and 1500 board feet of lumber (for coffins) on the first mailboat in June. Grenfell's anger over the government's callous disregard for the welfare of the Labrador people is raw.

With the help of Anne Grenfell, those portions of Gordon's journal dealing with the epidemic and events immediately after were published in order to raise funds for the Labrador Public School. Extracts have appeared in previous anthologies.

I understand that you have already had the gruesome details on the unimpeachable authority of an English university graduate who is in Holy Orders, who is known and loved from end to end of the Labrador, and whom I knew in England before he came out. At the request of the pathologists, especially Dr Rosenau of Harvard, I have appointed a special student from their medical school to get first hand accounts from the people, the traders, and all those who were present during the terrible period.

In Sandwich Bay, where we unfortunately had no medical officer at the time, one fifth of the population died, and some have died since of the aftermath. Wherever there were trained doctors and nurses, the mortality was enormously reduced ...

Gordon tells me that you expressed great personal interest in these unfortunate people. At the same time, I am shown for the first time the newspaper accounts of the action of the government at the time when those whom they are elected to care of might have been saved. The account of one of the ministers publicly stating that these people had better be left to die because there would be less for the government to feed would justify those of us who have devoted our lives to the service of these people in almost [any] extreme course of action we cared to undertake. The intolerable insult of sending down at the expense of the government, a doctor, an undertaker, a policeman, and fifteen hundred feet of lumber (with provisions for their own personal comfort and safety of a nature which, with your sense of humour, I leave you to surmise), really made the people nearly throw them into the sea when they landed, after they had refused to send help when it was needed [those many months before].

I am sure that you will acquit me of any intention of holding threats over the government, and understand that under no circumstances will anything be included in my report which would unnecessarily call attention to what we feel here has been so serious a mishandling of the welfare of the people. A long personal knowledge has created in our minds sincere affection for them. I should like to be able to add to my report the statement, that the government has seen its way to endeavour to prevent the otherwise unavoidable consequences during the coming twelve months, by the special appointment of a trained nurse for the district, to work in conjunction with our medical officers and staff.

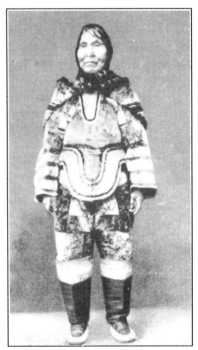

Inuit woman at Okak, 1894

Because of unfamiliar infectious European diseases brought by white men, the Labrador Inuit had been steadily declining in numbers since the mid-1850s. According to Moravian counts, the population between 1857 and 1907 dropped from 1172 to 894.

* PANL, GN 2/5, Colonial Secretary's Office. Special Subjects Files. File 862A

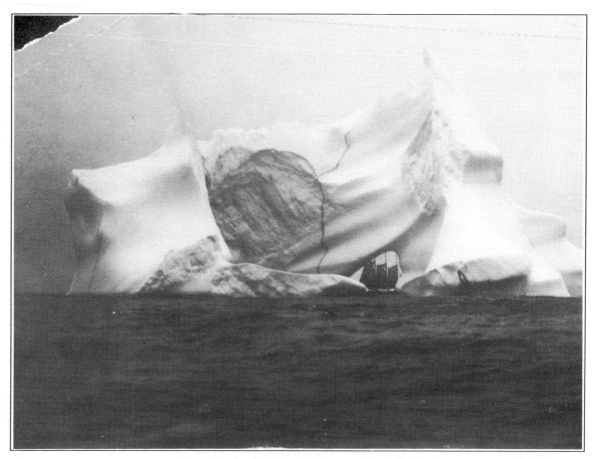

Mission supply vessel
George B. Cluett
seen through the arch
of an iceberg

DON'T SCOLD THE CHILDREN WHEN THEY
TEAR THEIR STOCKINGS*

*Le Petit Nord, or, Annals of a Labrador Harbour by Anne Grenfell and
Katie Spalding was a collection of pseudo-letters ostensibly written by the
incoming superintendent of the St. Anthony orphanage for the purpose of
raising funds for a new orphanage building. In order to achieve this, the IGA
mustered its considerable array of propaganda tools. Wilfred Grenfell illustrated the book.*

*Spalding gave ten years' voluntary service as head of the orphanage, having
replaced former superintendent Eleanor Storr in 1916. When in 1926 Grenfell
formed the Grenfell Association of Great Britain and Ireland and opened an
office in London, he placed the loyal Katie Spalding in charge of it.*

July 6

I have at last arrived at the back of beyond. We should have steamed right past
the entrance of our harbour if the navigation had been in my hands....

The ship's ladder was dropped as we came to anchor opposite the small
Mission wharf....We scrambled over the side and secured a seat in the mail boat.
Before we knew it four hearty sailors were sweeping us along towards the little
dock. Here, absolutely wretched and forlorn, painfully conscious of crumpled
and disordered garments, I turned to face the formidable row of Mission staff
drawn up in solemn array to greet us ...

* Anne Grenfell and Katie Spalding *Le Petit Nord, or, Annals of a Labrador Harbour* (Boston and
New York: Houghton Mifflin 1920)

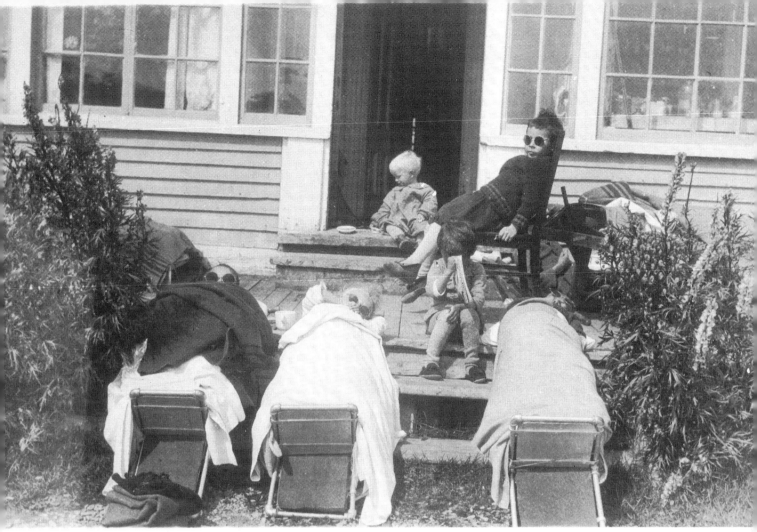
Sick children

How perfectly dear of you to have a letter awaiting me at the orphanage. Regardless of manners I fell to and devoured it, while all the 'little oysters stood and waited in a row.' Like the walrus, with a few becoming words I introduced myself as their future guardian, but never a word said they. As, led by a diminutive maid, I passed from their gaze I heard an awe-struck whisper, "It's gone upstairs!"

In answer to my questions the little maid informed me that the last mistress had left by the boat I had just missed, and that since then the children had been in her charge, with such help and supervision as the various members of the Mission staff could give. I therefore felt it was 'up to me' to make a start, and I delicately enquired when the next meal was due. An exhaustive exploration of the larder revealed two herrings, one undoubtedly of very high estate. As the children looked fairly plump, I concluded that they had only been on such meagre diet since the departure of the last 'mistress.' The bareness of the larder suggested a fruitful topic of conversation with which to win the confidence of these staring, open-mouthed children, and I therefore tenderly asked what they would most like to eat, supposing it was there. One and all affirmed that 'swile' meat was a delicacy such as their souls loved—and repeated questions could elucidate no further. Subsequently, on making enquiries of one of the Mission staff, I thought I detected a look which led me to suppose that I had not yet acquired the correct pronunciation of the word. We dined off the herring of lowly origin, and consigned the other to the garbage pail. Nerve as well as skill, I can assure you, is required to divide one herring into thirty-six equal parts....

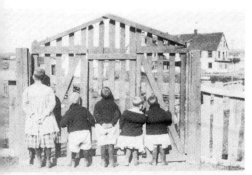

Orphaned children

I started to write this to you in the morning, but the day has been one long series of interruptions. The work is all new to me and not exactly what I expected, but the spice of variety is not lacking. I find it very hard to understand these children and it is evident from their faces that they fail to comprehend my meaning. Yet I have a lurking suspicion that when it is an order to be obeyed, their desire to understand is not overwhelming. The children are supposed to do the work of the home under my superintendency, the girls undertaking the housework and the boys the outside chores. Apparently from all I hear my predecessor was a strict disciplinarian, an economical manager, an expert needlewoman, and everything I should be and am not. The sewing simply appalls me! I confess that stitching for three dozen children of all sizes had not entered into my calculations as one of the duties of a 'missionary'!... [And] the food problems ... This country produces nothing but fish, and we have to plan our food supplies for a year in advance. How much corn-meal mush will David eat in twelve months? And if David eats so much in twelve months, how much will Noah, two months younger, eat in the same period of time? If one herring satisfies thirty-six, how many dozen will a herring and a half feed?

A little mite has just come to the door to inform me that her dress has 'gone abroad.' Seeing my mystified look, she enlightened me by holding up a tattered garment which had all too evidently 'gone abroad' almost beyond recall. Throwing the food problems to the winds I set myself with a businesslike air to sew together the ragged threads. A second knock brought me the cheerful tidings that the kitchen fire had languished from lack of sustenance. Now I had previously in my most impressive tones commanded one of the elder boys to attend to this matter, and he had promptly departed, as I thought to 'cleave the splits.' Searching for him I found this industrious youth lying on his back complacently contemplating the heavens. To my remonstrance he somewhat indignantly remarked that he was only 'taking a spell.' A really magnificent and grandiloquent appeal to the boy's sense of honour and a homily on the dignity of labour were abruptly terminated by shrill cries resounding from the house. Rushing in, I was informed that Noah was "bawling" (which fact was perfectly evident), having jammed his fingers in trying to 'hist' the window. In this country children never cry; they always 'bawl.'

I foresee that the life of a superintendent of an orphan asylum is not a simple one ...

August 15

You complain that I have told you almost nothing about these children, and you want to know what they are like. And I wish you to know, so that you will stop sending dolls to Mary who is sixteen, and cakes of scented soap to David who hates above all else to be washed. I find these children very difficult in some ways; many of them are mentally deficient, but it appears that no provision is made by the government for dealing with such cases, and so there is nothing to do but take them in or let them starve. Some are very wild and none have the slightest idea of obedience when they first arrive.

One girl I have christened 'Topsy,' and I only wish you could see her when she is in one of her tantrums, which she has at frequent intervals. With her flashing black eyes, straight, jet-black hair, square, squat shoulders, she looks the very embodiment of the Evil One. She is twelve, but shows neither ability nor desire to learn. Her habits are disgusting, and unless closely watched she will be found filling her pockets with the contents of the garbage pail—and this in spite of the fact that we are no longer dining off one herring. She says that

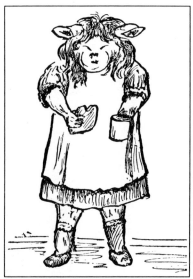

The rebellious Topsy, one of Grenfell's many sketches

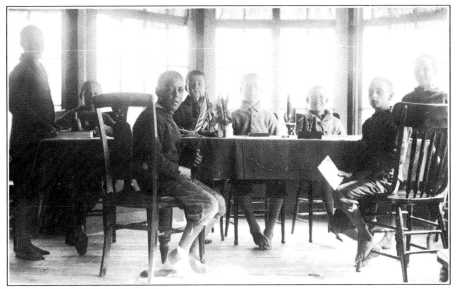

One of a number of postcards the IGA produced to raise funds for a new orphanage/children's home

On the table are binoculars and a microscope.

her ambition in life is to become like a fat pig! Last night, when the children were safely tucked in bed and I had sat down to write to you, piercing shrieks were heard resounding through the stillness of the house. A tour of investigation revealed Topsy creeping from bed to bed in the darkness, pretending to cut the throats of the girls with a large carving-knife which she had stolen for this purpose. To-day Topsy is going around with her hands tied behind her back as a punishment, and in the hope that without the use of her hands we may have one day of peace at least. Poor Topsy, kindness and severity alike seem unavailing. She steals and lies with the greatest readiness, and one wonders what life holds in store for her.

We have just admitted three children, so we now number more than the three dozen. One little mite of five was found last winter in a Labrador hut, deserted, half-starved, and nearly frozen to death. She was kept by a kindly neighbour until the ice conditions allowed of her being brought here. The other two, brother and sister, were found, the girl clothed in a sack, her one and only garment, and the boy in bed, minus even that covering. This is the type of child who comes to us....

September 25

I want to tell you something about our babies. They are four in number. David, aged five, considers himself quite a big boy, and a leader of the others. His father was frozen to death in Eskimo Bay some years ago whilst hunting food for his family....

Last month I went to Nameless Cove to fetch to the home a little boy of three. Nameless Cove is about twelve miles west of St. Antoine. I have never seen such a wretched hovel—a one-roomed log hut, completely destitute of furniture. The door was so low I had to bend almost double to enter. A rough shelf did duty for a bed, upon which lay an old bedridden man, while at the other end lay a sick woman with a child beside her, and crouched below was an idiot daughter. Altogether nine persons lived in this hut, eight adults and this one boy. Ananias is an illegitimate child, and has lived with these grandparents since his mother lost her reason and was removed to the asylum at St. John's. The child was almost destitute of clothing, and covered with vermin. He has the face of a seraph, and a voice that lisps out curses with the fluency of a veteran trooper....

Drusilla ... is three and comes from Savage Cove. The father has gradually become blind and the mother is crippled. Drusilla keeps us all on the alert ...

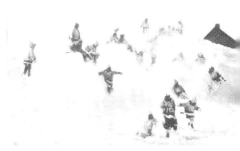

A second postcard, as endearing as the first

85

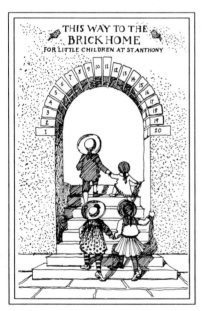

And a third ...

This is Lizzie Lucy of Labrador, a child at the home.

THIS WAY TO THE
BRICK HOME
FOR LITTLE CHILDREN AT ST. ANTHONY

Each Brick in Place costs 25 cents.
Will you help by sending 20 Bricks?

MARK OFF EACH BRICK IN RED
AS YOU COLLECT THE MONEY.

Another fund-raising strategy

The real baby is Beulah, just two years, and she exercises her gentle but despotic sway over all ...

February 28

Of one thing I am certain, we must have a new home, for this house is not fit for habitation, and it is not nearly large enough. Even after my recent return from living in the tiny homes of the people which one would fancy to be far less comfortable, this is forcibly impressed upon me. We simply cannot go on refusing to take in children who need shelter so badly. So please spread this broadcast among the friends in England. This home has been enlarged once since it was built, and yet is not nearly big enough for our present needs. We have no nursery, and I only wish you could see the tiny room which has to do duty for a sewing-room. It is certainly only called 'room' by courtesy, for there is scarcely space to sit down, much less to use a needle without risk of injury to one's neighbour. The weekly mending alone, without the making of new things, means now between two and three hundred garments in addition to the boots, which the boys repair. As you can imagine this is no light task and we are often driven almost distracted. I think the stockings are the worst, sometimes a hundred pairs to face at once! I fear we must once have been led into making some rather pointed remarks on this subject, for later, on going into the sewing-room, we found a slip of printed paper, cut from a magazine, and bearing the title of an article: "**Don't Scold the Children when They Tear their Stockings.**"

This building rocks like a ship at sea; the roof continually leaks, the windows are always 'coming abroad,' and the panes drop out at 'scattered times,' while even when shut, the wind whistles through as if to show his utter disdain of our inhospitable and paltry effort to keep him outside. On stormy nights, in spite of closed windows, the rooms resemble huge snowdrifts.... The building heaves so much with the frost that the doors constantly refuse to work, because the floors have risen, and if they are planed, when the frost disappears, a yawning chasm confronts you. Our storeroom is so cold in winter that we put on Arctic furs to fetch in the food, and in summer it is flooded so that we swim from barrel to barrel as Alice floated in her pool of tears. But far above all these minor discomforts is the one overwhelming desire not to have to refuse 'one of these little ones.'

One's heart aches when one remembers all the money and effort and love expended on a single child at home ... But in this land are hundreds of children, our own blood and kin, who must face their crushing problems often with bodies stunted from insufficient nourishment in childhood, and minds unopened and undeveloped, not through lack of natural ability, but because opportunity has never come to them....

You ask whether these kiddies have the stuff in them to repay what you are pleased to term 'such an outlay of effort.' My emphatic 'yes' should have been so insistent as to have reached you by telepathy when the doubt first presented itself. The home has been established now long enough to have some of its 'graduates' go out into life; and the splendid manhood and womanhood of these young people are at once a sufficient reward to us and a silencing response to you. Many of them have been sent to the States and Canada for further education, and are now not only writing a successful story for themselves, but helping their less fortunate neighbours, in a way we from outside never can, to turn over many a new leaf in their books.

HE PLAYS THE GAME*

Authors and journalists perceived Grenfell as a model of manly behaviour wedded to personal commitment. At least thirty books set out to represent the details of his life. Many were aimed at a juvenile audience, and nearly all portrayed him as the adventuring, Christian hero of the north. Fullerton Waldo, like most of the others, wrote 'heroic' biography with heavy Christian overtones.

As the doctor goes about St. Anthony he does not fail to note anything that is new, or to bestow on any worthy achievement a word of praise, for which men and women work the harder.

To 'The Master of the Inn' he expressed his satisfaction in the smooth-running, cleanly hostelry. "He is one of my boys," he remarked to me after the conversation. "He was trained here at St. Anthony, and then at the Pratt Institute in Brooklyn."

Then he meets the electrician. "Did you get your ammeter?" he asked. And then: "How did you make your rheostat?"

He points with satisfaction to a little Jersey bull recently acquired, and then he critically surveys the woodland paths that lead from his dooryard to a tea-house on the hill commanding the wide vista of the harbour and the buildings of the industrial colony. "Nothing of this when we came here," he observes. "The people seem possessed to cut down all their trees: we do our best to save ours, and we dote on these winding walks, which are an innovation."...

The house itself is delightful, and it is only too bad that the doctor and his wife see so little of it.

It is a house with a distinct atmosphere. The soul of it is the living-room with a wide window at the end that opens out upon a prospect of the wild wooded hillside, with an ivy-vine growing across the middle, so that it seems as if there were no glass and one could step right out into the clear, pure air. There is a big, hearty fireplace; there is a generously receptive sofa; there is an upright Steinway piano, where a blind piano-tuner was working at the time of my visit.

Lupins, the purple monk's hood and the pink fireweed grow along the paths and about the house. A glass-enclosed porch surrounds it on three sides, and in the porch are antlered heads of reindeer and caribou, coloured views of scenery in the British Isles and elsewhere, snowshoes and hunting and fishing paraphernalia, a great hanging pot of lobelias, and—noteworthily—a brass tablet bearing this inscription:

To the Memory of
Three Noble Dogs
Moody
Watch
Spy
whose lives were given for
mine on the ice
April 21, 1908
Wilfred Grenfell
St. Anthony

It is the kind of house that eloquently speaks of being lived in....

Nearly all our foremen were children whom we first educated on the coast and then got scholarships to technical or business or agricultural colleges.

W. Grenfell 1935

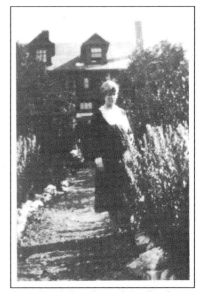

Anne Grenfell on the path leading from Grenfell House

---

* Fullerton L. Waldo, *With Grenfell on the Labrador* (New York: Fleming H. Revell 1920)

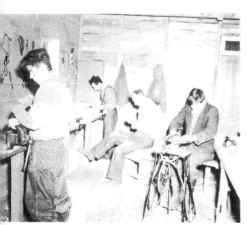
The machine shop at St. Anthony

Sometimes of an evening the doctor brought out the chessboard and I saw another phase of this versatile entity—his fondness for an indoor game that is of science and not blind chance. The red and white ivory chessmen, in deference to the staggering ship, had sealegs in the shape of pegs attaching them to the board. Two missing pawns—'prawns,' the doctor humorously styled them—had as substitutes bits of a red birthday candle, and two of the rooks were made of green modelling wax (plasticine).

"I love to attack," said the doctor, and his tactics proved that he meant what he said. He had what Lord Northcliffe once named to me as the capital secret of success—concentration.

When he had once moved a piece forward he almost never moves it back again. He likes to go ahead. He seeks to get his pieces out and into action, and a defensive, waiting game ... is not for him.

Once in a while he defers sufficiently to the conventions to move out the king's pawn at the start, but often his initial move is that of a pawn at the side of the board. He works the pawns hard and gives them a new significance. His delight is to march a little platoon of them against the enemy—preferably against the bishops. Somehow the bishops seem to lose their heads when confronted by these minor adversaries.

If you get him into a tight corner, the opposition stiffens—the greater the odds the more vertebral his attitude.

"I make it a rule to go ahead if I possibly can, and not to be driven back." This remark of his over the board of the mimic fray applies just as well to his constant strife with the sea to get where he is wanted—as on the present occasion when we were threading the needle's eye of the rocky outlet at Carpoon [sic].

The doctor has the real chess mind—the mind that surveys and weighs and analyzes—with the uncanny faculty of looking many moves ahead, of balancing all the alternatives, of remembering the disposal of the forces at a previous stage of the game. He becomes so completely immersed in the playing—though he rarely finds an antagonist—that it is a real rest to him after the teeming day, where many a man would only find it a culminant exhaustion. "Isn't it queer," he observed, "that most men who are good at this game aren't good for much else?"

His use of the pawns in chess is like his use of the weaker reeds among men in his day's work. Since he cannot always get the best (though his hand-picked helpers at St. Anthony, Battle Harbour and elsewhere are as a rule exceptionally able), he learns to use the inferior and the lesser, and with exemplary gentleness and patience he keeps his temper and lets them think they are assisting though they may be all but hindering. He gives you to feel that if you hold a basin or sharpen a knife or fetch a bottle or bring him a chair you are of real value in the performance of an operation—even if the basin was upset and the knife was dull and the bottle wasn't the one and the chair had a broken leg.

"Christ used ordinary men," he remarked. "He was a carpenter, and I try to teach people that he was a good sportsman."

All through his chess games, too, runs the Oxford principle of sport for its own sake: he wins, but the strife is more than the victory. He is never vainglorious when the checkmate comes; he is neither unduly elated by success nor depressed by adversity—indeed, his enjoyment is keenest when he is beset. He shows then the same strain that comes out when the ship is anchored and mate Albert Ash [sic, Ashe] pokes his head in and says: "If she drags, we've got but one chain out!" Then he will say nothing, or with a humorous twinkle he will cry in mock despair: "All is lost!" or "If you knew how little water there

Strathcona's mate, Uncle Albert Ashe

was under her you would be scared!"—and then he will go on with what he is doing. Whether it is the chessboard or life's battlefield, he plays the game.

So good a playmate and so firm a master—so rare a combination of gentleness and strength, of self-respect and rollicking fun, is difficult to match.

THE PROTEGE*

Warwick Kelloway was the son of a fisherman. After graduating from high school in St. John's in 1916, he worked for nine months as an itinerant teacher in Labrador and then joined the Royal Flying Corps (later, the RCAF). Still in pilot's training when the war ended, he was released from the forces. His story begins at this point.

Kelloway in the following selection acknowledges that while Grenfell judged others too quickly (being quite capable of accepting the most unsuitable volunteers, who were the bane of his staff and others like Reverend Henry Gordon), he inspired self-confidence and was a strong motivating force.

What now for me? I wanted to go to college, but first I would have to earn more money. To this end, I worked in Grand Falls for the winter and spring and then the next June found myself again on the coastal boat, this time heading for work in Notre Dame Bay.

We learned as we went along the coast that Dr Grenfell was attempting to raise money to build a much-needed hospital in this northern part of Newfoundland—it was to be built in Twillingate. Some of us passengers got the idea that it would be a fine gesture if we organized an informal concert on the ship and took up a collection for the new hospital. Since Twillingate was not a port of call, we decided we would have the concert when we docked at Pilley's Island, the nearest port. There was only one place where the show could be held, in the ship's lounge, but unfortunately passengers leaving or boarding the ship would have to pass through the end of the lounge on their way to their staterooms on the deck below.

We were about half way through the program when a pleasant and dignified-looking man entered, and, noticing that there was a meeting of some sort going on proceeded on down to his room. It was Dr Grenfell no less. I made so bold as to go after him and, after explaining the purpose of the gathering, asked if he would not come and explain to the audience the plans and purpose for the new hospital. He readily assented, and, by this good chance, a rather mediocre, though well-intentioned, project was changed into a very interesting and dramatic event to be remembered by all, and which for me in particular turned out to be the beginning of one of the most important relationships of my life.

When saying good-night, I said to Dr Grenfell, "How would you like to have a three-mile walk tomorrow morning?" "I would like that very much indeed, but how is that possible?" I explained that the next port of call was New Bay and while the ship was going the long way around the headland to the next port it was possible to go on foot by the three-mile road across the isthmus.

As we walked along the road, he showed an interest by asking many questions about my work in Labrador and in the Flying Corps. Then suddenly he said: "I have just had a great idea. How would you like to finish your flying course and then come to Labrador with me as a pilot?" When I recovered from my surprise I said "that would indeed be something, but I am convinced that

The Notre Dame Bay Memorial Hospital at Twillingate, opened 1924

Grenfell raised funds for the hospital and the IGA staffed it, but the hospital was run by a local committee.

---

* Warrick F. Kelloway, "Memories of Labrador and Dr Wilfred Grenfell" *Newfoundland Quarterly* 70, no. 2 (1973): 11-4

the first thing I must do—before I decide on anything else—is to go to college and get a college degree, and, as I have been delayed two years already, I feel if I don't go now I never will." He was silent for a moment and then he said: "You are right, you know. You should go to college before you do anything. But do you have money enough?" "I have $100 saved," I said, "and I am owed another hundred; I still can earn some this summer, and for the rest I expect to get work on the side while I am at college." I tried to make it sound optimistic, but it didn't come out that way.

Then came the biggest surprise: "You could perhaps borrow some," he said. "I don't have any to spare myself, but I know many people who contribute to our mission who do. I tell you what: I like your spirit—you go to college and do everything in your power to keep going, and, if you still get absolutely stuck, write or wire me and let me see what can be done."

Something happened inside me: from having just a hope, I suddenly had a confidence that it could be done. I now had the courage I needed to make the venture.

When we were coming in the port (Fortune Harbour) we saw a man—obviously a fisherman—coming toward us. When he got to us he stepped humbly to the side and removed his cap. "Good day doctorr!" he said with a pleasant Irish brogue. "And good-day to you," the doctor replied. "I 'spose ya don't rememberr me now, doctorr." "No, I can't seem to," the doctor admitted. "Have we met before?" "Do you rememburr a man on a ship who com t' your hospital las' summer with a crushed hand?" "Yes, I do remember now. How did you

'Good day doctor!'

In this photograph, the man in a sweater with his back turned is the Mission's newly arrived Dr Charles Curtis.

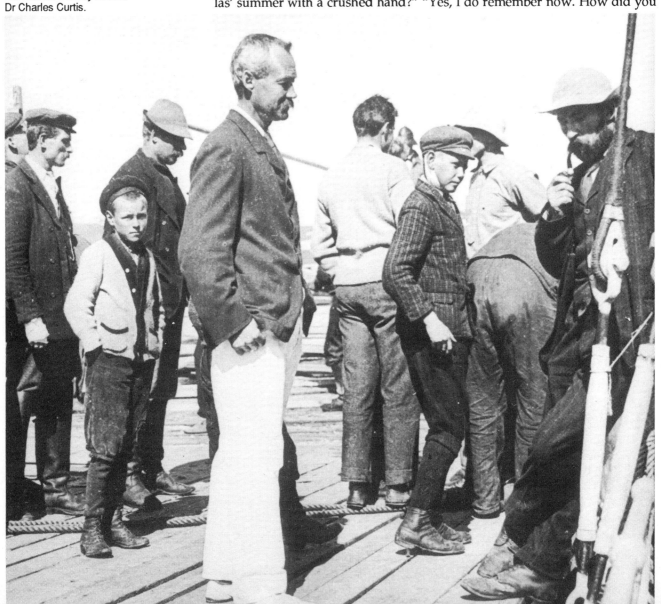

get along after?" "Foine, doctorrr—foine—an' I'm not furgitttin I owes the havin' me hand to work wi' to you, doctorr!" Dr Grenfell reached for the man's hand and examined it. "It has done very well indeed, but you must still be careful with it—don't put too much strain on it when you are pulling rope and things." "I will, doctorr, and t'ank ya again."

Just then the ship's whistle blew—she was obviously entering the harbour and giving warning to the people of the village. So we said "Good-bye" and moved along. The man still stood on the side of the road and I noticed two big tears rolling down the furrowed face, symbols of a common fisherman's gratitude. In one brief walk this benefactor had shown in practice his philosophy of religion: he had given new courage to two persons—a middle-aged fisherman and a young uncertain son of a fisherman anxious to start life.

I entered McGill University in Montreal that fall as planned. I found work teaching three nights a week and I worked every week-end. It was rough going, but I managed financially that year and the next. In the third year, however, I reached an impasse and faced having to give up college. I wired Sir Wilfred, as he had asked. Within a short time I received from him an encouraging letter with a cheque enclosed. The crisis had been met and in the years it took me to reach my goal I did not have to apply again for a loan.

Sometime during my term at McGill, Sir Wilfred came to lecture one evening in the interest of his work in Labrador. In the course of his lecture he happened to make the claim that, though students in Newfoundland did not have a basic pre-college education equal to many places, if they had the privilege of college they measured up. When after the lecture I went to say "Hello," I found him being interviewed by a lady reporter for one of the newspapers. I heard her say "Dr Grenfell, you spoke of your students from Newfoundland, in spite of handicaps, doing as well as those from other places if given a chance, do you have any of your students in McGill at present?" The question obviously caused him some embarrassment. He could not be expected to remember what New-foundland and Labrador students would be at any particular college. I saw a chance to pay him back in a small way for his service to me, so I took a step nearer to them and said "Yes, here is one: I consider myself a protegee [sic] of Sir Wilfred." The pleased, relieved look that spread over his face was something I shall never forget.

My next brief interview was in New York when I was attending Columbia University. I was fortunate in seeing an item in the *New York Times* that Dr Grenfell had arrived in New York in the interest of his Labrador medical missionary work; he would, during his stay, be the guest of a well-known citizen on Park Avenue. I looked up the telephone number and called him. He was the same genial person: after asking how I was doing and a few other things, he said "When can you come to see me?" We arranged a time.

At the number on Park Avenue I was taken to the top floor and ushered into a most lavish penthouse apartment. When we settled to talk he said, "I suppose you are wondering what I am doing in a place like this—well, there is a very interesting story behind it," and he told me the following: "My host had been a generous contributor to our work for several years and then one year he told me about his son who was very intelligent and promising, but who had lost his grip and was surely and rapidly going downhill. He ended by asking me if, in God's name, there was anything I could suggest he could do about it—he had tried everything he could think of and it had reached a hopeless situation. I said 'Yes, I have a suggestion, but you must do what I ask.' 'Anything,' he said, 'anything to save my son.' 'Let me take him to Labrador with me,' I said. I took him to Labrador and put him to work; driving dog-teams, chopping wood, going for and bringing patients to the hospital, scrubbing floors—all kinds of

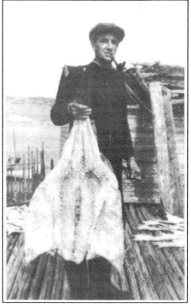

Labrador salt cod

A regular flood of visitors descended on us and this meant a lot of entertaining. Most of these were people who had been enthused by Grenfell and were doing the rounds of his various stations. Occasionally we got 'Problem men.' These were chaps who had got into trouble and had been sent to Grenfell for reformation. As often as not Dr Paddon or I were the Residuary Legatees of such. We received one of these a day or so after our return from south, and I promptly passed him on to [my assistant] Charlie Bird for some really strenuous work.

H. Gordon 1972

things—the only work he had ever done in his life. He came back a changed man, and is now making a great success. As a consequence his father can't do enough for me. Whenever I come to New York he insists that I must stay here, with a limousine and chauffeur to drive me wherever I need to go. What a change from Labrador! But it gives him so much satisfaction, I haven't the heart to deny him."

So two more lives have been helped by this advocate of practical service—a millionaire father and his lost son—taking a place beside two others, a common fisherman and the son of another fisherman.

SAMARITAN OF THE NORTH*

Dulcie Lear was one of three daughters born to Ernest and Caroline Lear of Hibb's Hole, Conception Bay, where her father fished. In 1923 he decided to try his luck at Lear's Room, Batteau, where Dulcie and her family spent the next thirteen summers. In 1936 Ernest Lear moved to fish at nearby Five Islands, and she went as cook. Dulcie Lear married Walter Spracklin and lived in Conception Bay.

Dulcie Spracklin here conveys the impressions of Grenfell she formed as a child.

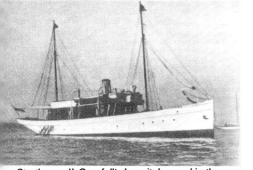

Strathcona II, Grenfell's hospital vessel in the twenties and thirties

I shall never forget the day I saw him. His twinkling blue eyes were set in a ruddy face surrounded by a fringe of thinning white hair. I stood and watched his good ship the *Strathcona II* slowly steaming into the land-locked harbour.

As soon as she was near enough for recognition, the men, women and children, with glad cries came flocking to the wharf the harbour boasted to greet their beloved friend.

The past winter had been an extremely hard one. Furs had been extremely scarce as had also the seal catch been very low. As a result, only enough skins had been found to provide boots for the fathers and older brothers whose needs must be first met in order that they would be able to go out to procure fuel and the other necessities of life for themselves and their families.

Most of the children flocking to the wharf that day were shoeless, their poor bare feet reddened by the rough rocks and cold mud which oozed up over their feet and between their scratched and bleeding toes.

I can see him now as his tiny launch reached the wharf, his whole being filled with compassion and pity for these poor, neglected souls, with his hand extended out to the smallest child, or the lowliest and dirtiest person, the same as to a king or lord.

What a contrast that following evening as all gathered in the little church on the hillside—the children no longer with poor cold and bleeding feet but clad in new clothing, new socks and shoes, all of which had been graciously supplied by his willing workers.

Many times it has been my humble privilege to sit in that little church and listen enthraled as his deep voice poured forth an earnest prayer on their behalf and told them of the Eternal Love. Here was a man who, while ever ready to supply the needs of the body, by words and actions clearly taught them that "Man cannot live by bread alone." ...

* Dulcie Lear Spracklin, "Samaritan of the North," *Newfoundland Stories and Ballads* 9, no. 1 (1962): 46-7. Reprinted by permission of the author. Copyright, Dulcie Lear Spracklin

Small wonder that a man possessing such a high Christian character should be content to leave the land of his birth, his home, friends and loved ones, to give his life in service and sacrifice to the poor and needy struggling souls of this rocky land.

IT WAS VERY INFORMAL*

Born into a wealthy Philadelphia family, Mary Williams graduated from the Presbyterian Hospital School of Nursing in 1920. She worked in Philadelphia as a visiting and industrial nurse among the poor, then joined the Grenfell Mission as a summer volunteer. She was at Battle Harbour for one summer and afterwards served as a missionary nurse in Alaska and other parts of the world.

Mary Williams Brinton was struck by the casualness of the Mission as well as by its ability to cope with chronic shortages of staff, equipment and supplies. In her experience, this brought out the best in its workers.

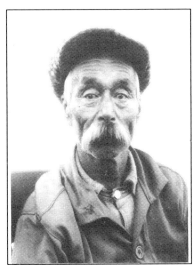

The *Maraval*, Dr Paddon's latest vessel dwarfed by an iceberg

When the steamer stopped outside the 'tickle,' we were taken ashore by motor boat, and deposited with baggage on the pier in front of the fish drying stage. The doctor, a dentist and two nurses greeted us, and grabbed the mail we brought, completely ignoring us while they looked at it. From there we went up the little path to the hospital on the edge of a rock, overlooking the harbour. So we had reached our island and were in Labrador!

I was immediately struck by my primitive surroundings. The frame hospital, a ramshackle affair, was surrounded by a few wooden houses, and a wireless station. The patients were natives—Indians, Esquimaux, and Anglo-Saxons— few of whom could read or write before the Mission was established in isolated communities. As it was early in the season, the management was not organized and was very informal. So we all drifted into the type of work in which we were most proficient.

"How would you like to run the operating room and give the anaesthetic?" I was asked the first day. The operation, a leg amputation for which the proper instruments were lacking, made me realize how absolutely on our own we were. If the needed supplies were not on hand, there was no way of getting them—we had to improvise. After searching we found a saw in the kitchen, which, to my horror, we decided to use, but we could not find the instrument pan and wondered what last year's staff had done with it. Finally, we unearthed a new fish kettle in the storeroom, and at ten o'clock I put the strange assortment of instruments in it and made a blazing wood fire beneath it. Then I returned to the operating room where we battled with blow torches on the dry sterilizer that made such a fearful noise I thought they were about to explode. The instruments were exasperating—they would not boil—and it was noon before we were able to start.

Samuel Pottle of Cullingham's Bight, a typical hospital patient

This photograph was taken by Professor Fred Sears in the early 1930s.

During the years of my training, I never dreamed of meeting a situation like this. The operation took place in a cold corner room under the most extraordinary conditions. It was the doctor's first experience on his own. I was a novice in giving ether, and we were so short-handed, in desperation the dentist was called upon to help. The patient, half Indian and half white, was sure she was going to die, but seemed perfectly resigned to her fate, which made me even more squeamish. To make matters worse, as the surgeon worked it started to

* Mary Williams Brinton, *My Cap and My Cape: An Autobiography* (Philadelphia: Dorrance 1950)

rain. The roof leaked and the water dripped so perilously near the patient we had to move the table to keep our field sterile. At the same time one of the 'Wops' who was trying to be useful turned green and had to be led from the room. Harrowing as it was, there was a sense of freedom which we all felt. No one to tell us what to do! We were on our own, and it brought out the best in us. Whatever skill and initiative we had, counted. Even the saw from the kitchen proved remarkable for its purpose.

When the operation culminated successfully, we felt strangely elated.

A TRUE KNIGHT*

When the new St. Anthony Hospital officially opened in 1927, Grenfell was at the pinnacle of his career, his best years at an end. Governor Sir William Allardyce used the occasion to announce that, in recognition of a long and distinguished record of service, Grenfell had been knighted by King George V. The British, Canadian and American press responded to this news with an enthusiasm reserved for only the most pre-eminent, respected men and women of the day, employing all the familiar themes and images associated with the Grenfell name. The following appeared in the Newfoundland Quarterly.

On July 25th, while at St. Anthony at the official opening of the new Grenfell hospital, erected and equipped last year at a cost of over $150,000, His Excellency the Governor read a message of appreciation from His Majesty the King, and announced that His Majesty had marked the occasion by promoting Dr Wilfred Grenfell to be a Knight Commander of the Most Distinguished Order of St. Michael and St. George.

The honour was stated by His Excellency to be in recognition of thirty-five years of devoted service given by Dr Grenfell to Labrador and northern Newfoundland, during which he had built and maintained four large hospitals, seven cottage hospitals, two orphanages and three public schools, and had substantially endowed the same, and in addition had erected and equipped at St. John's the Institute Building which bears the King's name and which was recently transformed into the YM and YWCA.

The *Quarterly* heartily congratulates Sir Wilfred Grenfell upon the well-merited distinction conferred upon him by His Majesty. As the *Telegram* has pointed out, to try to visualize what Sir Wilfred has accomplished, during the years in which he has conducted his mission of mercy among the fishermen and settlers of the north, one must first consider the number at present receiving treatment in the Grenfell hospitals, the educational institutions that are being conducted, and the numerous sick cases dealt with during visitations by land and sea; and then one must attempt to picture how deplorable the conditions would have been without the Grenfell Mission. The work has grown to such proportions that, according to a statement made recently in the public press by Hon. R. Watson, Vice-President of the International Grenfell Mission [sic], there is expended in this colony, in the medical and educational services referred to, a yearly sum of over $140,000, nine-tenths of which comes from outside, being the gifts of warm-hearted friends of Dr Grenfell in England, the United States and Canada. During the last year alone the various hospitals received over 600 patients while the number of out-patients treated exceeded 4,000....

With regard to the honour recently bestowed by His Majesty the King we venture to say that never has there been a knighthood which has received such

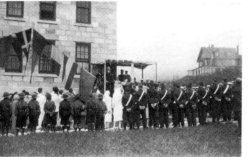

The opening of the new St. Anthony Hospital in 1927, Grenfell House visible at right.

---

* "Sir Wilfred Grenfell—a True Knight," *Newfoundland Quarterly* 27, no. 2 (1927): 25-7

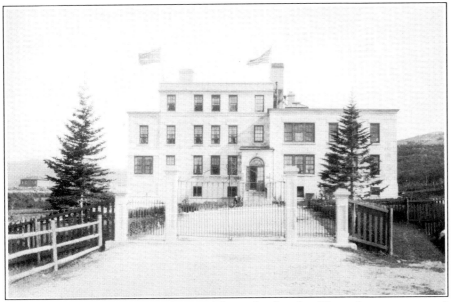

St. Anthony Hospital

Its architecture, accommodation and equipment were the most up-to-date in the country. Staff lodged in a connected building.

universal acclaim. The British press, from the *London Times* down, was most eulogistic, while in the United States and Canada, from the Atlantic to the Pacific, there was hardly a newspaper, city or provincial, that did not contain an appreciative reference. They all show the esteem in which Sir Wilfred Grenfell is held by his fellow-men, and the pleasure which his knighthood has given the English-speaking people of the world. The following excerpts, taken at random from papers published on this side of the water, are selected for publication here:

St. John's Daily News

"That the honour conferred by His Majesty King George upon Dr Grenfell is a well-merited one, is beyond question: and coming as it does, at a time when his life work is being crowned by the opening of the new hospital at St. Anthony, where for so many years his services to the people of Newfoundland have been centred, it is peculiarly opportune. The hope will be that the recipient of the honour may not only long live to wear it, but that his active interest in, and devotion to, the work of the International Grenfell Mission may continue for many years to come."

St. John's Evening Telegram

"The knighthood conferred by His Majesty the King upon Dr Grenfell on the occasion of the opening of the new hospital at St. Anthony is an honour well deserved. Coming as it does at what the prime minister [W.S. Monroe] aptly describes as 'the climax of Dr Grenfell's great personal efforts,' this recognition by the King is the reward of service which, it is certain, will as fully be appreciated by the recipient as it will be learned with gratification by his many friends."

Toronto Globe

"Dr Grenfell has been invested by the King with the insignia of a Knight Commander of the Order of St. Michael and St. George in recognition of his labour among the fisher folk of his lonely mission field in Labrador. If ever such recognition has been nobly earned it is in the present instance. In recent days the alleged 'buying' of titles has been severely condemned. In the case of Dr Grenfell, however, the purchase price paid is a lifetime of meritorious altruistic service that has few parallels in the missionary annals of modern days."

Toronto Labor Leader

"The knighting of Dr Wilfred Grenfell is an instance of conferring honour where honour is greatly due. Thousands will heartily rejoice at this timely

Our latest hospital was built entirely by Labrador boys trained under our care. It is fireproof, central-heated, electrically lit and with all the amenities of running water and good plumbing right through the Arctic winter. It has also most of the modern hospital special equipments, and has been standardized [ie. accredited] by the College of Surgeons of America.

W. Grenfell 1930 (2)

Edgar (Ted) McNeill, truly the versatile genius of the Grenfell Mission, was in charge of the hospital's construction. Among the first of the Mission's 'boys' to train at Pratt Institute, he was the Mission's general manager and overseer of all outside activities at St. Anthony. He constructed the majority of the Mission's buildings at St. Anthony, several Mission-owned houses, a number of its nursing stations, water systems at both St. Anthony and Cartwright, and the new hospital at Harrington Harbour. Retiring in the 1960s, his association with the Mission spanned fifty-seven years.

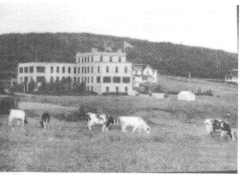

The hospital: side view

recognition of a true hero. The age of the heroic has not passed, and heroism is finding expression in the alleviation of human suffering."

Montreal Gazette

"Dr Grenfell's friends—and these are legion—will everywhere note this distinction of knighthood as a thoroughly deserved award made unto a faithful and devoted servant in the mission field. Work such as his may well remind us that knightly chivalry is by no means confined to the battlefield."

Calgary Herald

"Few careers have so appealed to the imagination of the public as that of this doctor of the Labrador coast, a man of simple nature, of great courage, of unusual organizing ability, a helpful worker among humble folk. The order of knighthood is, indeed, ennobled by the inclusion in its ranks of Dr Grenfell, who has been called the best loved missionary in the world."

New York World

"Dr Grenfell has been known as a knight ever since he went to Labrador in 1892 to start his hospitals and his orphanages, his schools and industrial enterprises. Since then he has slain more dragons that St. George could have counted; he has been more of a guardian to the fishermen of the Far North than St. Michael ever was to Israel. There are people in that region—thousands of them—who would say that he was their ideal of both a knight and a saint. Wherever throughout the world courage, devotion and high and altruistic purposes are admired his name has become an inspiration to men."

Boston Herald

"The knighthood conferred on Dr Grenfell has been honourably earned and everybody rejoices at this recognition of his toil and devotion. He has built hospitals and founded industries, and has revealed the pioneer qualities of an empire builder. Personally, he is the simplest of men and one of the most heroic. His country honours itself in the honour it bestows on him."

Springfield [Mass.] Union

"The story of Dr Wilfred Grenfell, who has just been made a knight by King George, is strangely like those tales of the Knights of the Round Table such as Sir Percival and Sir Galahad, who went forth and performed marvellous deeds of heroism and devotion, succouring the weak and laying low those who oppressed them. Knighthood is a fit reward for this doctor who has gone forth and performed great deeds of mercy."

Washington Post

"Many of England's great men have been described as empire builders. Few have built upon a more solid foundation than Sir Wilfred Grenfell, whose services to the British Crown have just been recognized in the form of knighthood conferred by the King. He has been the practical missionary, giving all in behalf of those he served. Labrador itself is a lasting monument to Sir Wilfred. The recognition of his Sovereign is deserved."

Manchester [N.H.] Leader

"The knighting of Wilfred Grenfell is the attachment of a badge of chivalry where it belongs. Seldom has an honour been more appropriately assigned or more richly deserved. Doctor Grenfell's work stands far up at the head of the list of the world's benefactors. Here is undoubtedly a true knight of chivalry, and the King of England does well to bestow upon him an honour so well merited."

Chicago Post

"If the spirit of a gentle and courageous chivalry be the qualification for knighthood, then never was it bestowed more worthily in modern times than when conferred on Grenfell of Labrador. His Britannic Majesty has made many knights to whom the title gave distinction, but now it is the man who brings distinction to knighthood."

Baltimore Sun

"Sir Wilfred Grenfell's fame may not encircle the earth, but it reaches as high towards Heaven as man's vision can follow it."

THE DENTIST*

B.J. Banfill was born on a farm in Richmond, Quebec, and trained as a nurse at Sherbrooke Hospital. Employed in 1928 as resident nurse at Mutton Bay, which came within the Harrington Hospital district, she found that frontier nursing suited her. A missionary course at the United Church Training School in Toronto prepared her for subsequent nursing assignments in the Canadian West.

The Grenfell Mission had been employing dentists since 1910. They did rounds of the hospitals and nursing stations, as Banfill explains.

On September fifth, suddenly, my subconscious mind told me that someone was hovering over me. Sleepily, I dragged my eyes open, then wakened to confront an apparition. [My aide] Annie was bending over me, enveloped in her oversized flannelette nightgown. Her corkscrew rag curlers stood upright as if with urgency. "Oh, Sister," she wailed. "The doctor's boat shes comin into the harbour. What'll Ise do? The fire bes not lighted. My curlers! Who'll go to the door?"

Before she finished her lamentations my feet struck the floor, "Hurry, we can be downstairs before they get here."

Never tell a coast person to hurry unless you wish to invite disaster. Annie jumped back, tipped over and upset my water jug and water coursed in all directions.

I grabbed my wrap-around uniform, twisted my hair into a sort-of tidiness and buttoned my Hoover as I went downstairs. When the doctor opened the door I was there to greet him. With him was a stranger, whom he introduced as the travelling dentist, Dr Morris. No, they had not eaten breakfast. Would it be long? No, fifteen minutes at most.

We hurried to make coffee and toast for them, as the doctor was in great haste to be gone. As soon as breakfast was over, he left for his eastern trip and Dr Morris began to unpack his equipment.

I had thought my office crammed to capacity. Now with treasures from the fathomless depth of the dentist's bag, it overflowed. Plaster, impressions, spatula, mixing bowl, basin, rubber sheet, forceps and novocaine were everywhere. He held up a handful of forceps, uppers, lowers, molars, syringes and sponges. With consternation on his face, he gazed at the bulky equipment bag which sagged at his feet and back to the overflowing tables, then, he raised his foot and shoved his bag under the table, while, with his empty hand, he contrived a clear space on the table.

Annie brought a teakettle full of boiling water. The dentist turned to her. "Get a wide-topped spittoon because they spit wide." Not being a tobacco chewer, I had no spittoon, but after scratching her head for a moment, Annie disappeared and returned with a wide-mouthed, enamel slop pail. Soon, I discovered that they also spit high as well as wide. In front of the slop pail, Dr Morris arranged a low-back chair, took out his syringe and commenced to mix up some novocaine. As I had never worked with a travelling dentist, I did not know what to expect. Suddenly, Dr Morris turned and announced. "Ready." I went to the hall and shouted, "First!"

Dr Morris, thickset, chubby, muscular, stood waiting. Mr Galliway, the first victim, six foot tall, bony and straight as a ramrod, stalked through the door, strode to the chair, hung his grey cap on the chair knob and sat down.

It is remarkable to note the excellent medical results which our nurses have accomplished. Professionally they have attempted almost everything ...

When visiting specialists have come along, these nurses make special clinics possible, even if the beach had to be commandeered for an operating theatre. This I remember was the case at Forteau Bay station, when I chanced in there in the hospital boat and found Dr Eves on the beach at work!

W. Grenfell 1930 (2)

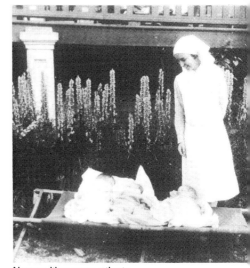

Nurse with young patients

---

* B.J. Banfill, *Labrador Nurse* (London: Robert Hale 1954)

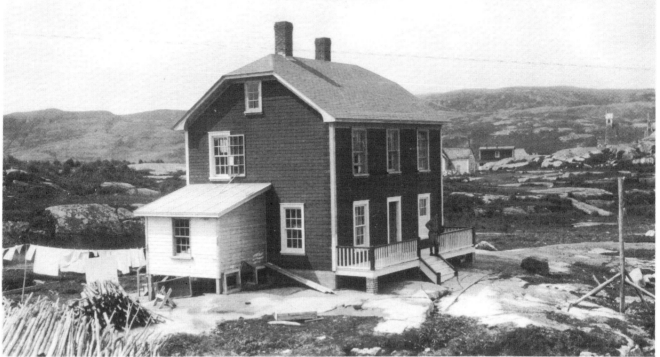

Mutton Bay nursing station on the Canadian Labrador

Although I adhered to the most rigid technique for minor operations and surgical dressings, sterile technique problems were multiple and many times the field was far from sterile. Just as I needed them one grandmother ran her hands over my sterile forceps exclaiming, "Ise jist wants to make sure yous will'nt burn Dorothy." Another mother stuck her finger into my basin of sterile water, "Jist to see that it is not too hot." I explained to her the necessity of keeping everything absolutely sterile and turned to the patient who asked for a drink. Her mother gave it to her, then before I could stop her spilled the rest of the drinking water into my sterile basin just as the baby made a quick debut into the world.

B. Banfill 1954

Dexterously, he curled his long legs around the chair legs, threw back his head and opened his mouth. I stood in front of Mr Galliway and gazed into that awful, yawning cavity. Rows of blackened stumps, with gaping, rotten holes in the centre, confronted me. I could think of nothing but fire-charred tree stumps, with decayed cores. I could picture a squirrel popping up from the bottom of one of these black stumps with what he could carry of his winter store of nuts.

They were terrible teeth—or rather, remnants of teeth—and the next fifteen minutes or so were terrible for all three of us. I marvelled at the dentist's dexterity and strength but more I think at the patient's endurance. After one brief interval when he got rid of the blood in his mouth he inquired calmly:

"How many more, Doc?"

(I thought he had reached the end of that remarkable endurance. Myself, I felt as if I could not stand another tussle followed by the sickening crunch of decayed bones.)

"Four more."

"Go ahead, Doc."

When four more blackened hulls were safely out, Mr Galliway cleansed his mouth, stood up, took his cap off the chair and remarked, "Ise mustn't keep yous because there be lots waiting. How much?"

"Fifty cents," replied Dr Morris.

Mr Galliway dragged out a dogeared, homemade, sealskin purse, tipped it upside down on the palm of his hand and out fell four pennies, two nickels, three dimes, two quarters and a handful of rank smelling tobacco. Carefully, he sorted out the two quarters, wiped off the tobacco, handed them to the dentist and muttered, "Much obliged." Relieved and satisfied, he walked out.

"Next" called the dentist. I stepped to the door and repeated, "Next." Annie in the kitchen echoed, "Next." Before Mr Galliway reached the outer door, the next victim was in the chair.

All day long, with half an hour off for lunch, we hauled out teeth. Men, women and children, who had suffered tooth troubles for months or years, came from harbours round about. Darkness set in so we kept on pulling by the light of a coal oil lamp. At last, all the patients requiring tooth extraction had been relieved of their offending teeth. All except Donnie. Screaming at the top of his lungs, this four year old fisherman-in-the-making had been brought by his father to the dentist. Mr Benny and I managed to inveigle him into the dentist's chair but to keep him there until Dr Morris could remove the offending member was another task. As Dr Morris reached for his forceps, Donnie streaked from our grasp like a greased pig and with a leap was out of the chair, through the door, and, like a flash of lightning, headed for home. Arrived there he crawled through a small hole in the foundation under their house. There, beyond our reach, he huddled until late that night when, tired and hungry, he crawled out, but early the next morning he darted back to his safe haven and stayed there until the "tooth man" left the harbour. At four Donnie already showed signs of the patience and endurance I had observed in so many of the patients that day, although it was unfortunately misdirected, for it would be at least one year, possibly two, before a dentist again visited Mutton Bay.

A CROSSROADS OF THE UNIVERSE*

Elliott Merrick was born in Montclair, New Jersey, in 1904. In 1929, graduated from Yale University and struggling to become a writer, he came to Indian Harbour as a summer volunteer. That fall he moved to North West River to teach at the IGA's Yale School. There he met and fell in love with the Australian nurse, Kate Austen.

After they returned to the United States in 1931, Merrick became a writer of some note, his reputation owing mainly to his skill as a writer of wilderness tales. One of his best books, Northern Nurse, *is the story of Kate Austen Merrick, which they wrote together, telling the tale in her own words as follows:*

A jagged island of black rocks lying in the ocean—that was Indian Harbour, the place where I was to be stationed for the summer. Across the black was a bank of green slope, topped with more black rocks and blue sky. No buildings were visible from seaward. We rounded the point and dropped anchor off a harbour sheltered by this island and another high one to the north. A few schooners, ice, some boats coming off, dotted the water. It was the first day of July.

The mission motorboat came alongside to load freight, tons of it, six heavy drums of gasoline, and me. Everybody knew Doctor Paddon, the silver-haired Englishman who was chief here. Twenty years he had been working for the mission, and as he hurried about the deck in his sou'wester and worn canvas coat, he seemed to have a smile for all his friends.

On the way in I met his crew: Jack Watts, a capable Newfoundlander in his twenties … Joe Kullinuk, an Eskimo … Graham Blake, a young Labradorman, expert hand with motors …

We went into the hospital part which was cold as a morgue from its winter vacancy, and half dark with most of the shutters still on.…

The ground floor consisted of dispensary, doctor's office, a bath, and a ten-bed men's ward. Mattresses were piled in a huge mound on one bed, covered with canvas. The roof had been leaking. Upstairs was a ten-bed women's ward, operating room with skylight, a couple of single rooms, another bath, an oilstove, kerosene sterilizer.…

I had expected to find a primitive shack here, and had brought soap and towels in case there shouldn't be any; also many pounds of sweet chocolate for an emergency ration. The size of the place consequently staggered me. There

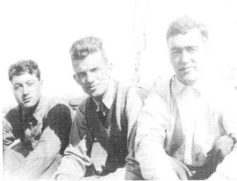

Young patient at a nursing station

Sid Blake, Jack Watts and Graham Blake

* Elliott Merrick *Northern Nurse* (New York: Charles Scribner 1942). Reprinted by permission of the author. Copyright, Elliott Merrick

99

were mountains of sheets and towels. In the storehouse were four cases of soap, ten barrels of flour, boxes, crates, food enough to feed an army. In another few weeks more staff, I learned, would arrive. The place was open for only two and a half months per year, but I could see that it hummed in the short summer. Soon more Newfoundland fishing schooners would arrive. As many as 150 were known to have anchored in the harbour at once.

I put the linen outside to air in the bright wind. I scrubbed and swept and dusted.... The mattresses had to be distributed, and medical supplies unpacked ... the dispensary set to rights, blankets aired, the beds set up....

At bedtime, too tired to tackle another job, we sat around the stove a few minutes and had a mugup of tea, and ship's biscuit....

"It's been a big day," said the doctor, leaning back in his chair....

As I looked at the four men, it struck me we were quite a conglomeration. Doctor Paddon had back of him a traditional English classical education, with medical training at London's famous St. Thomases, relatives who lived on estates, and now for many years his job had made him sailor, dog driver, hunter, surgeon, builder and Heaven knows whatnot.

Jack Watts had already been a sailor, fisherman and sealer. He'd been radio operator at several of the lonely Labrador stations, including Smokey, could build a house or a boat, lay cement foundations, and thought nothing of running-in a new main bearing for a motor or repairing a Delco generator. Having spent his life in and out of the sea, he couldn't swim, of course, and in a land where the snow is more than half the time neck deep, he couldn't snowshoe either, but he blithely tackled such chores as knocking together a dog's sledge, breaking a balky horse, salvaging a schooner or stepping up milk production on the mission's growing farm at North West River.

Joe was a pure-blooded Eskimo and owed his life to chance. Doctor had found him on an island, everybody else dead from the influenza scourge that decimated communities along this coast in 1918. Only six years old then, Joe had been living on seal fat and nothing else for a month. His sealskin boots were shrunk so hard and small they had to be snipped off with scissors. He'd grown so wild in his solitary state that he ran away and hid. It took them half a day to catch him. "If it hadn't been an island, you'd be loose yet," Jack said to him.

Graham had been such an outstanding student in the mission's schools that a well-to-do-American had taken him out to the States for further education, as well as training in a machine shop. After four years as protege of the American, Graham got lonesome for his country—which nearly always happens—and returned, bringing among his other effects a tuxedo and wing collar.

Englishman, Eskimo, Labradorman, Newfoundlander, and Australian, we were an assortment....

Mrs Peters — As soon as they knew the hospital was open, people came from all over. Hidden away in the jagged coast, in spite of its undiscovered look, were coves with hundreds of people. One of our visitors was a woman with three small children, set ashore by a motorboat which immediately steamed away and left them.

Here comes another patient, I said to myself as I hurried down the walk to help her with her big bundle. One of the children could walk, but the other two were in her arms. They were bedraggled-looking, and their yowls made the place resound as tears streaked their dirty faces. Their hair was long and oafish, and they were wet and thin. They looked utterly destitute.

"Can I help you? Here, let me take your bundle," I said. "Is some one sick?"

"Oh, no" Mrs Peters beamed. "We ain't sick. Us just aims to stay awhile. We're on a cruise."

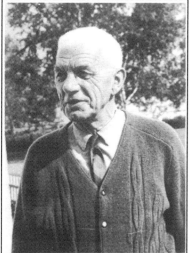

Mission veteran Jack Watts

Dr Tony Paddon said of him: "Jack's steadfast devotion to his duty and his employers, as well as his high humour, reckless courage and kindness, more than compensated for an occasional quick temper, and he earned the respect and confidence of the Mission and the people of Labrador."

They were going on what was apparently an annual visit to Brother Evan's at Horse Harbour, and they had come from Ragged Islands. Three different fishermen, just happening to pass by, had brought them various stages of the journey.

"How will your brother know you're here?" I asked.

"Oh, we got it all arranged," she answered. "He said he'd come soon as he hear'd the hospital was open. He'll hear pretty soon, likely."

"Well, come on up and get warm anyway," I asked her. I was a bit non-plussed, though I didn't let on. I hadn't yet realized that the mission hospitals serve also as hotels, and that that is part of their purpose.

Right away I took to the children. For all their travelworn grubbiness, they were cheery as larks once they got moderately warm and dry. The mother bustled around helping us set the hospital to rights as though she'd been there all her life. Between the two of us we finished rescreening the back porch. I told her she might as well take advantage of the hot water and tub while she was here to scrub the kids and get organized. She set right to it, washed them all till they glistened, and then went off to the laundry to wash their clothes. To dress them meanwhile, I got out pink wrappers and sweaters and things from the clothing store, cut their hair, set them in cribs on the back porch in the sun, tied ribbons in their locks and fancied them up till they were the handsomest youngsters you could imagine. Their mother had a good hot bath too, and finally washed and dried and ironed every rag they owned.

In the three days before Brother Evan came, Mrs Peters helped me cook and clean no end. "I believe I'll buy them pretties for the children," she said one day, indicating the finery in which her young were dressed. She opened up her bundle to disclose quantities of handwork she'd been manufacturing all winter: sweet-grass baskets, hooked rugs, knitted mittens, sealskin moccasins and beaded bags. The industrial worker was not here yet to value such products, but Mrs Peters said she'd leave them and settle all that on the way home from Evan's. Pay for handicraft work was very good, whereas our clothing store material was cheap, so I knew she'd have a substantial balance coming to her.

She went away as unexpectedly as she had appeared. I got up early one morning and she was gone. That was the way here; people came and went, and the hospital was open house to any one travelling the coast or waiting for the steamer. Some of our useful work never appeared in the in- and out-patient casebooks. Sometimes there were five or six fishermen bunking in the mission room waiting for some boat or other. They always pitched in to help us while they stayed. I soon became accustomed to it and thought it the best system that ever was, but at first it seemed strange to be actually living in a land where any one is welcome anywhere at any time. In many hundreds of miles' travel you would be asked to spend the night in every house you passed. They mightn't have a whole blanket in the house, but you could have what they had....

More staff — More staff came on the next steamer. The housekeeper, Martha Gibbons, a grand red-haired woman from Philadelphia, had been here other summers and knew every one for miles around. She also handled the clothing store business. Martha worked in collaboration with Annie Baikie, a pretty Labrador girl who was [the] industrial worker. Annie had been out to the States where she was trained in weaving, designing, sewing, carving and native arts. These skills, added to her natural ability and taste, as well as her intimate knowledge of local conditions, made her an ideal boss of handicraft activities in this region. She gave out materials, criticized and demonstrated techniques, made patterns and suggestions, and bought finished products from people who were all her friends and relatives and acquaintances. Over the course of years the mission had built up a large market for rugs, embroidery work, fur-trimmed

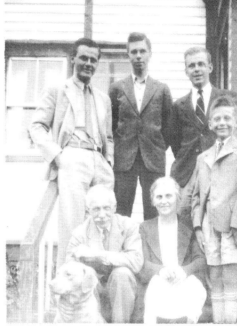

The Paddon family: Dr and Mrs Paddon, Tony, Harry, Dick and John

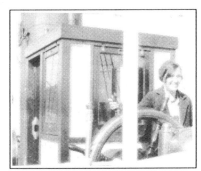

Eleanor Cushman, secretary of the Grenfell Association of America, at the wheel of *Strathcona II*

Phinney, an eye specialist from Cincinnati, did rounds of the Mission's stations during his summer vacations. In the 1920s and 1930s so did orthopedic surgeons Mackenzie Forbes of Montreal; Russell and Andrew MacAusland of Boston; Torrence Rugh of Philadelphia; Fremont Chandler of Chicago; and Joel Goldthwait of Boston. Harry Mount, a surgeon from Ottawa who had worked at the Mayo Clinic, was another. He later took a permanent position at St. Mary's River, such being the calibre of staff the Mission was still able to attract.

Doctor Mount had time for everything and was never busy. This was his 'vacation.' The most difficult cases along the coast, or operations so big one surgeon couldn't handle them, were saved for him. A dozen tonsils here, a thoracotomy there and he breezed north. A day or so ashore catching salmon, and then a stop to mend up another six or eight broken lives. It sounds debonair. Watching him do a plastic operation on a bad shotgun leg wound, I knew it was miraculous. In the case of a surgeon like that, the hand is not just a hand but the visible concentration of centuries of learning, a natural aptitude and a lifetime of training.

E. Merrick 1942

slippers, etc., which enabled men and women here to earn some cash in their winter evenings. The two outdoor workers, or wops, who were to chop wood, run errands, stoke stoves, dig graves, man boats, were Bill from Princeton with leanings toward the ministry, and Hoppy from Yale with leanings toward laughter and girls. Even as they came ashore they were ragging Mabel, the Chicago Junior Leaguer slated for the doctor's secretary: "Two evening dresses! Ho, ho, she brought two evening gowns ..."

The jolliest of them all was a young intern named Dudley Merrill from Boston, who had been here before as [a] wop several times. "How's the water system behaving?" he wanted to know. It seemed that he personally had carried several tons of cement and sand up to our high rock reservoir when the dam was being built. Medically he was keen for experience, interested head over heels, marvellously trained, with a strong sense of responsibility. We got on famously and worked well together, which was fortunate, as Doctor was often to be away in that battered little ketch *Yale* on medical trips, and Indian Harbour hospital might soon be full to the brim. Even in that steamer came our first TB's, beriberi children, septic hands and rotten teeth....

Strathcona II *arrives* — Hardly had Doctor Phinney left us when the little black steamer *Strathcona* came in off the sea, tooting her shrill whistle. She was bound north, way north, perhaps even to Cape Chidley, on a combined medical and charting cruise. They had two dories nested on deck, one of which Sir Wilfred had overboard and was rowing ashore almost before the anchor was down. He was bursting with energy and ideas as always, and had all kinds of plans for more cooperative stores along the coast, more schools, a new mission boat, and improved greenhouses at St. Anthony to provide the whole coast with cabbage plants.

The crew, with the exception of a Newfoundland mate and engineer, was composed of college boys from Harvard and Yale and various other places. The cook was a stockbroker's son from Princeton who had never so much as boiled an egg before in his life, so most of the ship's company, including Sir Wilfred's secretary, Eleanor Cushman, weren't long in ferrying themselves ashore in the remaining dory. They had a hungry look which Martha understood. They were full of fun, dressed in boots and sweaters and flannel shirts, and had already been through some exciting days of fog and storm and difficult passages in and out of the little harbours that Sir Wilfred dared even when fishermen wouldn't. The *Strathcona* has a wrought-iron bottom lined with cement, which has many times stood her in good stead. It is well dented, mate Sims told me. "They do say that *Strath* has been ashore more than she's been afloat, but that's not true."

Sir Wilfred's bronze face and white hair were everywhere at once, and everybody who talked with him felt useful and happy. He scoured the island, he crawled under the hospital and looked at the props, he chatted with the patients and held long consultations with Jeff and doctor, and with Annie on industrial goods. Then before you knew it he was out back of the hospital on a little flat patch of ground setting up a deck tennis court, and had a game in full swing....

[*All too soon*] *our days at Indian Harbour came to an end* — I lay in my bed and thought about the summer. You would suppose that on such a lonely isle as Indian Harbour nothing could ever happen. You'd think to look at it that it must be a sad place with its rocks and surf, the crying gulls, the salt grass blowing in the wind. All around was the sea, with nothing but a sail or berg whose point of white only made the distance longer. But out of those distances came people rich and poor, dilettantes, bunglers, whalers, Eskimos, sailors, sufferers, and miracle workers like Phinney, Mount, Paddon, Grenfell. A thousand stories and heartbreaks and happinesses had filtered through here in one short summer.

Instead of being bleak and sad, life had been warm and bright. On this remote chunk of rock there'd been so many comings and goings the place was like a crossroads of the universe.

ETHEL*

In the fall of 1928 Kate Austen moved from Indian Harbour to North West River. She had barely arrived when Dr Harry Paddon had a gall bladder attack, went to St. Anthony for surgery, and was sent from there to recover in the States, where Mrs Paddon was already with her sons. Kate Austen faced the winter on her own.

From the very first I had been surprised at the size of the hospital, a white, frame three-story building. In many respects it was amazingly modern, with hardwood floors, roller beds, linoleum in the kitchen. The big difficulty was that the ward was on the second floor and no bathroom was there, no sink, no water facilities of any kind. In the huge cellar was a broken hand pump, but the water wasn't good. "Do you mean to say," I asked Doctor Paddon, "that you built a $4,000 hospital here, and no water?"...

There were sixty children in the mission's grade school, most of them from two- and three-house settlements twenty or thirty miles away. They lived in two boarding cottages, one of which was run by Annie Baikie, the other by a Newfoundland housemother named Miss Pye. Polly from Massachusetts and a lonesome soul known as Miss Winette, from an Alberta homestead, were the teachers. Joe as chore boy, Jack as foreman, a dogteam driver and a laundress, me as nurse, Sarah Jane as cook, Pearlie wardmaid ... completed the staff. I was housekeeper at the hospital, where most of them lived. I managed all food stores, requisitions for next year, shortages for this, all bookkeeping, and was in charge of the clothing store, an immense proposition in the hospital attic where twelve huge cases of coats and apparel from the States sat waiting for me. Not the least of that problem was the fact that people paid for the clothing with salmon, trout, firewood, partridges, berries, moccasins, baskets, hooked rugs and labour. Are two salmon, a bearskin with some holes in it, three Arctic hare skins and a hooked rug the equivalent of four sets of woollen insides (underwear)?...

[In the summer of 1929] Sir Wilfred was going through the hospital admission and out-patient books with me, which contained a record of all cases, their treatment, and results obtained. This man of many parts whose small medical mission for fishermen had grown so vast that he could not personally manage it all any more, who spent his winters in England and America lecturing, writing, deciding policies, put his finger on one name after another in the big book. Here was Wilfred Grenfell, MD, and never mind the 'Sir.'

"Si Turner, axe cut, eh? General anaesthetic, stitches, tendon uninjured. You were lucky. In hospital three weeks. Can he snowshoe all right?"

"Yes, perfectly."

"This Broomfield, I arranged about his pension, and put his wheelchair ashore at Rigolet this trip. H-m, May Shepherd, she was operated on at Indian Harbour last summer, if I remember. Is she well now? Good. Goudie, Goudie, which Goudie is that? Oh, yes, his father was with me when we ran on a reef

* Elliott Merrick, *Northern Nurse* (New York: Scribner 1942). Reprinted by permission of the author. Copyright, Elliott Merrick

So instead of being the helper-nurse to a veteran doctor who had spent twenty years in this forest-rimmed settlement, I suddenly became, at the beginning of our long isolated winter season, head of the station and the only medical authority on the eastern edge of this continent between Belle Isle Strait and the North Pole.

E. Merrick 1942

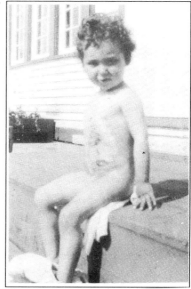

Ethel

I was constantly running into examples of the wonderful work Doctor and Mrs Paddon had done here in their twenty years of service. They loved this bay, and it was their true home. Mrs Paddon had raised four sons of her own here, and women were always telling me that they had learned more about feeding and caring for their children by imitating her than in any other way.

E. Merrick 1942

There were baby seasons, occurring nine months after the trappers' midwinter return from the woods and nine months after they came back in March from the spring hunt.

"Well, Miss," the mother would say about the second day, "you and me have borned him, now what'll we call him? I likes a strange name, like Arminius or Rhonora."

One of the strangest was Noti, given to a boy born when there was *no tea* in the house. I like simple names myself, so I suggested Kate for girls and Austen for boys until I began to fear that a whole generation of duplicates would hate me for an egotist.

E. Merrick 1942

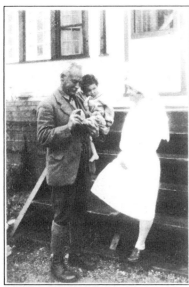

Sir Wilfred, Ethel and nurse Kate Austen: 'the most appealing picture he had ever used'

The hospital at North West River

Rebuilt after a fire destroyed the original structure in 1923, for twenty-one years it functioned without a supply of hot or cold water. Yale School, opened in 1927, is just visible at right.

off Okak once. Is he still living? Henry Jessup still has that chronic backache, eh? What did you do for that?"

"Well," I said hesitantly, "I didn't know what to do. I just gave him rhubarb and soda."

"Best thing. Used to give it to him myself. Poor old Sarah Gear has TB I see. Her husband's one of the best boat caulkers that ever was. Is he able to work?"

"He's a good help with the boats in summer, and very willing, but it's hard for him to get around in winter."

"Well, see that they get everything they need. M-m-m, you've delivered a lot of babies, haven't you? Placenta praevia, eh?" … "And this child Ethel, how did she get burned so badly?"

"Her nightdress caught afire from the stove."

"Who put it out?"

"Her mother tried to, but she caught afire too, and burned her hand and arm. Her ten-year-old brother, Chesley Shepherd, threw a bucket of water on them both."

"Oh, Shepherd, Valley's Bight. I know Peter Shepherd, went deer hunting once with him over back of Double Mer twenty-five years ago. A great talker. How is he?"

"He's fine, and still hunting deer. I spent a night there early in the spring."

"How large an area was burned?"

"About a third of her body. Her whole upper leg and side was a third-degree burn."

"Come, come, tell me about it. Don't make me question you … I have to lecture all winter, you know."…

[Austen proceeds to describe Ethel's burns and her lengthy course of treatment.]

"Come along," said Sir Wilfred. "I want to have a look at Ethel."

She was in her crib looking at a scrapbook. He examined her scars, and when I replaced the dressings, he said "You know, I think we ought to have a picture of Ethel, and us too."

He picked her up and carried her down into the sunshine, where we had several pictures snapped.

The following summer Sir Wilfred showed me one of them and told me he had used the lantern slide of it in all his lectures. He said it was the most appealing picture he had ever used, and that the response it had brought from people everywhere was going to save a good many other Ethels.

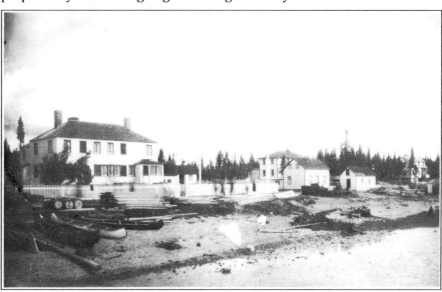

ALL THE TIME IN THE WORLD*

After his graduation from Cambridge University in 1926, Dr Donald Johnson signed on as medical officer with the Cambridge University East Greenland Expedition. Returning to London and entering a standard hospital practice, he discovered that the lack of adventure was not to his taste. In 1928 he applied to the IGA and was assigned to Harrington Hospital that fall. He was filling in for Dr Donald Hodd, who was going on a winter sabbatical. The following spring, working as a temporary house officer at St. Anthony, Johnson became disenchanted again. A disillusioned and fitful Dr Johnson in 1929 returned to England, passed his bar examinations, but practised medicine. He eventually left medicine to publish books.

In March, when I called at the Grenfell Association offices in Victoria Street for perhaps the seventh or the eight time, Miss Katie Spalding, the honorary secretary, had some news for me.

"Yes, Dr Johnson. Yes, we've had a telegram from New York this morning. Dr Hodd at Harrington Harbour is due for a winter's leave this coming winter and they may want a replacement. They'll confirm in a week's time," she announced excitedly.

I asked the obvious question. If I got married, could I take my wife?

"Of course," beamed Miss Spalding, the underlying benevolence of her nature overcoming the last traces of secretarial reserve. "Most of our doctors are married. You'll need your wife there, I expect. I believe there's a separate doctor's house at Harrington Harbour. We would want a married man."

This seemed too good to be true. This slightly brusque, elderly spinster became transfigured into a real life embodiment of the Good Fairy. Though, as I later found, Katie Spalding's brusqueness did in fact cover a rare goodness of character—at the end of a lifetime of devotion to active missionary work she was, during the time I knew her, giving her services for nothing to the London office of the Grenfell Mission, and living on a small private income—some said merely on the old age pension. A rare spirit indeed in times such as the present.

"We shall be wanting you to see Mr Rowley Bristowe, our staff adviser," added Katie Spalding, reverting to officialdom. "Then I expect that we shall know within ten days time."

I called on the late Mr Rowley Bristowe at his house in Harley Street for the appropriate 'vetting' and, after another ten days, I heard that the job was available and that I had got it. That was, it was mine for the mere signing of a pledge form that I would neither drink myself, nor condone the drinking by others, of any form of alcohol during my service in Labrador, or during my journey there.

"I'm afraid that Doctor—Sir Wilfred Grenfell—has very strict views on alcohol," said Miss Spalding apologetically, as she passed the form across to me. "He won't even allow brandy to be used in our hospitals."

I signed the form and was told that we were now due to report on the Canadian Labrador the middle of September ...

At Harrington — Hodd introduced me to my new duties. It was soon obvious that the routine duties of medical officer to the Harrington Harbour Hospital did not take up a large part of one's day.

Born in Ontario, Donald G. Hodd graduated MD from the University of Toronto in 1925. After interning at the Hamilton General Hospital he went to Harrington Hospital in 1926, intending to stay for a year or two at the most. Hodd left Harrington in 1944, returned in 1947 and retired in 1970.

The first doctor was Dr Hare, who had been there from 1906 to 1916, and then he went off to the first world war. Next, was a Dr West, he was there for two or three years. There were several other doctors including Dr Yates, Dr Frost and even a fake doctor for one summer ... By the time I got there in 1926, the place was starting to get pretty run-down.

D. Hodd 1979

---

* Donald McI. Johnson, *A Doctor Regrets ... Being the First Part of 'A Publisher Presents Himself'* (London: Christopher Johnson 1949)

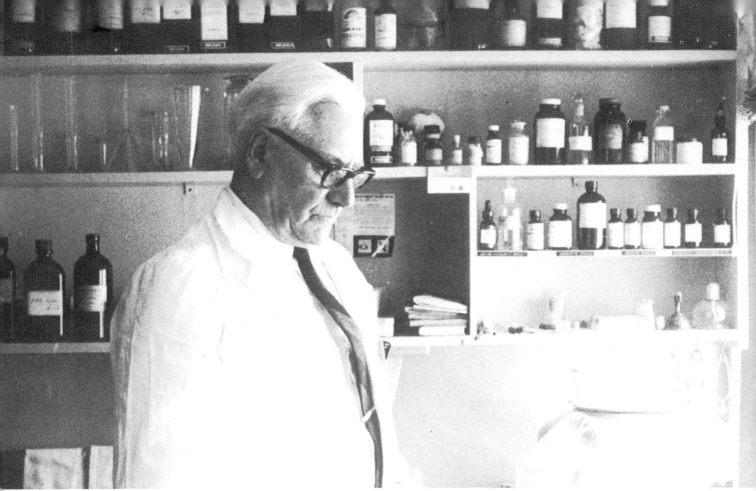

Donald Hodd

When I used to go out [on winter sabbatical] every four years or something like that, I did not go for a holiday, I went to work. I took courses, they were not actually courses, but I worked in hospitals as an intern or an extern, whatever you want to call it ... I spent one sabbatical leave doing surgical pathology at Hamilton General Hospital. I spent one winter at Toronto General Hospital in the sick children's ward brushing up on reading X-ray films ... Other years I worked in the sanatorium at Ste-Agathe and down in Montreal at the Royal Edward Laurentian Hospital. For a good bit of my work on the coast I had to learn by myself. I used to have some medical students in the summer time. I think I got more out of them than they got out of me.

D. Hodd 1979

"Of course, you'll have your winter trips to fit in," said Hodd encouragingly when the first morning we had looked at the two cases who occupied the female ward—both chronic pulmonary tuberculosis. The male ward was unoccupied.

My new practice, indeed, if not numerous (probably not more than 2,000 souls in all) and, if not busy as a routine, was a scattered one. It had length but not depth. It took in the whole length of coast with both English and French fishing settlements, from Natashquan on the west to Blanc Sablon on the Newfoundland border to the east—a matter of some two hundred miles....

Harrington Harbour, with its four or five hundred English-speaking inhabitants, was in the centre of this stretch of coast and was by far its largest settlement. It ... was, during the time I knew it anyway, a prosperous settlement. The fishing and sealing seasons were short but both, in those days brought in good stable incomes.

Moreover Harrington benefited from the lion's share of the bounty of the Grenfell Mission ... [I]t was soon obvious that a generous helping of clothing was given in return for the comparatively small quantities of local products and even less work—a fact which the shrewd Harringtonians were not slow to realize. My arrival coincided with the time for stocking up the winter fuel for the hospital and 'cords' of wood (a 'cord' seemed to be a local measurement— and a somewhat arbitrary one at that!) were piling up unasked for, and frequently unannounced until after they had been deposited, at the hospital wharf! Five dollars was the recognized price of a cord of wood and for five dollars one got a very good supply of woollen clothing at the clothing store—a very good supply indeed....

Uncle Will — The most exasperating quality [of the natives] was their appalling slowness. Whether it was doing anything; coming to the point in conversation, or making a mental decision, there was all the time in the world at Harrington Harbour. It was inevitably so out of the nature of their life. Apart from their short six weeks fishing season in the summer, there was only one other occupation for the majority of the coast people and that was to cut sufficient wood in the fall … But during the long winter months there was nothing to do at all other than sit round the stove, tinker with the fishing gear, swap gossip, and spit about the place. Time on the Labrador coast was an ample commodity. It could be wasted *ad lib*; it could be spread on thick; it could be left lying about. For three-quarters of the year it presented only one problem—namely, what to do with it.

All the same, it was not easy for one coming from the busy hive of London to grasp this.… For instance, it had always been my custom (in those days before queues) when I wanted anything in a shop, to go in and ask for it, and come out again with a brief, perhaps perfunctory, "Good morning." But this pernicious habit was almost my downfall as far as Harrington was concerned. I was blissfully unaware of the anti-social nature of my behaviour until tackled one morning by Padre Le Moignan …

"Look here, doctor," said the Padre in mock horror. "What on earth have you been doing to Uncle Will?"

"Nothing," I said. "What's the trouble?"

"I couldn't say. But when I asked him how he got on with you, he didn't say much until I pressed him, when he just grunted 'I don't understand him.' It seemed to me as if he has taken umbrage at you for something. What **have** you done?"…

"I've only been into his store and walked out again," I protested.

"That's probably it," said Le Moignan … "I expect you moved too quickly for him."

That may or may not have been it. Anyway, I could take no chances. Uncle Will was a man who mattered. I must obviously mend my ways. A visit to his store, be it for a ball of twine or for half a yard of canvas duck, was for the remainder of my stay a morning's ceremony. It went something like this:

"Morning, Uncle Will." This was the opening gambit as one came up the stairs.

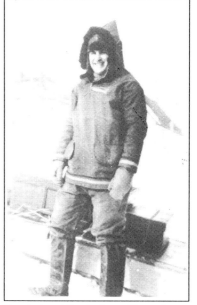

The doctor at Harrington setting out on a medical trip, Harrington Hospital behind

"Good morning, doctor."

Pause while Uncle Will, a portly figure with round florid face and walrus moustache, pottered about, weighing sugar or indulging in some similar occupation.

"What do you think of the weather, Uncle Will?"

Uncle Will would take off his cap and scratch his head: "Wonderful weather it is."

There was very little need for Uncle Will's indecision. The weather at Harrington was always wonderful. 'Wonderful' in Labrador jargon was an abbreviation for 'wonderful bad.' Yes, we certainly had wonderful weather at Harrington!

Pause for several minutes.

"Have you heard where Uncle Fred is, Uncle Will?" … Uncle Fred [w]as the mailman. His whereabouts was of prime importance; particularly when the weather became too uncertain for the *North Shore* to reach us.

"They say as he's waiting to Natashquan for the *North Shore*," said Uncle Will.

Pause again. But it was now Uncle Will's turn to make conversation.

"How's Lizzie Chislett?"

"Not so good, Uncle Will."

Pause again.

"And how's Aunt Maggie?"

"A little better."

So it went on. It was not until the well-being of the hospital patients, and any other sick members of the community had been discussed, the prospects for the winter's travelling gone into, with perhaps digressions concerning both Dr Hodd's adventures and those of other Harrington doctors ranging back over the past twenty years, that one could really get down to the business in hand—namely the purchase of a ball of twine, or half a yard of canvas duck, as the case might be....

It was surprising how easy it was to accustom myself, once broken in, to the easy-going tempo of Labrador life—the pottering about in general management of affairs which ran with a minimum of interference anyhow. Life had its disadvantages, but it was none of the things that we had feared it might be or had been warned that it would be. Above all it wasn't dull....

Uncle Esau — Uncle Esau, of the older generation of the Andersons, was the officially-appointed boatman-cum-dog-driver to the hospital doctor and during the four months under survey I certainly saw more of him than I did of either of my head nurses—and, for that matter, probably more than I did of my own wife. Genial, kindly, loyal and cautious, with almost every thoroughly decent trait of character that one can think of showing on his deeply-lined and weather-beaten face, Uncle Esau was, all the same, not always infallible as a guide. It was indeed no easy matter to be infallible in the circumstances of winter travelling when the sea froze and the ice settled along the coast, and then the snow came and settled on the ice, and the snow and the ice and the low-lying islands and the rocks and the spruce trees melted into each other in a continuous white sheet so that one island looked much like another island, one rock like another rock, and one spruce tree exactly like the next, and whatever landmark remained became finally obliterated by the misty clouds of drifting snow that stung one's face like fine sand. Anyway, when the occasion arose, Uncle Esau and I, clothed for our travels, he in his white canvas-duck suit, myself in Grenfell cloth, would perch ourselves on the square komatik box which was the traditional masculine mode of Labrador travel (only women and Roman Catholic priests used the more comfortable and protected 'coach-boxes') and he sitting in front, myself behind, we would set out behind the motley collection of dogs that formed the hospital team. So we would wander out into the unknown in the general direction of where we wanted to go ... and Uncle Esau would proceed to lose himself in the featureless landscape. He would seldom confess this to me, but one began to know that he was getting lost at the stage when, despite the climatic conditions, he would take his cap off and start scratching his head. We would then wander round aimlessly for an hour, perhaps two hours, or maybe three, when at last Uncle Esau's face would light up and a note of confidence would come into his voice as he exclaimed:

"Ah, now I knows where I'm to."

It was an uncertain method of progression, but we usually seemed to reach our destination where, seated round the fuggy cabin, whose warm haze was practically as thick as that of the cold drifting snow outside, Uncle Esau would relate our experiences to Pierre or Paul, Charlie or Fred (according to the nationality of the settlement we had arrived at), concluding with the inevitable dictum:

"Yes, sir, it certainly is wonderful weather."...

Nadir — What can I say of the remainder of my time with the Grenfell Association as house surgeon to the St. Anthony Hospital other than that it was an anti-climax? It was a return to a subordinate position. It was a return to the cooped-up conditions of hospital work. It was an endeavour to work as the only Englishman with an all-American staff—and though they are likeable people in many ways, I did not find Americans easy people to work with.

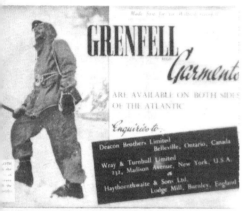

Marketing Grenfell garments: a modern brochure

The British weaving company Haythornthwaite & Sons produced a closely woven cloth of cotton gabardine that was so successful in repelling rain, snow and Arctic gales it was sold under the Grenfell label. The company in the late 1930s began manufacturing garments using the cloth: the slogan, 'Grenfell, a name with great associations.'

... The complex character of the late Sir Wilfred Grenfell himself demands a separate biography ... But it would be wrong to omit mention of his somewhat fleeting presence during that summer and of the undoubted privilege of having seen and known him in his old age amongst the surroundings which he had created and made famous. The Grenfell house on the hill at St. Anthony was now occupied for only some few weeks in each year during the summer when 'Sir Wilf,' together with the dignified and charming Lady Grenfell, would appear as the figure heads of the establishment. But with Grenfell, as so often with others of brilliant early fame, advancing years had already taken their toll. Now, at the age of sixty-four, though socially and publicly lionized in Great Britain and the United States, he was a potterer divested of real authority in the organization which he had built up during the hey-day of his powers. The whole latter part of his life had been devoted to platform appeals for funds in the big centres of population, while the work on the coast of Labrador had fallen into other hands—it was institutionalized and organized from the head office in New York.

After Harrington, after the roseate expectations I had formed in regard to the centre of the Grenfell work, St. Anthony was a disappointment. Though this must in fairness go on record as a personal reaction. That the St. Anthony Hospital did, and is undoubtedly still doing, splendid medical and surgical work under the superintendence of Dr Curtis, let there be no mistake.... But the zest of Grenfell's crusading spirit, manifested on his public platforms, seemed to have departed from the work. Amongst the summer volunteer workers, young college men and women, mainly from the Eastern United States, who had been induced by Grenfell's eloquence to spend their summer in doing the humbler tasks about the hospital, the result was disillusionment and a tendency for natural high spirits to find their outlet in horseplay of various kinds, most of it of such a kind as to lead to friction and misunderstanding with the more sombre-minded permanent staff....

We English types were, I fear, regarded as hopelessly frivolous and irresponsible by the very earnest brand of American who comprised the main body of the permanent Mission staff—and perhaps they were right.

"Why are you so late?" was the peremptory greeting of the stumpy, grumpy little man who awaited us on the [St. Anthony] dock. He had already been pointed out to me as Dr Curtis, the medical superintendent of the St. Anthony Hospital— my new chief. Without waiting for the explanation which I was only too willing to give, he turned on his heel and walked away.

This incident set the tone of our future relationship.

D. Johnson 1949

The American Dr Charles Curtis came to St. Anthony in 1915 as a summer volunteer. The antithesis of Grenfell, he was quietly competent, modest and unobtrusive, but brusque. Succeeding Dr John Little as chief of the St. Anthony Hospital in 1917, he proved to be an excellent administrator. Curtis served the Mission for nearly fifty years.

'Somber-minded permanent staff'

Head nurse Selma Carlson is seated behind Grenfell, Dr Charles Curtis to his right.

ST. ANTHONY THEN AND NOW*

In 1930, Jessie Luther revisited St. Anthony after an absence of sixteen years. She took pride in the tangible evidence of its progress and growth.

I have just returned from a short cruise on the *North Voyageur*, a small steamer of the Clarke Steamship Company, to St. Anthony, Newfoundland via Montreal, Quebec and the St. Lawrence River and Gulf ...

What a change since my last visit sixteen years ago!...

There was the old hospital at one time the largest building in the village, but now quite overpowered by the beautiful new concrete hospital near by. There was the old orphanage, unchanged in itself but now transferred to the industrial department and quite insignificant compared with the large substantial orphanage building standing on the top of the hill near the little Guest House, which I almost had to search for in the midst of other buildings.... Perhaps the greatest change was in the wharf with its coal pocket and overhead landing stage, a large storehouse and near by a real dry-dock. Derricks, winches and various landing equipment were in use unloading the *Cluett* which had just come in with supplies. A little railway ran down the wharf from the storehouse, and I could scarcely believe my eyes as a small truck rushed by with a most business-like air when I later started forth to explore what seemed almost like a strange community. What a change! In former days there were not only no trucks, but no roads to run them on....

The industrial department itself, grown out of all recognition is now a veritable workshop or factory, with a weaving room, a dye room with steam vats, a room for toy making, a room for ivory carving, groups of workers tearing long strips of outing flannel for hooked mats, another group cutting the tops off silk stockings and the legs into narrow strips for the finest grade mats. There was also a designing room, a group cutting stencils and marking the burlap used for hooking; and, in what was once the large orphanage playroom, deep shelves held finished products ready for shipping and quantities of materials in the process of preparation.

One of the rooms was a real office, with someone in charge, of course a necessity with an industry grown to such proportions; and Miss Pressley-Smith, the efficient young head of the department, took me to the supply building full of materials of all kinds, though mostly for weaving and hooked mats. The amount of material fairly took my breath away.

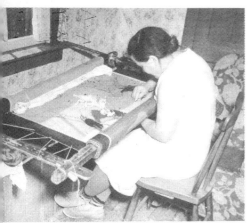
Hooking a Grenfell mat

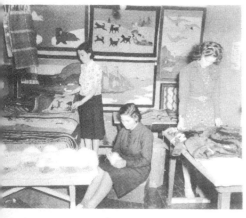
The handicraft shop at St. Anthony

Hooking mats: cottage production

Strips of brightly coloured rags, or used silk stockings, stripped, washed, dried out-of-doors and powder-dyed, pulled through burlap on a simple, four-sided wooden frame, produced a remarkable, tapestry-like effect.

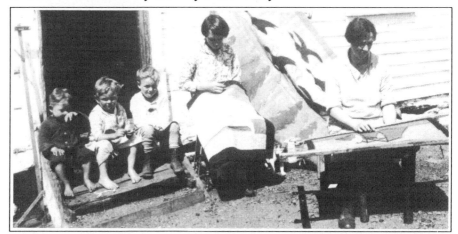

* Jessie Luther, "In Retrospect," *Among the Deep Sea Fishers* 28, no. 3 (1930): 112-24

110

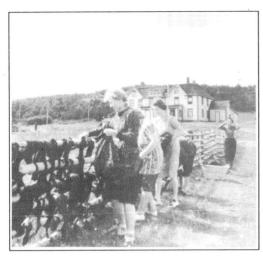
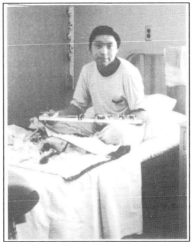
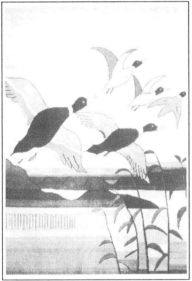
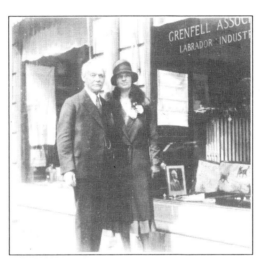

INDUSTRIAL WORK

Grenfell recruited administrators, teachers and artists from all over the British Isles and North America to run his Mission's industrial department. They interacted with indigenous craftspeople to produce a creative, though not always strictly traditional, product. The immensely popular Grenfell hooked mat, for example, was local in terms of colour and technique; designs, however, while depicting northern scenes, were dictated by New England tastes. The mats accounted for the largest part of the Mission's industrial output because they were eminently suited to cottage production. The toy industry was introduced chiefly to provide work for convalescent patients and permanently disabled men.

Marketing was the special concern of Anne Grenfell who co-ordinated a small army of willing volunteers, many of whom had worked on the coast before. They organized private sales in Canada, Great Britain and the United States; ran Grenfell Labrador Industries shops in New York and Philadelphia; and managed tearooms in the summertime—the Dogteam Tavern at Ferrisburg, Vermont, and the Connecticut Dogteam Tea House at Oxford, near New Haven. By 1930, cash proceeds were exceeding $50,000 a year and over 2,000 people were receiving income and clothing vouchers.

Although the industrial department was never truly self-sufficient, it served a variety of purposes. It provided skilled craftspeople with materials, markets and income; because it accepted products from the less skilled, it benefited them; and it provided occupational therapy.

From the top, left to right:
Used silk stockings for the mat industry, dyed and hung out to dry: 'When your stocking runs, let it run to Labrador'
Occupational therapy
Grenfell rug: a remarkable, tapestry-like effect
Lady Anne and Sir Wilfred Grenfell outside the Grenfell Labrador Industries shop in Philadelphia
Display of Grenfell products

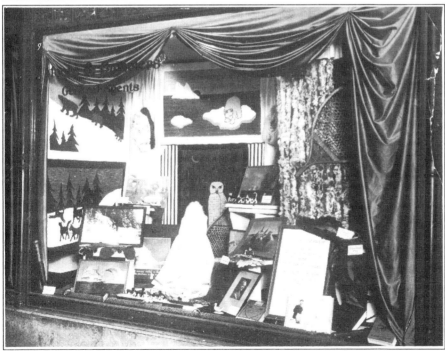

I BIT MY TONGUE*

Born at Rigolet, Labrador, Millicent Blake began her education at a one-room school run by the Church of England. She moved to the IGA's boarding school at Muddy Bay and from there to its school at St. Anthony, where she dreamed of one day becoming a nurse. Having finished grade nine, she worked as a nursing assistant at North West River, 1929-1933. The IGA at this point arranged for her to complete high school at Madison, Wisconsin, and to train as a nurse at Duluth, Minnesota. After an absence of seven long and lonely years, Blake returned in 1940 to work at the IGA hospitals at Cartwright and St. Anthony and finally, in 1943, to take charge of the small hospital (later, nursing station) at St. Mary's River. Here she met and married Sidney Loder, manager for Baine, Johnston and Company at Battle Harbour. The couple lived for seven years at Hopedale before moving to St. John's.

In 1969, after Sidney Loder's death, Millicent Loder returned to Labrador to work at most of the nursing stations operated by the IGA. At North West River, her spiritual home, she established the infants' home. In 1980 Memorial University awarded her an honorary degree. In 1982 she became a member of the Order of Canada.

Here Millicent Loder speaks eloquently of a cultural gap few could bridge.

The International Grenfell Association, in order to give educational opportunities to the more promising young people of the coast, and in order, as a remote eventuality, to eliminate imported workers, has for some years past sent a limited number of boys and girls to the United States, Canada, and England for supplementary education, chiefly along technical lines. Of the hundred students so far thus trained, some eighty-one have returned to their own country.... These returned students are now serving on the coast, some as plumbers, mechanical engineers, electricians, shoemakers, teachers, stenographers, dressmakers, trained nurses, dieticians; while we have at least one tanner, and one tinsmith, and two clergymen in the number!

Grenfell Association of Great Britain and Ireland 1930

The Mission's boarding school at Muddy Bay, the former Labrador Public School (shown on p. 80), accommodated from forty to fifty children each winter. Destroyed by fire in 1928, with no loss of life, the school was replaced by the larger Lockwood School built at Cartwright. The IGA received government approval to favour the teaching of practical and industrial skills at each of its schools.

Early in September the IGA hospital boat, *Strathcona* steamed into Rigolet harbour and I was rowed aboard after saying good-bye to the rest of the family, dressed in my Sunday best, ten years old and leaving my family behind. I was the only child on board so I was placed in the dispensary of the boat and told not to touch anything. The half door was barred for safety, and I was alone. As the houses of Rigolet faded in the distance, I became homesick and stood peeping above the door, crying and miserable. Finally Dr Grenfell himself came in and sat me on his knee. He started leafing through a magazine, telling me about the things and places pictured there. He came to one picture of a very grand lady. He told me that if I was a good girl, worked hard and got a good education I would one day be a lady. This was the one time in my life that I spoke to Dr Grenfell face-to-face, but I always remembered his kindness when he would come to visit the schools in later years. Like most of the children who knew Dr Grenfell, I loved him dearly.

When we arrived at Muddy Bay, the school looked monstrous to me. The staff and children of the school came down on the wharf to greet us. I was taken to the school and was handed over to the head mistress. She looked at me, then called one of the working girls over and said, "Take her upstairs and show her where she is going to sleep. Check her head, give her a bath and put some decent clothes on her." I was heartbroken. I was being treated like I imagined poor children were, and I knew that my mother had given me the best she could.

This being my first time away from home, I suffered severe homesickness for a long time at Muddy Bay school. Gradually, I made friends with the other children, but I still found school life very different from home. There were so many rules and regulations to get used to. You were not allowed to go into the staff room. You had to ask permission to go out and to come in. Eat everything on your plate. Make your bed before leaving your room. Button the clothes of the younger children. Take your cod oil without fussing. There seemed no end to the list of what you should and shouldn't do.

I soon learned to adjust....

We all had our chores to do; some peeled potatoes (when there were any), others swept and scrubbed the floors, or cleaned and trimmed the lamps. I

---

* Millicent Blake Loder, *Daughter of Labrador* (St. John's: Harry Cuff 1989). Reprinted by permission of Harry Cuff Publications Ltd., copyright Milicent Blake Loder

played with and minded the little ones, because I was ten and used to caring for my brothers and sisters. It was considered a great privilege to be allowed to dust and tidy the staff rooms, or to mend the teachers' clothing, darn their socks and perhaps to iron some of their things. The teachers had such nice things; clothes with lace on them, pretty beads, flowered hand mirrors — real treasures. Sunday was a special day at the school. There was no studying, so we spent the day reading, playing and having services. Each pupil recited the Bible text set for that week. For an extra special treat each Sunday, as we filed out of the dining room after supper, we were given a candy....

Whatever else I did at Muddy Bay, I learned a lot from my private reading. I read everything, good and bad, and made up my own pronunciations and meanings for words I didn't know. There may have been a dictionary around but I was not aware of one, nor had I been taught how to use one. Later I found that I had to relearn a lot of words and meanings; I also knew that much knowledge had been lost to me by reading without guidance. Apart from school, I learned about life in general at Muddy Bay. I learned that some of the people we were taught to regard as models had feet of clay. The staff was good to us, but always let us know that we were not their equals. The staff came from abroad and felt themselves to be missionaries, trying to bring a bit of England to the Labrador wild. In the same building, they ate apart from us, had different food and better living quarters. I'll bet there were some children, especially the boys, who had never seen the staff quarters. It was off limits. Worst of all was when you had been spanked, or otherwise punished, there was no one to put their arms around you to comfort you and let you know you had been forgiven.... In later years I have always tried to remember that children are very sensitive and intelligent people, and they must always be spoken to and treated with care and kindness. There were many good times to remember of my two years at Muddy Bay, and I left with some sadness, but I was full of joy to be going home....

I can recall quite clearly my first sight of St. Anthony. There was fog around and for some time we had been hearing a foghorn, the first one I had ever heard. As we rounded the Cape, St. Anthony was spread out around us. There were many houses around the harbour and I saw two churches, one on each side of the harbour. We tied up at a wharf, the size of which I had never seen before. Up from the wharf were several large buildings that belonged to the IGA. There was a large shed and farther up, enclosed by the fences, was a large yellow box-like building. This was the orphanage, where we were to live. Five Labrador girls and a number of boys had come to attend school that year.

We were met and warmly welcomed by a jolly, smiling, motherly sort of lady. This was Miss Karpik, the head mistress. Her greeting convinced me from the first that this school would be more to my liking than Muddy Bay. Miss Karpik took us around to our room. This was called the Labrador Girls' Room. Other children were everywhere in the halls and in the dining room. Some had been there for years, while others were newcomers as we were. The dining room had lots of tables and when we all filed in they were all full. It was like a big family. Miss Karpik and her helpers sat at the table with us, quite a change from Muddy Bay. Miss Karpik told us all about the rules and regulations. She told us that she would be glad to help us out with anything at any time. I loved her from the first. That night we were allowed to go out for a little while. There were swings at the front of the building, real swings with chains and seats. We spent the evening swinging up high and getting a good look all around St. Anthony. I told Eva I was going to like it here. After we got in bed we chatted about the place, the head mistress and expectations for the future. We fell asleep happy.

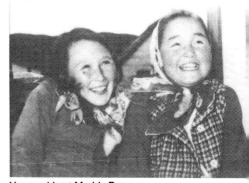

Young girls at Muddy Bay

At St. Anthony is located a large day school, run by the International Grenfell Association, and entirely undenominational in character and outlook.... It is intended to safeguard the education, not only of the children in the St. Anthony orphanage, but for the whole village. Its accommodation is utterly inadequate to the growing need, and already many of the younger children have to be refused admission, while those who do attend are packed like sardines. The casual visitor cannot fail to be impressed by the excellence of the work accomplished under such conditions. In a school accommodating nearly 200 scholars, there is not a drop of running water for drinking, cleaning, cooking for the domestic science class, or for the prevention of fire in a building whose only lighting system is the kerosene or paraffin lamp. The drinking water has to be carried daily from a distant house, and for cleanliness a nearby stream serves in summer— the snow filling that need during the winter months. A new school building is urgently needed.

Grenfell Association of Great Britain and Ireland 1930

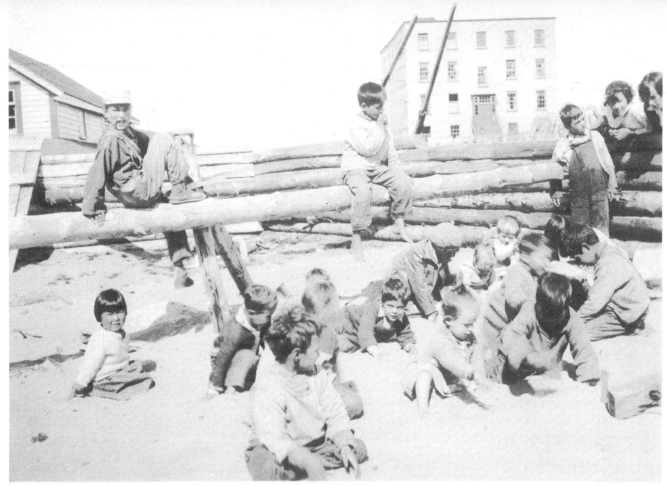

At play in the sandpile at St. Anthony

In the background is the new children's home achieved after years of fundraising.

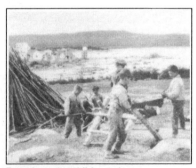

Boys from the children's home sawing wood

The next morning, on the way to school, I took a good look at the buildings. Everything was clean and neat. There were Bible verses on some of the buildings, which made me feel more at home than anything else. I had heard those verses many times. There was a building next to the hospital where patients who were not hospitalized stayed. On the building, in big black letters, was 'Faith, hope and love abide and the greatest of these is love.' On the school was 'All thy children shall be taught of the Lord and great shall be the peace of thy children.'

School at St. Anthony was an enchantment from that day. There were four classrooms with a teacher in each room. Each room had several grades. My teacher was Miss Frances Byers, an American. I would have done anything to please her and I believe most of her class would have done the same. After all these years I remember her with love and appreciation. She put us on the right track to gaining knowledge and understanding, to enjoy competition and success and how to accept defeat and profit from it. For the first time I felt that I could relate to an 'outsider' as a friend. Shortly after I arrived, Miss Byers asked me if I would help her clean her room and do up her clothes on Saturdays. I was very flattered. The first Saturday I cleaned, ironed and sewed some things for her, and I was surprised when she gave me twenty-five cents. I had my own spending money! While I stitched or darned, Miss Byers told me about other countries and other people. Soon I began to realize how small my world was.

Perhaps because I was older, I felt that I had a lot of freedom at St. Anthony. On Sundays we were free to go out after dinner and do what we liked, as long as we were back by mealtime. Sometimes you might be asked to have a meal by some of the townspeople and permission was always given. Quite often we walked across the harbour or up the Bight, and we would be invited into the homes. We would be given bread and molasses or jam, and sometimes a cup of tea or other tidbits. Some of the dearest friends I have today are people that I met at St. Anthony....

I don't recall being homesick at St. Anthony. Our days were full and there were so many new things to get used to. It was at St. Anthony that I saw electric lights for the first time. I saw the inside of a hospital. I saw nurses at work, learned what an X-ray was, and I visited the dentist. I began to understand why outside people were so different, for the world outside that I was being taught about was very different from Double Mer and the things and ideas that the Grenfell Mission had brought to St. Anthony were the wonders of the world compared to Rigolet....

In my dreams at the Labrador Girls' Room in St. Anthony I pictured myself dressed in white and working as the nurse in charge of the North West River hospital. I dreamed that I would pattern myself after Miss Carlson, the head nurse at the St. Anthony hospital. She was Swedish born, trained in the United States and had been in St. Anthony for many years. Miss Carlson was a very dignified, organized and fair person. I watched her admiringly as she went among the staff and patients. I saw how she handled them and saw the respect they gave her.

When I finished my grade nine my parents wondered what could be done with me. I was considered old enough to work, but there was little for girls to do in those days. I felt that I had learned enough at St. Anthony to be of great help to my mother and be able to take over for her when she went to deliver a baby or look after someone sick, but Ma knew of my ambition and tried to encourage it as best she could. Once again she put her pride in her pocket and approached Dr Harry Paddon at North West River to see if there was a job I could do with the IGA. Later that summer I got word that I could come to North West River to work as a servant girl in the hospital. I was overjoyed. Ma and I worked to get me ready. It was 1929; I was fourteen.

As I sailed up beautiful Hamilton Inlet toward North West River and my first job, I dreamed of what might come of this position. I hoped to earn enough to be able to go on to school and later become a nurse.... I felt grown-up and confident that I would see my dream come true.

Arriving at the hospital, the girls who worked there got me settled away and told me what to expect in the morning. I stayed with two other girls in one room. It was good to have their company and listen to their advice about how to handle the work, what the staff was like and how to please them....

My starting salary at the hospital was fifty cents a month. How I looked forward to my first payday! At that time the Grenfell Mission was financed entirely by donations. I suppose that was why our wages were so low. I do remember occasionally we would all be called together by Dr Paddon; he would tell us that the Mission was having a hard time and ask if we would be willing to work a month or two without wages. Of course we always did. We were still getting free meals and a bed to sleep in. As far as I was concerned I was learning something about my trade....

The three of us took turns at doing the cooking, cleaning the staff quarters and working as ward maids. In my second month at North West River it was my turn as cook. For me, cooking was a month to endure. Patients and servants ate the same food, while doctors, nurses, teachers and other outsiders had specially cooked foods, for they were not used to our kind of cooking.

The first time it came my turn to do a month as staff girl, I was very excited. I hadn't been in the staff quarters, except in the living room once or twice. Remembering the pretty things the teachers at Muddy Bay had, I was looking forward to seeing what the outsiders had at North West River. First thing I did every morning was to take a jug of warm water to the rooms of the doctor, nurses, teachers and other outsiders and awakened them. While they were dressing, I was preparing their breakfast. The cook would see to it that the coals

[In 1942] I was the only nurse from either Newfoundland or Labrador with the IGA. The other nurses and the doctors were all Americans, for there were few English people with the Grenfell Mission during the war. Sometimes it struck me how differently I was treated by the 'outsiders' now that I was considered staff, while some of my relatives or friends were looked down upon. I soon concluded that the Mission was missing a golden opportunity by sticking to their own group. As staff I was treated well by the Mission and the doctors and nurses all tried to help me succeed. But, generally, the IGA did not make the most of their opportunities to educate the people about health matters ... [to explain] the importance of these matters in layman's language, rather than medical terms.

M. Loder 1989

A young graduate of Cambridge University, J. Scott, was part of an expedition mounted by Professor Geno Watkins in conjunction with Grenfell to further the aerial mapping of Labrador. He was at North West River the previous winter (1928-1929), when he observed: "Like poor relations we were only waiting to be asked out to dinner and the hospital crowd were always ready to invite us.... At the hospital there were civilized meals, served on clean dishes and a white table-cloth, and eaten with fresh weapons for every course; and we had to bridle our tongues and make polite conversation about theatres and towns and far-off things."

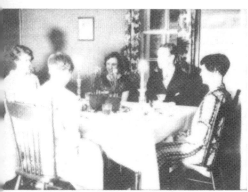

Grenfell staff at dinner

were just right for making toast, which was made at the last minute so that it would be hot. The table had to be set just so. When the staff assembled and were seated at the table, a little bell would summon the staff girl in with breakfast. After breakfast all the bedrooms had to be done—beds made, lamps trimmed and cleaned, everything dusted and tidied and the slop pails emptied and cleaned. I hated this part of the job. I didn't mind doing it for sick people, but I promised myself that when I got to be a nurse I would look after my own things. In addition to the normal daily duties there was one other job for the staff girl, making butter balls. There were two little wooden paddles with grooves in them and a pattern on one side. You dipped the paddles in ice water and placed a blob of butter on them, then rolled it around to form little balls with a pattern on them. I bit my tongue to keep from asking what difference it made. For supper the staff would all dress and the staff girl would have to wear a black dress with a frilly apron and a little white headdress. You lighted the lamps and built a fire so that everything would be warm and ready for supper. After the dishes were done and other chores taken care of, you had to turn down the staff beds and make sure there was water in their jugs. Sometimes, if it was really cold, a little kerosene stove was lit and moved from room to room to take the chill off the air.

For four years I went from one job to the other and back again. I enjoyed most of my work and endured the things I did not like, because I knew that some day I would get to be a nurse. I learned a lot and grew to think of North West River as the place I loved best. I became even more determined to come back when I eventually got through my training.

THE LOST RADIUM*

Hilton Willcox was a twenty-two-year-old medical student at Dunedin, New Zealand. Called by the 'Gods of the sea' from his final year of medical studies, he signed as a deck hand on the City of New York, *the vessel bringing Commander Richard E. Byrd back from the South Pole. Sailing with Byrd to the United States, he applied in 1930 to the IGA and that fall, commenced a one-year contract as house officer at St. Anthony. Here he developed an enduring respect for Dr Charles Curtis, his 'Chief,' who was an acknowledged raconteur.*

Willcox, despite his admitted wanderlust, eventually returned to New Zealand, completed his medical studies and became a medical officer with the RAF. Like many others who served the Mission, he was the adventuring, not missioning, type.

Ollie Davidson, who was in charge of the [clothing] store, showed us a letter he had received that morning: it read: "I am sending you two roosters and three laying hens. I want you to send me some clothes for a little boy and a little girl, and everything a woman wants." Dr Curtis capped this tale with the story of a letter he had received a few days earlier. It contained a twenty-cent piece, a lens from an old pair of spectacles, and requested a pair of spectacles with lenses of the same strength, "with gold over the nose and gold-coloured ear-rings." As Dr Curtis remarked, "Quite a bargain for twenty cents!"

H. Willcox 1986

In those days when winter was quietly creeping up on us there came one unforgettable day, the day we lost the radium: the only radium in the whole of Newfoundland and Labrador. It was worth a thousand pounds, or some four thousand dollars, and that was a lot of money in those far-off days. Also, being the only radium in the country, it was a lot of radium. Old John Smith or Brown or whatever his name was (we might forget his name, but none of those who were present there that day would ever forget the drama) had been sent to us from St. John's for radium treatment of a form of skin cancer situated behind the left ear. I myself had carefully fixed the precious tube to the tumour in the early afternoon; and had then gone off to walk around the harbour to visit a patient. I returned to find the nurses at panic stations: "The radium is missing,

---

* Hilton L. Willcox, *Beneath a Wandering Star* (Edinburgh: Pentland Press 1986)

Doctor! We've looked everywhere, and there is no sign of it anywhere!" The patient had not stirred out of bed; and no-one had removed the radium from him; it had simply vanished. I felt no real alarm about it; but after toothcombing the bed and its environs for the precious stuff, I did begin to wonder a little. I refused to worry; it was bound to turn up! It did not; but the Superintendent did! And the medical superintendent was not the sort of man calmly to receive the news that the colony's entire supply of radium was missing. It was tea-time, and he stormed into the lounge to order all nurses, on duty or not, to the ward, to join in the search; which meant turning the place upside down. "It's just goddam carelessness! If you want anything done here, you've got to do it yourself."

I had already stripped the patient, poor unfortunate fellow, of his shirt, vest and socks, with no sign of the precious radium. Now, amidst all the turmoil, I took him by the elbow, and said, "Come along with me." In the operating theatre I stripped him naked; and there, lo and behold, in his long underpants, the radium!

Next morning, Dr Curtis put the radium on the cancer area and pinned a large notice on his sleeve, intimating to the world in general, and to nurses and house physicians in particular, that the radium was behind the patient's ear, and that no-one was to touch the ear, or anything in the vicinity thereof until 11:30, when he would remove it himself; which he did.

A SUMMER'S VOYAGE*

In the summer of 1931, Hilton Willcox was released from the St. Anthony Hospital in order to go north on Strathcona II *with Sir Wilfred and a variety of helpers and friends. The vessel was to rendezvous with Dr Alexander Forbes, a researcher from Harvard who was conducting an aerial survey of the Labrador coast. The survey, known as the Forbes-Grenfell expedition, was undertaken over a series of years. It was one of Grenfell's last services performed on the coast. He hoped the large tourist vessels would thus be able to push beyond Battle Harbour and visit even more scenic fjords to the north.*

Willcox begins by introducing the crew, advisors and passengers of this typically Grenfellian voyage. He kept a log (extracts are given) and published his autobiography in 1986.

Sir Wilfred's second son, Pascoe, [was] an enthusiastic angler: on board *Strathcona* he helped Will Stiles in the engine-room. His brother Wilfred was assistant to the mate, Abe Mercer. Both of them were university students in the States. Hoyt Pease, a student from Yale, acted as assistant navigator. Bob Blake, a student from Harvard, was ... in charge of the galley. An Englishman named Goldman was a general factotum, giving a helping hand wherever it was required. He too had been blessed—or cursed!—with the restless spirit of the wanderer; and had, while still in his twenties, been four times around the world.

Before we sailed, we were to be joined by a number of people who would have no official duties on board; except, perhaps, Miss Eleanor Cushman, better known as the 'Sphinx' (a soubriquet not bestowed upon her for any serious devotion to the Trappist philosophy!), who acted as Sir Wilfred's secretary. She had given many years of devoted service to the Mission; and a cruise along the Labrador was but a partial recompense for all that she had contributed to the work of the organization. Professor Frederick Sears, of Massachusetts Agricul-

Around Levi Reid's log fire, Dr Curtis waxed reminiscent about his years on the coast.... [H]e said to me, "You'll meet old Aunt Jane Mugford one of these days: she lives in Pine Cove, between Eddy's Cove and Flowers Cove. She disapproves of dog-drivers eating with the doctor. On one occasion, I stopped at her place, and the driver came into her sitting-room and sat down. Aunt Jane commenced preparing lunch and setting the table, every now and then giving a questioning look at the driver. Finally, she could stand it no longer, and came up to me and whispered in my ear, 'Is he,' indicating the driver, 'is he allowed to eat with you?' "

H. Willcox 1986

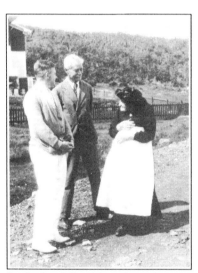

Curtis, Grenfell and Aunt Jane Mugford

Although Willcox described Aunt Jane as "a hunch-backed tiny creature with the features of Mr Punch of London" who "two hundred years ago would have been burned as a witch," he also said she was "the soul of kindness and wonderful friendly hospitality."

---

* Hilton L. Willcox, *Beneath a Wandering Star* (Edinburgh: Pentland Press 1986)

A Grenfellian crew

Seated in front, left to right: H. Willcox, P. Goldman, Hoyt Pease, Eleanor Cushman.
Seated behind: Pascoe Grenfell, engineer Will Stiles, Bob Blake, Sir Wilfred, Fred Sears, mate Abe Mercer

tural College, was a regular annual visitor to the north, primarily as an adviser to Grenfell staffs on matters agricultural, and on the possibilities of their gardens. When opportunity offered, he was a fountain of wisdom and encouragement to those fishermen ... who had initiated their own schemes for producing edible wealth from the soil as well as from the sea. He was a little, balding, grey-haired old man who was, in Kipling's words, a 'little friend of all the world.' At every Mission station he was ashore, inspecting, advising, ever looking to the future.

Noel O'Dell had no official duties on board. He came from Cambridge University, where he was professor of geology; and he hoped to pit his mountaineering skills (he had been a member of an earlier British Mount Everest expedition) against the mountains of north Labrador, to study their geology, and to report on the suitability of the area as a tourist attraction....

The voyage of the *Strathcona* began on a calm sea on 27th July ... At Battle Harbour, Grenfell had established the first of his chain of hospitals; and it was this one, which, together, with a large store, had been burnt down the previous year. Grenfell blamed some unfortunate smoker's cigarette; and we unfortunate smokers in his ship shared, in his eyes, some portion of the universal blame for all fires everywhere. As expected, we all received, while in Battle Harbour, new threats and restrictions on the subject and I became second assistant engineer, or, more usually, stoker in Will Stiles' engine-room, where I could smoke without fear of the wrath above. Great men all have their little foibles, and lesser men must respect them—within limits!

The fire [I wrote in my log] *made a complete job of it. Pascoe Grenfell and I inspected the ruins after supper, to find only a great heap of ashes, and bent and twisted and tangled iron and wire. Exploring further, we found, at the top of the island, a small radio station; ... Some medical work still goes on here, with a staff of one nurse, one medical student and an American dentist, who works along the coast during the summer. They have their headquarters in a reasonably comfortably furnished house. A new hospital has been built at St. Mary's River, about eight miles west of Battle Harbour; and Dr Moret, who was medical superintendent of Battle Harbour until its demise, is already established there.*

Cruise ships were already operating along the Labrador in 1931: the *North Voyageur* we had met in St. Anthony; and now, on our second morning in Battle Harbour, we awoke to find another ship of the same line anchored quite near to us. She was the *New Northland*, about whose coming we had known nothing; but a call at 6 a.m. to 'All hands' to clean up the ship soon enlightened us. About 8 o'clock we went alongside the cruise ship, and took on board some seventy

Our people are poor people, but things are opening up steadily. Already a splendid steamer from Montreal offers for about $125 a fortnightly round-trip as a weekly service during the summer. It touches various points around the Gulf of St. Lawrence, the west coast of Newfoundland, and visits at least four of our stations. It is a thrilling tour. The northern fjords and rivers are magnificent, and an air excursion to the Grand Falls—twice the height of Niagara!—only awaits the completion of our coast survey.

W. Grenfell 1935

of her passengers, amongst them Lady Grenfell's mother ... We promptly set
out for the new Mission station at St. Mary's River, where they all went ashore
amidst rain, fog and mosquitoes: they were probably very glad to return to the com-
fort of their own ship. Strathcona, having taken them back to that comfort,
returned immediately to St. Mary's River, where we all spent the evening with the
Grenfell staff. The new hospital has twelve beds, a modern operating theatre,
electricity, but as yet no running water. Dr Moret, who is a Swiss, has a staff of
two nurses, one Canadian, the other Australian, and an industrial worker, an
American—the International Grenfell Association thus well and truly living up to
its name. When the new Mission school, now being built by summer volunteers, is
completed, the staff will be increased by at least one teacher. I am sorry for the
'wops' building the school; they work, amidst mud and mosquitoes, like the prover-
bial Trojans. I only hope that some day, maybe on a cruise liner, they will return,
and, pointing to the school, say with justifiable pride, 'We built it.'...

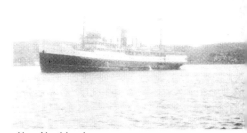

New Northland

On the last morning of July, I was called at 5:30, after two hours' sleep (more
mosquitoes and stifling heat below decks!) to take the wheel, 'because Goldman was
making tea.'

It seemed rather odd, and very unprofessional watch-keeping; but I took the
wheel, and soon began to enjoy the sheer beauty of the early morn. We were
passing island after island, the scene ever changing; Square Island, ragged-look-
ing Dead Island with some schooners sailing south, Venison Island and beyond
it Venison Tickle, through which we ran to make the narrow entrance to
Hawke's Harbour on Hawke Island; where we tied up at the wharf of the
Newfoundland Whaling Company to take on 3½ tons of good coal. This
precious fuel in our bunkers, we sailed past Red Island lighthouse; and veered
off our course towards a gigantic, pinnacled iceberg, 100 to 120 feet high, whose
majestic proportions lured two of our enthusiastic cameramen away in the
jolly-boat to secure photographs and cine-film of *Strathcona* against the background of this white monster of the northern seas.

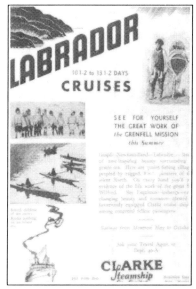

From a contemporary brochure of the
Clarke Steamship Company: 'Grenfell
Labrador Cruise'

We steamed around the berg, a little too close to it, I thought. Perhaps Sir
Wilf shared my critical thoughts; for he told us how, many years ago, he was
steaming towards a giant berg, and decided to sail through a high arch in it; but
while he was about 500 yards from it, it foundered, breaking up with a terrific
roar into thousands of miniature bergs and lesser fragments, churning the sea
about it into a wild turbulent maelstrom. For the benefit of ardent photo-
graphers, we were, I thought, much too close to this one....

Sunday, August 2. — Sir Wilf conducted a simple, impressive service on the
afterdeck with a few local people, including one fine old couple, 'Uncle' Mark Crid-
land and his 'woman,' adding to the numbers. We sang a couple of hymns, Sir
Wilf read a chapter from St. Luke's Gospel, then preached a simple direct sermon,
comparing our little service with the open-air gatherings of fisher-folk in Galilee to
whom Jesus preached, oftentimes from a ship, and in just such a manner as this.

We departed about noon, sailing through the 'run' between outlying islands
and the mainland, crossing Blackguard Bay, and beyond Sandy Island seeking the
narrow tickle leading into Batteau harbour. Nearly twenty schooners were
anchored there, and inevitably there would be much work ahead. Most of the work,
however, came from the 'liveyers', the permanent inhabitants of the bay. They are
poor people about here, living in rude-built shacks which paint had never seen.
They are people who expect everything for nothing, and are horrified if asked to pay
a few cents for medicine. I was working most of the afternoon, and until 11 o'clock
this evening. Many of them had very little wrong with them, and when one youth
of 17 produced almost every symptom in a text-book of medicine, and a thorough
examination revealed nothing abnormal, I am afraid that I forgot Sir Wilf's sermon
of the morning, and was exceedingly rude to him. Indeed, I find it difficult to be
polite to any of them. I do not like these Labradormen as I do the Newfoundlanders;
although the general opinion, certainly in St. Anthony, is quite the opposite.

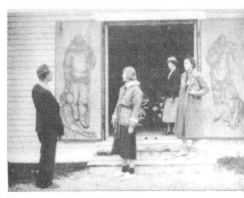

Tourist attraction at St. Anthony
—the handicraft shop near the wharf

August 3 — Patients were aboard by 7 a.m., and I had to go ashore to see
several more. It was a relief to sail from Batteau for Spotted Islands; but, before we

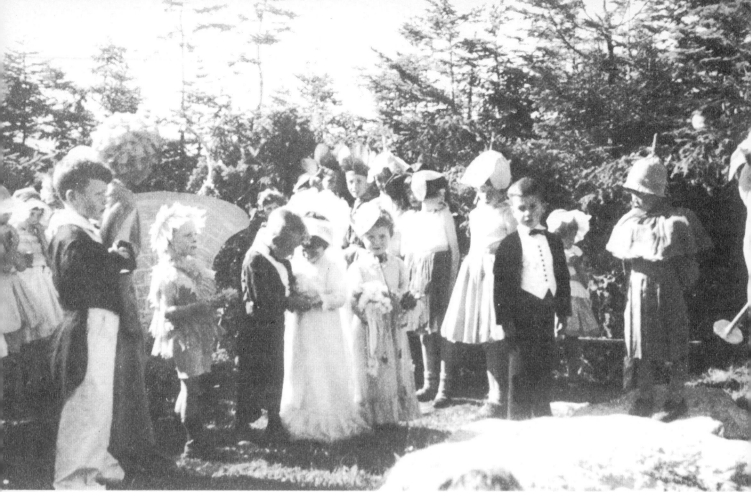

Children from the Mission's home preparing for the operetta staged each day a cruise vessel arrived at St. Anthony

They raised $1,100 to purchase new laundry equipment.

reached it, we were hailed by a motor-boat from Salmon Bight, and I had to go off to see a young man who, they thought, was seriously ill, but who had no more than a minor stomach upset. The motorboat took me the nine or ten miles to Spotted Islands, where Strathcona had anchored to permit Sir Wilf to visit the nursing station and its staff of one nurse and one 'wop.' The people here are worse than those at Batteau; they are lazy, good-for-nothing beggars. One man told the nurse (and she a new arrival!) that if she charged for medical work, she could be fined and jailed. They refuse to bring supplies from the mail-steamer unless they are paid $1.50 a trip. They charge ten cents for a small bundle of sticks for the Mission. They ask for money for medicine bottles (empty) for medicines for themselves, and then expect the medicine free. Sir Wilfred gathered them together this afternoon and told them what he thought of them; but it seemed to me that he was filled with just a little too much of the spirit of Christian love and compassion. Dr Moret wants to pull down both nursing station and school and remove them to some other place, perhaps Batteau; but after my own experience of Batteau, I would be all in favour of moving both stations somewhere else. These people would be helped far more by their having to stand on their own feet.

August 5 — Threading our way through tickles and channels we came ... to Cartwright, the most imposing settlement we have seen thus far. The Hudson's Bay Company have their largest Labrador post here; and four miles to the west, at Muddy Bay, they run a silver fox farm ...

Many years previously Grenfell had established, at this same Muddy Bay, a Mission post; but, four years before our visit, a schoolboy with few educational ambitions and little love for the Mission had burned down the school. Grenfell decided to rebuild at Cartwright; and, against strong opposition within the organization, had gone ahead, raised the money, and had the satisfaction of seeing his scheme come to fruition during the time of our visit. During the previous year, a school and an orphanage had been built; now, thirty 'wops' were digging a mile-long trench for pipes to convey water from a dam then under construction by workers from St. Anthony to the Mission buildings.

Waterpipes, to withstand the winter frost, had to be many feet deep ...; and the work these 'wops' were doing was hard labour of the most appallingly difficult kind. Much of the mile was rock, requiring blasting; the rest was swamp, and it was not yet, on the Labrador, the age of mechanical shovels. On our last evening at Cartwright, Sir Wilfred gathered the whole Mission staff together; in the course of a two-hour talk, which covered some of the history of the Mission and some Grenfellian philosophy, he thanked the 'wops' for the work they were doing.

They certainly deserve the greatest possible credit and thanks [I wrote that night].
To pay their way here, to pay for their food, to work under the conditions as they
exist here, and to work for nothing, is indeed worthy of the highest praise.

They would not complete their task that year, but many would return in 1932, to see the taps turned on in orphanage, school and staff quarters.

Grenfell's plans for Cartwright included a new hospital, but there was no definite date for its commencement. Grenfell said he thought that Cartwright would become the Capital of Labrador.

The 'wops' had a holiday, of sorts, during the second day of our visit, when *Strathcona* took them all on a cruise to Sandwich Bay, some 15 to 20 miles west and somewhat south of Cartwright. It was, however, scarcely a holiday from work; for when *Strathcona* returned, her decks were piled high with logs for her furnace.

Goldman and I did not go on the 'holiday,' but remained at the Mission, and in the afternoon rowed Miss Wilson, a charming Virginian who was in charge of the industrial department for the summer, across the harbour to the Hudson's Bay post ...

August 9 — After a dawn start we sailed north through the channel between
the mainland and Tumble Down Dick Island to reach the open sea beyond George's
Island. About 11 a.m. off one of the Herring Islands, we dropped anchor and
lowered a boat for the photographic enthusiasts to go ashore and take pictures of the
thousand of puffins now nesting there. The shore was rocky and steep, and landing
from the jolly-boat called for swift and accurate judgment; but there were no casual-
ties, and I rowed the boat back to the ship, where Will Stiles, Pascoe Grenfell and I
jigged for cod.... With the exception of a few cod we kept for our own table, we
gave all our catch to people in Indian Harbour, into whose calm, sheltered waters
we sailed in the late afternoon. It is a rocky, rugged treeless place, the harbour real-
ly a winding channel between several islands.

Grenfell built a hospital here in 1894; but it is now used only in summer, this
summer in charge of a Dr Walcott, from Boston. Two volunteer nurses complete
the staff. It comes within the parish of Dr Paddon, who is there at the moment on
his ship Maraval to meet Sir Wilf. We shall not be visiting his hospital at North
West River, Sir Wilf being anxious to reach as far north as possible. Mr Willmer,
Chief Executive of the International Grenfell Organisation [sic], is here with Dr
Paddon on Maraval; he offered to find me a position on the coast this winter if I
want one; but I need my medical degree before I indulge my wanderlust any fur-
ther; so I said, 'Thank you, but no!'

Next day was Sunday, and we stayed at Indian Harbour. A party of us went exploring far enough along a creek to bring us to trees. Will Stiles looked at the load of wood we brought back, and he said to Sir Wilf, "That wood won't burn, Sir." "And why not?" asked Sir Wilf, a little tersely. "That's Sunday wood, Sir."

A thin fog enveloped Indian Harbour when we sailed next morning about 6 o'clock; and as we were burning logs, not coal, I went down to help Will Stiles in the engine-room. After about an hour, the speaking-tube from the bridge whistled, and captain informed engineer that owing to increasing fog, he was going to make harbour. The engine-room telegraph rang for 'Half Speed,' and we cruised quietly along for about half an hour, when suddenly there came a great shuddering thump, followed by a series of lesser bumps and scrapes along

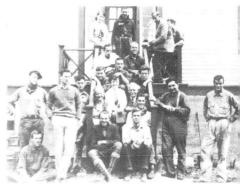

Wops at Cartwright, 1930

They were thoroughly advised ahead of time on travel arrangements, what to wear and how to behave.

In the last quarter century over 2,500 young men and women from both sides of the Atlantic have come to Labrador and given to the country the advantages which 'civilization' has afforded them. However, they all agree that the little they have been able to give is not to be compared to what they have got.

W. Grenfell 1938

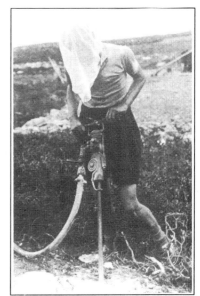

Scottish 'Wop' in a mosquito net builds a road at St. Anthony, 1935

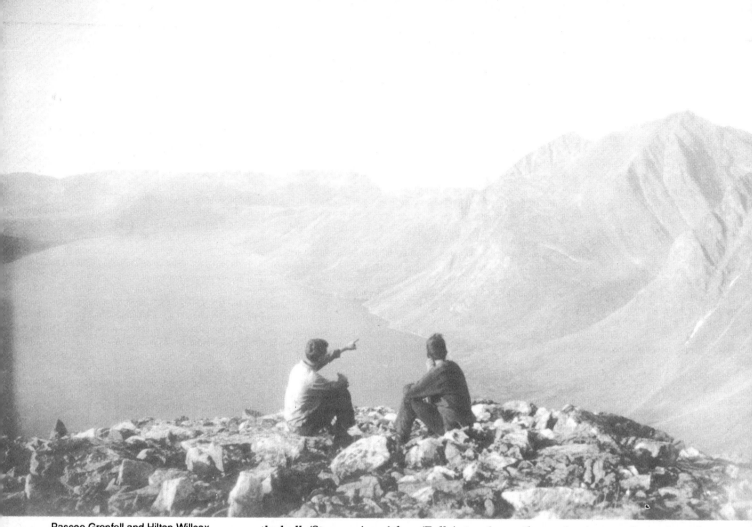

Pascoe Grenfell and Hilton Willcox
overlooking Ryan's Bay

the hull. 'Stop engines,' then 'Full Astern' sang the engine-room telegraph; and I left poor Will and clambered up onto the deck and the bridge to see what was happening. We were aground in a narrow tickle between a small cape of Brig Harbour Island and Sloop Island ... and our captain was greatly perturbed: "I've lost her, I'm afraid; I've lost her!" But the good ship struggled valiantly to free herself from the reef, bumped and scraped her keel this way and that, and finally slid astern into the deep water. There was always a guardian angel around whenever Grenfell's 'By Guess and By God' style of navigation landed him in trouble....

We rounded Sloop Island to run in via the northern tickle and to anchor ... Soon afterwards the fog cleared before a rising northwesterly wind, and it was decided that we should continue. The wind, however, steadily increased in strength; and off Holton Harbour Sir Wilf decided that it would be wasteful of our hard-earned logs to attempt to go any further. We turned into Holton Harbour, and remained there all day. "A pity that we ever started at all," said Will. "We've burned 300 pieces of wood to travel eleven miles and hit one rock!"

> We have made, and still make, mistakes. To say that we are far above criticism would be to say we are far from human. But, after forty years, we continue to keep our flag flying on the hospital steamer, and to get an immense pleasure and satisfaction out of life.
>
> *W. Grenfell 1930 (2)*

122

A LEG UP*

Lester Burry (1898-1977) was a United Church minister born in Safe Harbour, Bonavista Bay. Serving at St. Anthony and on the west coast of Newfoundland, he spent a further twenty-six years based in North West River. An avowed Confederate, in 1946 Burry was elected to represent Labrador in the National Convention, and he was among the delegates chosen to negotiate terms of union with Canada. The 'Jim' to whom he refers below was in fact Jim Tucker, head of the Mission's agricultural department.

One of the great thrills and blessings of my life was to meet the world famous Sir Wilfred Grenfell. My first appointment after graduation at Mount Allison University in 1923 was the St. Anthony charge. I arrived there on board the S.S. *Prospero* late one afternoon. The next morning while eating breakfast in the home of Mr and Mrs Ford Pike, where I lived as a bachelor for four years, Sir Wilfred walked in. I don't mind saying that I was just about frightened out of my wits but before we had the first cup of coffee finished I was completely at ease. After he had given me a very gracious and generous welcome to St. Anthony he told me what was especially on his mind and how he thought that perhaps I could help him.

A day or two ago he had returned from a trip along the shores of the Strait of Belle Isle and among the many needy families he met was one that he thought called for special help. He had plans to help them all but this one was especially on his mind now. There was a man with a large family making a brave effort to support them under the circumstances, but he needed some help and that could best be given him by bringing him and his family to St. Anthony to work in the Mission garden. "I am going to build a house for them," Sir Wilfred said, "but the Mission has no land on which to build it." This is where he thought I could come into the picture. The Church at that time had some extra land and he wanted me to try to get a piece for him. This was a fair and just request and I went to work on it but I regret to have to say that I did not succeed then. Later the Church shared with those in need every square foot not in use. However, the land was found and the house built for this man by the Grenfell Mission. Sir Wilfred was high in his praise of what he could do for this man [*sic*] if only he was given a chance to do

it. I will always remember a phrase Sir Wilfred used. He said "I want to give Jim 'a leg up' and I am positive that he will lift the other by himself." I have known Jim ever since and have watched him making a great success in rearing and educating his family. After his family was settled in St. Anthony Jim was sent by the Mission to the Truro Agriculture College, Nova Scotia and his training there enabled him to bring a tremendous contribution to the gardening work of the Mission at St. Anthony, and hundreds of people in northern Newfoundland and Labrador depended on his early grown house plants for the success of their gardens. It must be said of this man that he was and still is one of the all-time great laymen of the Church. I relate this story to indicate the first impression Sir Wilfred made upon me. My association with him through the years did more than anything I can think of to lead me to dedicate most of my life to the north.

We have tried to meet the problem of deficiency diseases by animal husbandry and agriculture. David Lloyd-George gave us some two years ago eleven little pigs—now multiplied many times. Later he and Angus Watson met the need still further by sending to Labrador a highly pedigreed boar. Other friends have made gifts of splendid cows. The original herd was presented by a surgeon friend who shipped these pedigreed Holsteins to Labrador in the late autumn. When they arrived, the doctor in charge [Curtis] wired me: "What am I to do with these cows with winter coming on and nothing to feed them?" Before I could think up an answer, a second telegram came: "Don't worry about the Holsteins. Grain steamer bound Montreal to Liverpool gone on shore close to hospital." Her load had to be lightened before she could once more be floated and enough grain was removed to feed the cattle.

W. Grenfell 1938

In addition to the reindeer, Grenfell had earlier attempted to introduce a breed of Scottish sheep that could be fattened on heather, but they ate all the wild vegetation in sight. Eight highly bred milk-producing goats worth in the vicinity of $500 apiece were imported from the States. They ate all the local gardens.

*   Lester Burry, "Memories of Labrador," in *The Book of Newfoundland*, J.R. Smallwood, ed., Vol. 4 (St. John's: Newfoundland Book Publishers 1967): p. 59

CABBAGES*

Having long recognized that dietary deficiencies among the local population were pronounced, the Mission commenced an energetic nutrition campaign in the late 1920s. It developed an agricultural program and promoted the more effective use of existing food resources, launched new child welfare programs and renewed its anti-tubercular efforts.

As given below, Grenfell's rather simplistic version of the beginnings of the agriculture department ignores the contribution of a number of outstanding researchers and nutritionists, American as well as British, who worked for the Mission in the north. They focused attention on nutrition, deficiency diseases and remedial measures in general. Teams of volunteers, university students, taught the principles of health and hygiene and conducted child welfare clinics.

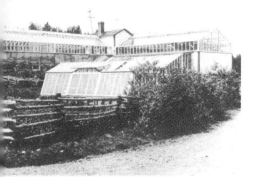

Greenhouses at St. Anthony

In a small motor boat we were visiting the villages along that shore, journeying inside the ice-floes which were just loosening their grip on the land. An old fisherman welcomed us warmly. He was in sore distress. This fishing season was just opening; there was endless work to be done; and his two big sons of twenty and twenty-two years old were lying on the floor paralysed and only able to move their heads! "What can you do, Doctor? Can they be saved?" cried the old man. "Cabbages!" was my answer. He looked at me almost in anger. "Cabbages," I repeated. The two young men were suffering from beriberi, due to lack of vitamins. Already on the coast I had seen deaths from blackleg scurvy—three grown men in one family. What could have saved them? "Cabbages," or "potatoes, eaten in their skins." They had no cabbages, and the few potatoes which the merchant had allowed them they had chipped raw, fed the peels to the chickens, and ruined the remainder by long boiling.

So our agricultural department came into being, and is steadily becoming a more constructive influence all around the coast. Formerly seeds were placed in the frozen ground after the snow had gone in early June. Young plants could not put their noses above the soil before July, and our very early fall frosts caught the vegetables unripened. Meanwhile, cutworm, root lice, and caterpillars destroyed unchecked the vitally important food supply. Today many fine little hothouses in widely separated centres are appearing, so that the seeds sown under glass in March enable the little plants to go into the ground in early June with so good a start that the fall frosts have not arrived before the vegetables are matured. As one result, new gardens are coming into existence. Many thousands of young plants, two months ahead of time, are now sold, or 'worked out' each spring, by the poorest families, and acres of land have come under cultivation. A professional volunteer agriculturist visits the coast each summer. Exhibitions are held and prizes given for the best results, where once a native potato was unknown, and miserable turnip tops, cut in summer, were the nearest thing to a green vegetable many families ever knew. The champion cabbage so far weighed nineteen pounds; and a steady average of ten-pounders has been maintained.

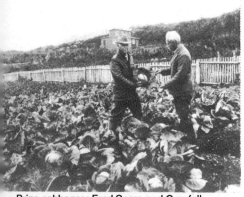

Prize cabbages: Fred Sears and Grenfell

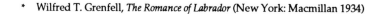

> The unanimity of opinion of my medical colleagues on this branch of our work, and at St. Anthony the real genius of James Tucker, leave one deeply regretful that we did not years ago divert some of our hospital resources for the development of the agricultural department.
> *W. Grenfell 1932*

* Wilfred T. Grenfell, *The Romance of Labrador* (New York: Macmillan 1934)

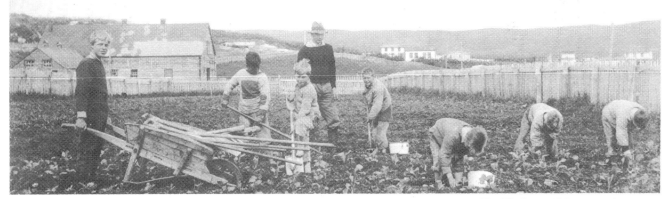

The Mission's children at work

THE 1933 GARDEN CAMPAIGN*

To professor Frederick C. Sears, a horticulturist at Massachusetts State College, the Mission's agricultural efforts owed much of their success. Sears initiated the gardening program in 1928; by 1933 it was well under way. Between 1928 and 1939, Sears made in all eleven trips north.

There have been some right interesting developments in the Labrador garden work during the season just past. Almost every settlement where there is soil enough to make gardening possible is exerting some effort to grow vegetables; and some of the villages with better conditions have really done remarkably well....

Some of the most interesting work was done at Flowers Cove by our very efficient nurse, Effie Mansfield. With the help of a capable wop, Jack Wright, she has cleared and drained with ditches about four acres of land. The method of handling this work was original and very interesting. The land was staked off into small blocks. Each block was then examined, the relative difficulty of clearing it estimated, and a fair price reached for the job on the block. Then a contract for clearing and draining the block was let to some man who wanted work, and the work was paid for in second-hand clothing or food. This has given us a fine lot of land for gardening, and was a tremendous help to the people of that section....

At Forteau the work has come along well, with a lot of good gardens, an excellent garden contest, and, best of all, the installing of one of our hot-bed heaters in a neat little building ... This will make certain our having early cabbage plants for the gardens of that section—a big factor in successful cabbage growing. The garden at Forteau attached to the Mission's nursing station has one of the best soils on the coast....

At Red Bay several large, fine, new gardens have been cleared which, with the large areas already under cultivation at Moore's Point ... puts that village in an enviable position as to vegetables. I was much gratified to receive in the late autumn a letter from Minnie Pike, who has charge of the Mission station there, saying that no potatoes would be imported into Red Bay this year—a new record for the village.

At North West River, under the able leadership of Dr and Mrs Paddon, a number of very interesting and hopeful developments have occurred. To begin with, we had the most successful garden contest, in point of the numbers of exhibitors and of the interest shown, than we have ever had anywhere on the coast. Excitement ran so high that some of the leading contestants would go to each other's gardens to measure the largest cabbage heads they could find, and

It is a small satisfaction to return a patched up patient to the conditions which caused his disease, particularly with regard to deficiency diseases and tuberculosis. Social service, in its various branches—education (including domestic science, home nursing, first aid, etc.), the development of community agriculture, occupation[al] therapy and the inauguration of any auxiliary industries which can increase the earning power—these are the necessary allies of hospital treatment in a frontier practice.

H.L. Paddon 1936

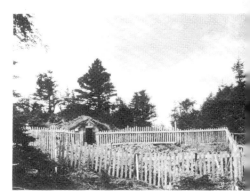

A small garden on the coast, fenced to keep the dogs out

---

* Fred C. Sears, "The 1933 Labrador Garden Campaign," *Among the Deep Sea Fishers* 32, no. 1 (1934): 8-12

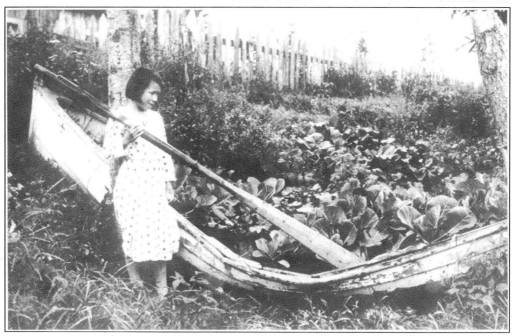

Gardening in an old boat
at Mud Lake

Following on the agricultural work, invaluable efforts for better feeding have been started. Community canning enables women to bring their own salmon, cod, herring, rabbits, and partridges, greens or berries, to a central kitchen and preserve them for their own use. Anything which cannot be sold or used at once is thus turned to account, and thousands of cans have been placed in homes against the long winter which often only saw dry 'loaf,' molasses and tea in days gone by.
W. Grenfell 1934

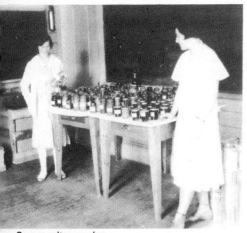

Community canning

then, having measured their own best, would report, " 'Bill's' best cabbage is only twelve inches, and I've got one that's fifteen." The contest was won by Bert Blake ... and it was really worth winning, for to the winner not only went a special set of garden tools for the village but also a prize of $5.00 offered by professor George L. Farley of the Junior Extension Department, Massachusetts State College, for the best garden on the coast.

Another development at North West River was the clearing of more land for garden purposes. This was done by man-power, ... providing employment. Dr Paddon has made a survey of the gardens of North West River to find out the total area under cultivation; and we are planning to get enough commercial fertilizer this spring to give a good application to each garden. This should give the owners big additions to their crops, and at a very small outlay. Fertilizing material is often difficult to get in the north.

Another move which we have made in that section is to provide sets of garden tools—a good spading fork, a heavy rake and a hoe—to be used as community equipment and passed on from one person to another. It is hard for anyone who has not been down there to realize the pitifully meagre equipment most of those people have for their garden work.... There will be from one to five sets in a village depending on the number of families in it. We plan to let these folks pay for the tools with labour or with such products as grass baskets, seal-skin boots, etc., and re-invest any money we receive for these products in some phase of our garden work....

Miss Sims, the teacher at Flowers Cove, conducted a very interesting garden contest, or *two* contests, among the children there. One was a potato-growing contest for the larger boys; the other a contest in general gardens for the younger boys and girls. In each case the children were required to go to the local dealer and secure their seeds or seed potatoes, making a contract with him to pay for them when the crop was harvested. This is good training not only in gardening but also in citizenship. I hope we may try it out in a few other villages this coming summer. The prizes which I furnished were in both contests little hand weeders to each winner, designed to help out garden work in the future, and three candy bars to the winner of the first prize, two to the winner of the second, and one to the winner of the third, designed to cheer these youngsters on their way.

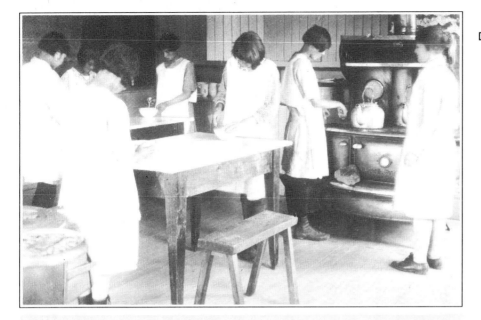

Domestic science class

The child-welfare work has done much for the scattered communities. It has taught the danger of the nailed-up window, the value of clean teeth and clean bodies, of sunshine, of games, of kindness to animals. The director of humane education of the Animal Rescue League of Boston visited the coast as a volunteer and started what she called 'Sir Wilfred's Crusaders,' giving to each of the members a much-valued button. One day a nurse saw a 'crusader' taking pot shots at a songbird. "I thought you were a crusader," she said. "Oh, I am, but I done took off the button before I shot."

W. Grenfell 1938

GARDEN CONTESTS FOR NEWFOUNDLAND AND LABRADOR
I. Rules and Suggestions

1. Each garden entered in the contest must contain at least 150 square feet; ... but the larger the better.

2. The following vegetables should be the leaders: beets, cabbage, carrots, lettuce, potatoes, spinach, turnips.

3. Other vegetables which might be tried are: chard, peas, radishes, chinese cabbage.

4. The gardens will be judged on the basis of the quantity and quality of the different vegetables produced, on the care taken of them, and on their general appearance.

II. Prizes

1. For each garden entered in the contest which makes a creditable record, an award of one package each of cabbage, carrot, lettuce and turnip seed will be given.

2. In addition, the following prizes will be awarded in each community:

   1st Prize-One hand weeder, one ounce each of cabbage and carrot seed, and one package each of beet, lettuce, spinach and turnip seed.

   2nd Prize-One ounce of cabbage seed, and one package each of beet, carrot, lettuce, spinach and turnip seed.

   3rd Prize-One package each of beet, cabbage, carrot, lettuce, spinach and turnip seed.

3. A prize of $5.00 presented by the Junior Extension Department of the Massachusetts State College will be awarded for the best garden on the coast.

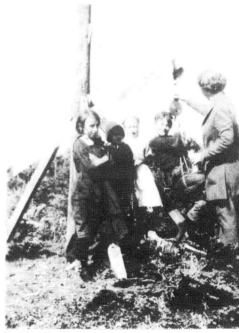

Child welfare clinic

THE NURSE FROM FLOWERS COVE*

Anna Kivimaki was at the Flowers Cove nursing station in the mid-1930s. She writes here for an American nursing audience in hopes of recruitment, but makes clear that only strong, resourceful, independent women need apply to the International Grenfell Association. Its staff selection committees were based in New York and London.

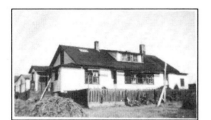

Flowers Cove nursing station

The nursing station itself was a small frame house. Upstairs there were two bedrooms and a storeroom; downstairs, a small ward for the occasional inpatients, a dispensary, bath, kitchen, and sitting-room [for the nurse]. Usually a volunteer community worker lived with her; two local girls did the housework.

A. Kivimaki 1937

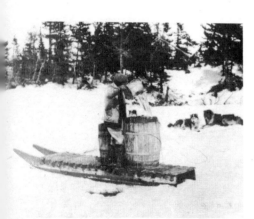

Getting water in winter

The wind beat at the walls of the little frame houses like waves pounding a ship at sea. It drove sharp needles of snow against the window panes. It fought every living thing which ventured out. But the fisher folk in northern Newfoundland knew and respected the power of the elements and were staying under shelter until the weather 'eased up.'

The Grenfell nurse at the Flowers Cove nursing station always had a list of tasks waiting to be done during the blizzards which to her meant 'spells of peace.' All morning she and the girl who did the cooking had canned the seal meat somebody had given her for delivering a baby. The canned seal meat would be very welcome in the summer when meat was hard to get.

In the afternoon, she had gone over her dispensary shelves. On fine days when the 'going was right good,' there would be a constant stream of people in and out all day long. They came to her for all their ailments—accidents, sores, colds, frostbite, pregnancy, itch, snow-blindness, beriberi, tuberculosis, or if they just felt 'wonderful bad all over.'

By supper time the storm had let up considerably, but it was still 'shockin' dirty outside' two hours later when she heard the familiar stamping and brushing going on in the little shed outside the kitchen door, warning her of the arrival of a caller. It proved to be Uncle Noah Biles from Eddy's Cove, sixteen miles north, who had come to get her to see his sick son. She knew Uncle Noah for a man of good common sense who would never come for her after dark on a bad night except in a serious emergency, so while she asked questions, she got out her bag.

While Uncle Noah had a cup of tea, she dressed for the trip. Over woollen underclothing, she pulled on a sweater and trousers; then over several pairs of socks, the sealskin boots which looked like moccasins with leggings sewn on them, tied with tape below the knees. Over her head she pulled a 'dickie,' a hip-length jacket with hood attached, made in one piece and fitted so that when she pulled the tape in the hood, only the middle of her face showed, framed in the fur trimming. Skin mitts over woollen ones completed the costume. The whole outfit weighed very little, was wind-proof, allowed perfect freedom of motion, and was the only costume warm enough for the bitter climate.

By the time the nurse was ready and had given a few parting instructions to the community worker who lived with her, Uncle Noah had the traces straightened out and, with shouts to the dogs, they were off. It was a good team—nine of the lean, short-haired, nondescript mongrels which all the local people kept—and they raced as hard as they could go as Uncle Noah kept yelling "Home! Home! Home!" It was too dark to see a thing, but all had faith in the lead dog ...

It was ten o'clock by her watch when they got to Uncle Noah's house. Eight of the children were sitting up in the kitchen. The arrival of the nurse was an

---

* Anna Kivimaki, "Nursing with the Grenfell Mission," *American Journal of Nursing* 37, no. 6 (1937): 593-8

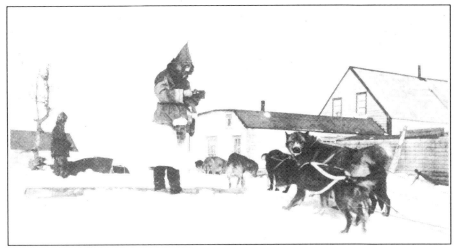

Nurse on her rounds

exciting event not to be missed. She climbed the ladder leading to the loft where the sick boy was. He certainly looked as if he were suffering.

"Feels like they'd poured hot gravy all over me insides, Nurse."

She applied an ice pack and waited. St. Anthony Hospital and the nearest doctor were over forty miles away on the other side of the long narrow peninsula which forms the northernmost tip of Newfoundland. At midnight the pain was no better. She told the father they'd have to get the boy to the hospital and every minute counted.

Uncle Noah had crossed the peninsula before. "I'll call you soonest we can start," he said.

So the nurse stretched out with two of the other children on a bunk in the same room with the patient. The child whose place she took went to sleep on top of the box of hens in the kitchen.

At four o'clock she heard dogs barking in the exciting way they do when straining at their traces. The wind and snow had stopped. There was a full moon, so although it was cloudy, it was now just possible to see, and two teams and drivers were just about ready, each sled having a 'woman box' on it. They put the patient in one, wrapped like a mummy in blankets. The nurse addressed a telegram to Dr Curtis at St. Anthony, "Left Eddy's Cove four a.m. with probable ruptured appendix," asked somebody to send it from Flowers Cove during the day, got on the other sled, and then the two teams set off ...

Not until long after dark, when humans and dogs were utterly weary did they sight the welcome lights of St. Anthony, especially bright in the operating room, where the patient was immediately taken and cared for.

The nurse from Flowers Cove, after having a bath and supper and the excitement of talking to everybody at the hospital, started to think of everything she should remember to do while in St. Anthony. She didn't get the chance to come very often. Could the clothing store spare some baby diapers and send them over by the next team going back? And could she get a few seeds from the greenhouse for her window boxes? Could the hospital spare some Blaud's and rhubarb and soda pills? By the time she had several little parcels together, the doctor came down from the operating room.

"Just got him here in time," he said. "Touch and go, but I think he'll pull through. How's everything in your district?"...

The doctor knew every family in his district, and it was long past midnight before he had all the news from the Flowers Cove region....

She had been back [at Flowers Cove] only two days when she was fetched for a delivery thirty miles south. While there, she took the opportunity to visit the other eighteen families in the place because she didn't know how soon she

Selma Victoria Carlson, who has been in charge of the nursing service at St. Anthony for the past ten [sic] years, nursed in Boston before her appointment in the Grenfell Mission. She is also housekeeper and anaesthetist and is assisted by an operating room nurse and two general staff nurses. During the summer the staff is increased by three to six nurses who volunteer their service for the busiest season, May to November....

The hospital nurses are often sent out by boat or dog team to see post-operative cases, deliver babies, or to look after a settlement if an epidemic breaks out.

A. Kivimaki 1937

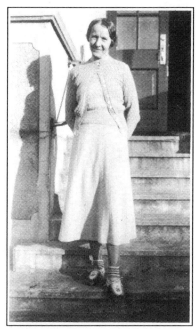

Selma Carlson

After twenty-five years as matron of the
St. Anthony Hospital, Carlson retired in
1948. When she died in 1968, her
ashes were deposited in the rock on
Fox Farm Hill.

In the summer of 1937, the 45th
anniversary of Grenfell's coming to
Labrador and three years before his
death, the Mission's assets included six
hospitals; seven nursing stations; four
hospital vessels; four boarding schools;
fourteen industrial centres; three
agricultural stations; twelve clothing
distribution centres; the King George
the Fifth Institute; the supply schooner
George B. Cluett; a co-operative lumber
mill; and a haul-up slip for schooner
repairs. It had a permanent staff of
about sixty doctors, nurses, teachers
and social workers, and a supplementary summer staff of approximately one
hundred volunteers. The Grenfell
Alumni Association numbered
nearly two thousand.

could manage to get there again. Every one of the thousand or so people in her
district was in her charge, and she saw them all as often as she could. During
chats in the kitchens she tried to get the conversation around to bread baking
and advise them to use brown flour instead of white to avoid beriberi; she
always took a great interest in their gardens.

Every day was a busy one. In the summer time the people came for her in
boats instead of by dog teams, and she was very busy with her own garden and
her supplies which were brought by a large steamer from the States to St.
Anthony and distributed to the other stations by schooner. When the schooner
came, she had to check in the food, drugs, fuel, and sewing machine parts to be
sure she was stocked with all necessities before navigation closed. During the
dull periods in the spring and fall when dog team travel had either broken up
or not begun, and when boats couldn't get through the ice, she made up her
requisitions and arranged for the most needy and deserving people to do the
work of hauling her coal from the boat when it came, and digging up the garden,
in return for clothing....

The nurses on the Labrador coast are women whose main objective in going
north is a desire to render service. The salaries offered do not entice others.
Nurses who go for a minimum stay of a year at one of the hospitals receive $300
a year and their living and travelling expenses; those at the outport nursing
stations receive $500. Each has a three-month holiday every three years. The
summer volunteers who sign up for six months receive their living and travelling expenses only.

SPEAKING TO OLD FRIENDS*

*On 9 December 1938 Lady Anne Grenfell died of cancer in the United States.
That summer her husband, in poor health himself after a series of heart attacks,
brought her ashes to St. Anthony to be placed in the rock on Fox Farm Hill,
alongside those of Dr John Mason Little. This was Sir Wilfred's last trip north.
Reverend Lester Burry of North West River, who tells the following story, was
party to it because in order to broadcast religious services he had built a radio
transmitter, assembled receivers and distributed them. He was at Cartwright
when Grenfell arrived.*

*Harry Paddon, the Mission's chief presence in Labrador, died suddenly on
Christmas Eve, 1939, while on a winter sabbatical in the States. His ashes were
returned to North West River to be buried on the side of a small hill overlooking
Groswater Bay. Sir Wilfred Grenfell died on 9 October 1940 at his home,
Kinloch House, in Vermont. Truly it was the end of an era.*

I am told that the last time Sir Wilfred Grenfell ever spoke in a microphone
was at one of my broadcasts on board the *Glad Tidings II* at Cartwright. In the
summer of 1939 he came to St. Anthony much against his doctor's orders. While
there Dr Charles Curtis, the medical officer in charge, watched him very closely.
He wanted to go to Labrador but Dr Curtis put his foot down with a definite
no, only to discover that when the mail boat S.S. *Kyle* pulled out of St. Anthony
enroute north it had on board its most famous stowaway—none other than Sir
Wilfred. A message was sent immediately to Dr Forsyth at Cartwright to stop
him from going farther north, which he succeeded in doing but not without
firm action. I was at Cartwright at the time in the *Glad Tidings II* on a regular

* Lester Burry, "Memories of Labrador," in *The Book of Newfoundland*, J.R. Smallwood, ed., Vol.
4 (St. John's: Newfoundland Book Publishers 1967): pp. 58-63

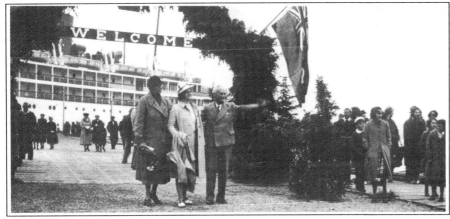

Sir Wilfred and his daughter Rosamond being welcomed at St. Anthony, 1939

Harriot Curtis is on the left; the cruise vessel *North Star* is in the background.

trip. I remarked casually to Sir Wilfred one day that I was broadcasting to my parishioners every evening at seven o'clock and would like him to share the program with me tomorrow. "You could speak to your old friends," I said. That struck a responsive cord and he consented readily. That evening I told my listeners that I would have a special treat for them tomorrow as Sir Wilfred Grenfell would be with me on the program. I was no sooner off the air when Dr Forsyth stepped on board, all excited. "You can't do that," he said, "I have orders from Dr Curtis to keep him away from all excitement." After consulting together in all seriousness, knowing how anxious he was to speak to his friends, we agreed on a five or six-minute period for him but no longer. At the appointed time the next evening he came on board with Dr Forsyth. After a few preliminaries, I gave him the microphone. He plunged right into reminiscing with his old friends as though they were in the cabin with him, calling them by name as if he had them listed on a paper before him. To Uncle Johnnie Ukepilruck he says: "Do you remember the time you first piloted me into Mullatartok Bay. I have made it on my own several times since, thanks to your good piloting." To Johnnas Iglolionte he remarked: "I hope, Johnnas, you are not too busy these days at your special trade (*which was coffin making*) but that you are busy building houses." He reminded Austin Flowers of the great catch of salmon they made one day in the Tomluskum River. And so on for five minutes, ten minutes with Dr Forsyth getting red in the face and looking daggers at me. After another minute or two I secretly pulled a switch and put the transmitter off the air. Dr Forsyth quietly took him on shore. I went back on the air and explained what had happened. The fan letters following that broadcast were many. I have been assured that his death in the States a few months later was not related to that event.

In passing I must say that I have been distressed and very much annoyed on a few occasions of late years, when freelance writers after a few days visit to the north upon their return use their pens to blast the Grenfell Mission on something they apparently picked up in passing, which if they had taken time to investigate, the truth would have given them a different slant on the whole matter.

I know the Grenfell Mission doesn't need me to defend them but to one who has been so closely associated with the fine work they have done over the years and are still doing, I find it hard to take.

L. Burry 1974

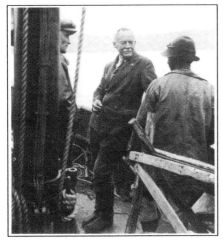

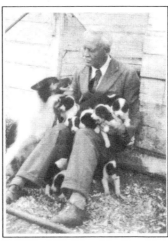

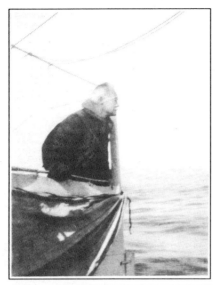

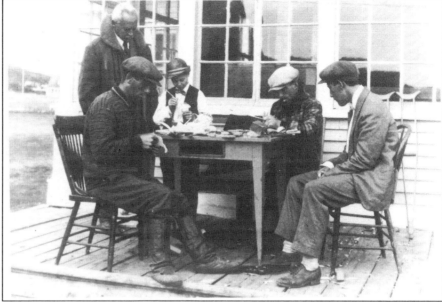

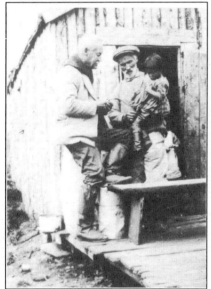

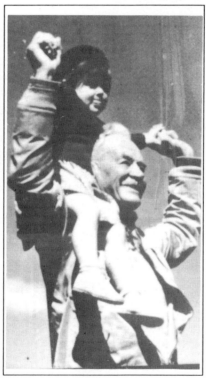

THE FIELD OF HONOUR

Having spent his last winter at St. Anthony in 1918–1919, Grenfell since 1920 had lived in the United States. Though he came north each summer, during the twenties his visits had grown shorter, more disruptive to his staff, and his influence had waned. Gradually he lost touch with the activities of his Mission, the leadership of which passed into new hands: Grenfell had ceased to be in control. Yet in the early thirties he remained nominal superintendent of the IGA and, with Anne, continued to travel, lecture and raise funds as his health declined. In 1934, when under the new Commission of Government he was offered the governorship of Newfoundland, he refused to consider it. In 1936 he reluctantly resigned from the Mission's active management while resisting suggestions that he retire completely; finally resigning as superintendent in 1938, Curtis replaced him. Returning to St. Anthony with Anne's ashes in 1939, when all but two of these photographs were taken (with notebook at sea, *c.* 1933, and with stethoscope), Sir Wilfred Grenfell came as the Mission's founder—a saintly figure unwillingly removed from the scene of past heroic deeds, a veritable St George, slayer of dragons.

In his lifetime, Grenfell's honours were legion. In 1906 he was named a companion of the Order of St Michael and St George and in 1927

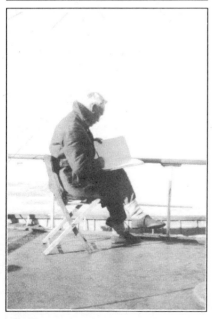

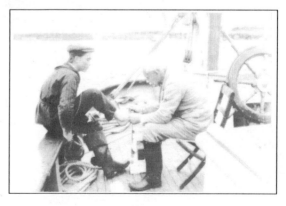

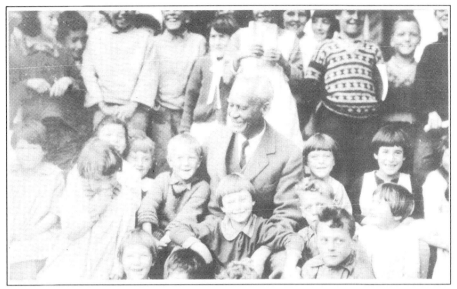

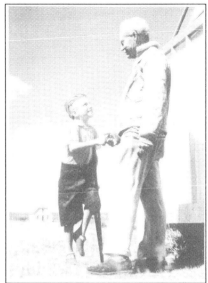

he was knighted. He was an honorary fellow of the College of Surgeons of America and a fellow of the Royal College of Surgeons. Among the many universities awarding him honorary degrees were Williams College, Harvard University, the University of Toronto, the University of New York, McGill University, Princeton University, Bowdoin College in Maine and Middleburg College in Vermont. In 1911 the Royal Geographical Society awarded him the Murchison Bequest for his geographical work. In 1920, the National Academy of Social Sciences (American) gave him a gold medal. From the Royal Scottish Geographical Society he received the Livingston Medal. The Council of the Royal Empire Society, in recognition of his services to Empire and the excellence of his book, *The Romance of Labrador*, in 1935 awarded him its gold medal. From 1929 to 1931 he was Lord Rector of St. Andrews University in Scotland. The American Geographical Society of New York made him an honorary member in 1939, the year before his death.

In the summer of 1941 Sir Wilfred Grenfell's ashes were returned to St. Anthony and, on 25 July, were sealed in the rock on Fox Farm Hill beside Anne's. A simple brass plaque bears his epitaph:

Life is a field of honour

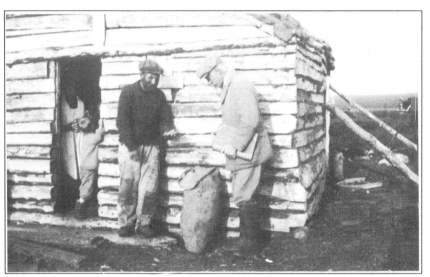

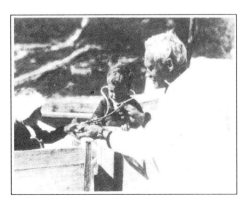

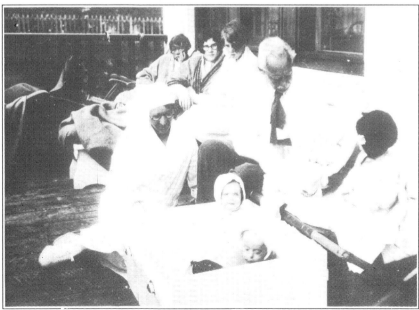

NOT MANY WILLINGLY GIVE IT UP*

In 1929 Indian Harbour had been reduced from the status of hospital to nursing station. A variety of economic factors over which the Mission had no control had by that date reduced the size of the Newfoundland schooner fleet to perhaps sixty per cent of what it had once been. Dr Harry Paddon estimated that the number of shore fishers had been reduced by as much as seventy-five per cent. The Mission responded by focusing its attention on the settlers of Labrador, whose economic situation, if anything, grew progressively worse. As stations at Indian Harbour and Battle Harbour were gradually phased out, medical, educational and industrial activities in Labrador were concentrated at North West River, Cartwright and St. Mary's River.

The old station at Indian Harbour has gone.... Its passing, hard on the heels of the old Battle Harbour Hospital, has marked the closing of a picturesque and romantic phase of the Mission's story. We no longer spend our summers on the windswept outer isles, right in the heart of the fishery, but in the relative comfort and shelter of the deep bays, where we can keep open all year round.

For this purpose the new station at Cartwright is ideally situated, being at a sort of crossroads between summer and winter settlements.... The busy summer season, when there may be twenty to thirty in-patients at a time, is comparatively short. In the winter season, the average complement is not above ten.

C. Forsyth 1943

In the fall of 1931 Dr Garth Forsyth joined the Grenfell staff as house officer at St. Anthony with a one-year contract. The following winter, 1932-1933, he replaced Dr Donald Hodd at Harrington for several months; in the spring he returned to practise in Norfolk, England, little suspecting how Labrador had 'got into his blood.' Soon he was asking for a permanent position on the coast. Forsyth returned to St. Anthony in the fall of 1934 and the following year replaced Dr Moret at St. Mary's River. In 1937 he married Clayre Ruland, an American nurse stationed formerly at St. Anthony, Spotted Islands and Mutton Bay. In 1938 the IGA decided to station a doctor permanently at Cartwright, and the Forsyths moved there. They retired from Cartwright some time after the Second World War.

Forsyth here conveys the unorthodox nature of a Mission practice and, by the same token, the unconventional kind of person it would attract.

To the average Englishman, Labrador is a *terra incognita*. There is an impression of a cold, bleak, barren land, somehow associated in the mind with the name Grenfell. There is no especial reason why anyone should know much about it. Labrador has few inhabitants, and no important men. But these few inhabitants are the proud possessors of a great wild country of half a million square miles. Admittedly their homes are restricted to the coast line, but their trapping grounds honeycomb the country, and still further back are the hunting grounds of the Montagnais and Nascopie Indians....

The qualifications required to be a successful [settler] of the country are rather high. In the summer he must be a good seaman, a good fisherman, a good carpenter and, if possible, a good gardener, too, in his spare time. In the winter he must be a good trapper—a highly skilled profession—a good dog driver, and a good woodsman. The life is a hard one, and the returns slender. The Labradorman does not know enough of the outside world to know that there his astounding versatility would be regarded as something of a marvel....

[T]here is no denying the fact that most of the people are very well adapted to their environment, and lead happy, carefree lives. They are very clannish, and have a wholesome contempt for anyone who is not a Labradorman based on the inability of most 'outsiders' to perform a fraction of the tasks at which they are so proficient. They are a difficult people to work among, and those who have claimed otherwise have usually done so from ignorance rather than knowledge. None the less, because they are the world's super-realists, we do thoroughly enjoy working among them....

It would seem probable that a doctor with a practice several hundred miles long would spend the bulk of his time travelling. But this is not so. The people seldom come more than seventy miles for the doctor, but will occasionally bring a patient into hospital from a further distance by dogs, or from anywhere on the whole length of the coast in the summer by boat or steamer. Conditions in the homes are so adverse to sickness that they have gradually learned that their sick have a much better chance if brought to the hospital. Besides, in the winter, calls to the furthest limits of the practice can take days, and even weeks, of travelling. It is customary for the doctor [in winter] to make one routine trip throughout the whole district, covering the best part of a thousand miles and taking from one to two months....

*   C. Hogarth Forsyth, "Life and Work in Labrador," *Medical Press Circular* 204 (1940): 398-402

Taking an all-the-year-round average, actual medical work does not involve the doctor more than four hours a day. Station operation adequately fills up the rest of his time. The station centres around its hospital and boarding school, but accessory to the operation of these are the following: stores, farm, roads, drainage, machine shop, three motor boats, truck, tractor, generators. All supplies have to be ordered on one annual requisition. Heating and cooking throughout the year take sixty tons of hard coal and two hundred cords of wood. In fact, the doctor has to adapt himself to quite a number of occupations besides medicine. Needless to say, such a varied life is absorbingly interesting, and not many who have once entered upon it willingly give it up.

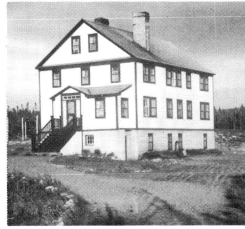

Cartwright Hospital

DR FORSYTH'S DOGS*

A good team of dogs was essential for winter travel until the Mission acquired aircraft in the early 1950s. Many of the Mission's doctors longed for teams of their own. Forsyth was one of them.

Dog-team travel on the coastwise trails, and trapping three hundred miles into the wilderness sound romantic, and possibly dangerous, but have a death and morbidity toll a mere fraction of that caused by automobiles outside. In fact, about the only way connected with dog-team travel that one can get killed is to be eaten by the dogs. About once every two or three years somebody gets killed this way, usually a child. Not that the dogs are outstandingly dangerous, but *any* dogs in teams or packs are potentially dangerous, and I think that, if the dog of the country was the Alsatian instead of the Husky, there would be a much higher death toll....

Once I was building up a dog team, and I wanted good dogs. Two small girls turned up to have their tonsils out. Their father had one of the best strains on the coast. So four tonsils were paid for by two excellent dogs....

Over a period of two years I gradually built up and trained a ten-dog team. The third year, shortly after they had been let out from their summer's penning, and were consequently in an excitable mood, they fell foul of a girl, who had committed the unpardonable sin of *running* by them. No matter how great the hurry you are in, you must never ran past or through a team of dogs. She got badly bitten, and by the irrevocable unwritten coast law, I lost my dogs.

I set to work to create another and better team. As a safeguard this time I castrated all my male pups. I put everything I knew into the rearing of those dogs. But in the early winter, when they were nearly grown and I had started to break them in, one morning early, when few people were about, a small boy started to play with them. He was discovered a few minutes later lying on the ground shrieking, with all the dogs over him. He was carried into the house and, on examination, found to have only one tiny nip. Obviously the dogs meant no harm, for they had plenty of time to eat him up entire. But the coast goes on circumstantial evidence only. I knew the talk and criticism this would evoke, so my second team, one of the loveliest I ever saw, had to go the way of the first. Since then I have given up having dogs. I could not go through that again.

The station foreman, Harvey Bird, was the Cartwright equivalent of Jack Watts—a splendid man on a boat, most conscientious, and a natural mechanic who could make missing parts of machinery and repair anything. He was the second of three generations of a family who devoted their lives to the association, and at the same station.
W. Paddon 1989

The staff members who stayed in Labrador during the [Second World W]ar deserved decorations for they ... carried on, despite shortages of equipment, help—almost everything—even when no one could be found to replace them during a vacation. Dr and Mrs Garth Forsyth were such a couple.... Dr Forsyth [was a] quiet man who deserved much more credit than he ever received ... together they did a fine job of promoting education as well as health.

W. Paddon 1989

*   C. Hogarth Forsyth, "Life and Work in Labrador," *Medical Press Circular* 204 (1940): 398-402

THEY CAME FROM EVERYWHERE*

Dorothy M. Jupp (1909-1986) was an immensely capable and resourceful woman, but a restless one. Raised in a Barnardo home in England, she became a nurse. Strongly inclined to missionary work, she trained further with the Church Missionary Society in north London. In 1938 Jupp came to Labrador as company nurse for an abortive cordwood venture; when the company failed in 1942, she joined the Grenfell staff. After a first, unhappy winter with Dr and Mrs Spicer at Cartwright while the Forsyths were away on leave, she took charge of the small hospital at St. Mary's River. Here she was a tireless gardener, kept a small herd of Toggenburg goats for milk, and became the archetypical Grenfell nurse, capable of anything her position required.

Though the Grenfell Mission, as a mission, ceased to exist in Jupp's time, she adjusted along with the rest of the staff. She moved to Nain around 1951, when the IGA was in the process of taking over health services from the Moravian Mission, and in 1958 travelled around the world. In 1959, the redoubtable Dorothy Jupp returned to Labrador to work at IGA nursing stations all along the northern coast. She retired in 1972 and died in Cornwall, England.

The hospital [at St. Mary's River] was a cheerful looking three-story building, and larger than it really looked from the outside. It had a woman's ward, a men's ward, an isolation room, operating room, four staff rooms overhead; a patients' bathroom; and the usual linen and service rooms. The staff living room, bedroom, office, dispensary, and two kitchens were on the ground floor. Furnace room, boiler room, laundry, workshop and store cupboard were all in the basement.

The view from the living room was one of great beauty. From it, across low hills and islands, one could see the spars of the Battle Harbour radio station, and at calm water, the land reflected back. The skies and clouds made a picture that artists dream about, but seldom see.

In the winter the house was warmed by a wood burning hot-air furnace. Goats and hens supplied the hospital with milk and eggs, and on occasions, meat; the gardens supplied the vegetables during the summer time.

In the spring and fall, men were employed to cut and stack wood, and other jobs for which they were paid in cash or by clothing from the clothing store, as they wished. A large general storage shed was on the wharf and near-by was a small shed for gasoline and kerosene; another for hay and lumber. On the strongly built wharf itself was a sturdy derrick.

The harbour itself was landlocked; trees grew on its northeast and southern shore, and houses were scattered along the northwest and north sides. The hospital was built beneath the hill on the northeast corner of the harbour; and the staff consisted of a doctor, nurse, aide, cook and a girl to do general work....

One day in the first week in January [1944], I received a telegram from the doctor [Forsyth] at Cartwright saying he would be visiting us first chance; this was to be the annual visit to us. It was the middle of January before he arrived, and we were glad to see him; it was so long since a doctor had visited us for any length of time, and there were so many medical problems awaiting him.

He arrived on a beautiful day and had a day's rest before the great rush started. Previously a message had been broadcasted announcing the doctor's expected arrival.

I will not say much about that winter at Cartwright. It was a nightmare from beginning to end. Everything went wrong. It would be very unfair to give one side of the picture, but I will say that too many sensitive people were living together that winter, and it was like living on the edge of a volcano at the time.

D. Jupp 1971

[In 1942 when the *Maraval* paid us a visit,] two things rather distressed me. The first came as a result of a conversation with the dentist's wife. We had been discussing the beauty and position of St. Mary's, and then passed to the methods of making contacts with people. I happened to remark that I thought it was a pity that the hospital was so far away from the rest of the settlement, also that I thought closer contacts made it so much easier for Church work to be done. The curt reply was, "The Mission does not bother about that any more, it's purely medical now." The second thing was that in the course of general conversation, and the prospects of the Mission generally, someone remarked, "The Mission is finished on the coast now, it is just a business venture." To anyone else it may not have had much significance, but to me, as one trying to find her niche in the Vineyard of the Lord, it was, to say the least, very discouraging.

D. Jupp 1971

---

* Dorothy M. Jupp, *A Journey of Wonder and Other Writings* (New York: Vantage 1971)

Two days later, teams began to arrive bringing people to see the doctor, but this was only a beginning. Next day the rush really began, and reached its peak two days later; teams came from north, south and west. People who wanted to get teeth 'hauled'; people who were sick; people who came to get advice; but even this was not the peak of the rush.

An emergency operation was performed on the Wednesday, after much debate and thought, as there was no other nurse around; but it was carried through to a successful conclusion. After the patient was put to bed with the aide to watch her, we went to the out-patients dispensary, and what a sight met our eyes! People were sitting on chairs, on the sofa, and in some cases on each other's knees, and overflowed to the kitchen and porch. There must have been fifteen or sixteen teams tied up around the hospital, and the noise made when all the dogs lifted up their heads and howled can be imagined.

For a while things were quite hectic with requests and demands from every quarter, "Do you want to buy some rabbits, Miss?" "I wants to pay my fee, Miss," or, "Can I see —— Miss?," or "I got toothache, Miss, wants Doctor to haul it." From upstairs came another call, and up I went two steps at a time. The situation there demanded the doctor's presence, and he was obtained by a call down the stairs. After settling the matter in hand, we both returned to the dispensary and the waiting people were now reinforced by the arrival of fresh teams. While the doctor was busy, I tried to clear up some of the other work—giving receipts for fees paid; issuing clothing slips for rabbits and other game brought in; answering questions about the conditions of patients; giving advice as to diet, etc.; helping the doctor to find medicines, etc., in the dispensary; running upstairs to look at the operative case; shake up a pillow; give a drink of water; fetch some books for a patient; and in between, assisting the doctor.

After a very busy day we watched the last team leave, and dropped into chairs for a rest. Our respite was short-lived as a scared voice at the door said, "Please, Miss, there is someone out here to see the Doctor." This someone turned out to be another emergency operation.

On Thursday the picture was repeated with another emergency operation, but gradually the teams lessened, and by the end of the week, the doctor left on his way north.

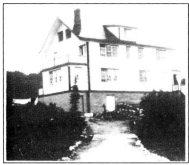
Nursing station at St. Mary's River

About this time [1943] the financial position of the Mission became critical, and it was felt that unless money was forthcoming, St. Mary's would have to close its doors. This, of course, caused no little anxiety to the local people and to me. After six years on the coast, I felt I was just beginning to know and understand the Labrador people, and I had great affection for them, and their hard struggle to live had my sympathy. I felt, however, that if the issue was put up to them they would respond. Accordingly, a letter was sent to each settlement, telling the people the situation, and asking for their help. The result was beyond my expectations; $680.70 was raised in a short time.
D. Jupp 1971

SHE BORNED A LOT OF BABIES*

Born at Makkovik in 1894, Mary Andersen at the age of thirteen was taken to Battle Harbour to see Dr John Grieve for a septic finger. The finger was amputated, forcing her to remain at the hospital over the winter. The following spring she travelled as far as Indian Harbour, where she stayed to go to school. For ten or more years, Anderson worked at hospitals at Indian Harbour and Battle Harbour and then moved to the St. Anthony Hospital for one year. The IGA at this point arranged for her to train as a midwife in Boston for a further two years. She then returned to work at St. Anthony, and several years later married and moved to Main Brook, in Hare Bay.

Mary Andersen's son, George Simms, vividly recalls what it took to be a frontier nurse.

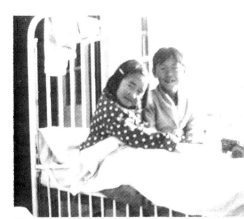
TB patients, St. Mary's River

* George Simms, "I Remember One Time in Particular," *Among the Deep Sea Fishers* 73, no. 3 (1976): 12-3

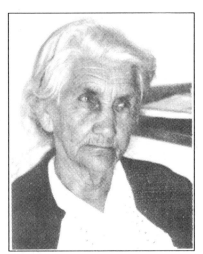

Mary Andersen Simms

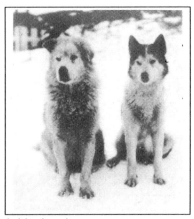

A dying breed

Dr John Gray, a travelling doctor on the Labrador coast, made one of the last trips by dog team around 1957.

Because of her previous work with the Grenfell Mission, she was called on by the people for every need, borning babies, extracting teeth, closing up cuts, attending scratches, bruises, burns, scalds, scabies and even setting broken bones which turned out to grow straight and in perfect condition. All this had to be done without the aid of a doctor, because there were times in the year when Main Brook was completely isolated, too much ice for a wooden boat to get through and not enough for a dog team to go on. All the people had to trust to were her experience and her strong belief in God.

She knew how to make linseed meal poultices. She gave cod oil and the odd drink of brandy to pull the sick through.

She travelled to Fishot, St. Julien's, Croque and Conche and to this day, the people of the area show their appreciation by visiting their Aunt Mary, as they all call her, and say that she was sent by God.

Only this past summer, I took her to Conche and then to Croque by car, and it would do your heart good to see the people from around the community coming to see her and talk of the hard times she had had travelling in that area.

The older men came and talked to her with tears in their eyes and told of the times they had to tie ropes around her so they would not lose her in the brooks that were cut out by the spring floods.

Around 1945-46, Bowater's came to Main Brook to set up wood operations and the Grenfell Mission asked her to look after the Bowater employees, which at that time had a work force of about four hundred men, and it was then that she was really kept busy. She worked for thirty dollars a month at first and the last two years she worked, she received fifty dollars a month, which was a big increase at that time.

I know what it is for Mom to go to Fishot Island for a day and be caught out there for a month due to ice conditions. I know what it is to come home from school and get my own meals or get up in the morning and get my own breakfast, Mom being called away in the night, and not knowing where she went.

I know what it is to see a man brought from Bowater's woods, taken to our living room, and watch Mom closing up a four to five inch cut or larger with an old half-moon-shaped needle and catgut.

I know what it is to be taken from my bed and patients put in, especially people from Englee and Roddickton that stayed overnight before travelling on to St. Anthony the next day by dog team.

I remember one time in particular. Six teams of dogs set out from Roddickton with six patients in coach boxes. Bad weather came on and they went astray. Four more dog teams set out from Roddickton to look for them. So about twelve o'clock that night ten teams of dogs (approximately 100 dogs) stopped by our door. Men, patients and dogs were half frozen and covered with snow. Our living room was divided into four small rooms by hanging up white sheets and four patients were put in there. The remaining two patients had to be brought into the kitchen by the wood stove, coach boxes and all. One of the patients had his right hand severed by a mill saw. Our family had to be taken from their beds and [had to] stay up all night to let the dog team drivers rest, so they could travel on to the St. Anthony Hospital the next day. We didn't dare venture outdoors because our chances of survival was nil with so many dogs out there.

Our home was used as a clinic for travelling doctors. People from all around the area would come for treatment.

Mom's worst and [most] frightening experience was when she had a boy about three years of age brought to her practically eaten by seven savage dogs in a community called Springs about eight miles from Main Brook. That was the first time I saw her look away from anything at first. I remember about eight o'clock that winter evening, a dog team pulled up to the door and without warning, the little boy was brought in kicking a blood soaked blanket from him; the sight of his body, face and head was frightening. After a few moments, Mom gathered up courage and bandaged him and made him ready for the long sixty mile trip by dog sled to St. Anthony. The child died in its mother's arms before reaching St. Anthony.

She always was a lover of dogs until that incident, and then she always said, "Dog is a good servant but a poor master."

She borned a lot of babies and in some cases up to the third generation. At that time, the charges for borning a baby was five dollars and all money collected had to be sent to St. Anthony Hospital. In most cases, she never did get paid, because people had no money and in some cases, she took off her own clothes to wrap the baby in after it was born. She kept the mother in bed for nine days after the baby was born and made a visit every day plus bringing the mother's clothes home to wash.

In her lifetime nursing, she travelled by boat, dog team, snowshoe, ski-doo, makeshift bosun chair over cliffs and hills and also [made] a few trips by plane.

She borned her last baby when she was seventy-six years of age.

TWO PHILOSOPHIES*

Tony Paddon, Harry and Mina Paddon's eldest son, every summer since 1933 had worked with his father on the Maraval, *first as a summer volunteer and later as a medical student. He studied to become a doctor in New York, graduated in 1939 and did a two-year residency at a New York hospital; in 1942 he joined the Canadian Navy. At the end of the war, Tony Paddon returned to northern Newfoundland and Labrador to work at St. Anthony, Cartwright and eventually North West River. Here he married Sheila Fortescue, a British Grenfell nurse.*

Tony Paddon explores in the following selection one of the central tensions of the Grenfell Mission—St. Anthony with its large, modern hospital, distant and remote, versus the smaller, outlying hospitals and nursing stations, attempting to cope at a grass roots level with problems the centre could hardly envision, much less understand. On another level, there were the tensions between the social service end of the Mission's work and its medical side. Such tensions had been with the Mission since nearly the beginning. They exist to this day.

The year is 1945 and Tony Paddon has just returned from war service.

At St. Anthony Hospital, there were three or four nurses; a couple of locally trained nursing assistants, who would compare favourably with almost any trained nurse; Dr Curtis and I; an excellent laboratory technician; and an X-ray technician who doubled as a dental assistant. No dentist was available and I had done several hundred extractions on the hospital boat *Maraval* before the war, so I undertook to do as much dentistry as time permitted. As well as extractions, which were—I think—of adequate quality, I also did fillings. Like a good Massachusetts General surgeon, Dr Curtis looked on this activity with some amusement, and a bit of condescension. But I persisted ...

From the beginning, I was needed as surgical assistant, and for this my training was quite adequate. We operated most days, and often at night. The nurses included the ageless Selma Carlson, who had been with my father and mother at North West River twenty-five years earlier; in St. Anthony, she

Tony Paddon on the deck of the *Maraval*, which he described as "arguably the best all-round medical patrol ship in Grenfell history"

* W.A. Paddon, *Labrador Doctor: My Life with the Grenfell Mission* (Toronto: James Lorimer 1989). Reprinted by permission of James Lorimer Limited, copyright W.A. Paddon

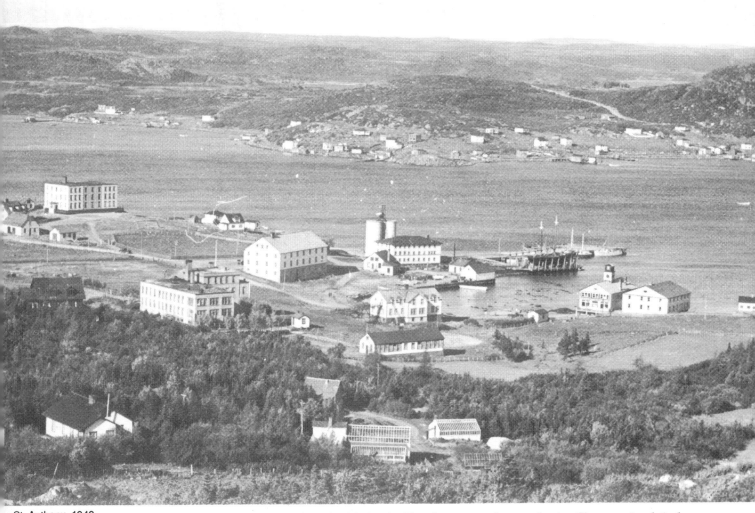

St. Anthony, 1942

Here we are, in that much dreamed-of, confused, interesting, stimulating, depressing, wonderful time which has been labelled 'the post-war era.' And here is the Grenfell Association, very much alive, busy, sound. We are planning—not spectacular expansion, but orderly continued progress.... The average size of contributions may have decreased [during the war], but we are very proud that the number of contributors has increased.... Income from patients' fees has increased from $6,700 in 1934 to $17,500 in 1945.... All IGA accounts are 'written in black.'

New England Grenfell Association 1946

carried the double load of head nurse and anaesthetist. She remained tireless, immensely efficient, and greatly respected, both in the hospital and the entire district of St. Anthony and the Straits.

The work of St. Anthony Hospital was of the highest quality, despite its relatively small bed capacity—somewhere between thirty-five and fifty beds—which varied according to demand. Dr Curtis expected from me a complete medical history and physical examination for each patient being admitted, although the process could be abridged for those who had recently had complete examinations. This made for long days, especially if we operated all morning, did treatments, histories and physical examinations all afternoon, and faced twenty-five new admissions from one of the steamers in the evening.

The chief method of getting to the hospital—except, locally, by motorboat—was on one of the coastal steamers. The *Northern Ranger* ran between Corner Brook on the west coast of Newfoundland, up around the tip of the northern peninsula, and into St. Anthony. She would then continue south to St. John's, and make the return trip in the other direction. The *Northern Ranger* called into innumerable small fishing villages and went up many of the deep bays. When she arrived—very often at night—her whistle announced her, and Dr Curtis and I headed for the wharf in the old association truck. Most of the patients were very poor and travelled in steerage ... Dr Curtis would line up all those who could stand; anyone more seriously ill or injured would be sent to the hospital in the truck. In half an hour, the steamer would be blowing her whistle

140

as a warning that she was about to cast off, although most captains would give us more time if we considered it essential.

Dr Curtis would go down the line, looking intently at each one, asking pertinent questions, and making quick decisions. Long and intimate knowledge of the people of the area made him seem almost psychic in his ability to diagnose. Malingerers, frauds, those with welfare passes or plans to shop in the stores of St. Anthony rather than undergo surgery or medical treatment, were recognized at first glance. His conversation became a series of rapid-fire questions and grunts of approval or disapproval, and it was not difficult to tell which were which....

The steamer *Kyle* always brought some people from the other side of the straits, in southern Labrador. Most of these patients, and those from the Cartwright area, were referred by the small hospitals of St. Mary's Harbour or Cartwright, where there were doctors. Very few came from anywhere further north: the Inuit were afraid to go to St. Anthony, perhaps because, after the death of my father in 1939, the patrols made by the *Maraval* were usually manned by doctors unfamiliar with the people or the area. These doctors always demanded that the acutely ill go south to St. Anthony, and they and other patients consequently came to view a trip south as a death sentence. It was obvious that someone was going to have to work on this problem; organize appropriate groupings of patients to travel to St. Anthony; and find other ways to dispel the fear felt by the Innu and Inuit about leaving their own districts. It was also obvious who that person would be, but it would have to wait until my year at St. Anthony was up.

A few Inuit did come to the hospital, and seeing a familiar face helped some of them get better. I think that, at the time, Dr Curtis judged the chances of a patient's recovery by the excellence of the diagnosis and treatment. This approach was fine for patients who were familiar with him and the hospital; these were people who knew that most patients get well in hospital. But such confidence was certainly not shared by either the native people or most of the white settlers north of Cartwright. The quality of care was probably of little interest to such patients, who arrived frightened and lonely, and who knew little or no English.

The hospital, none the less, was a very friendly and kindly place, and, with the exceptions noted, most of the people admitted had utter confidence in its staff. Dr Curtis was a massive father-figure, with a gruff kindness that suited the Newfoundlanders very well.

Operating with him was an experience in itself. He was a general surgeon of a sort no longer seen, taking on anything that he thought he could handle. His surgery was not as elegant as that of Gordon Thomas, the extremely able man who would succeed him, but it was invariably sound, and his versatility was boundless. When he performed a thoracoplasty, for example, his skill was astounding.... I saw him do two such collapses in a single morning, after which he put bone grafts into a patient with tuberculosis of the spine.... There was also time that morning for Dr Curtis to take out most of a thyroid gland and a gall bladder, although when it was all over, we were all a bit limp, and soaked in perspiration.

Sometimes, during a busy operation, Dr Curtis would walk a few steps away, toward the window, and ask what ship was just coming into the harbour; or who the woman was, passing down the road. Since he seldom did anything without a good reason, I think that these apparent lapses were, in fact, a way for him to take the stiffness out of his spine and his cramped, weary muscles. There was also the pipe: he was an inveterate smoker, but Miss Carlson's

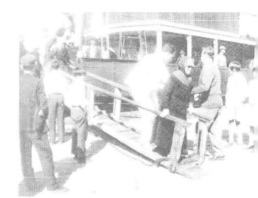

Dr Curtis, in sweater, meets the *Kyle*

My father ... did try to elicit from Dr Curtis some interest in the Innu and Inuit of Labrador, but was not very successful.

W. Paddon 1989

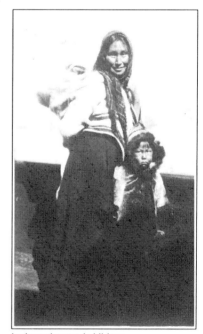

Inuit mother and children

This photograph was taken by Professor Fred Sears in the 1930s.

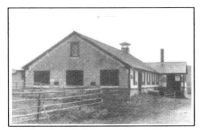

The Jessie Goldthwait Dairy at St. Anthony: 'Dr Curtis was passionately fond of his ... cows'

After my father's death, things had become very difficult for my mother. During the war years, she carried on as best she could, with very little money or staff, or support from Mission superintendent Dr Charles Curtis at St. Anthony headquarters. She was responsible for everything: the medical supplies; the yearly food supplies; the school, teachers and house mothers; the requisitions; the planning; and, above all, the hospital and patients. In addition, there were the displaced settlers and Inuit who had uprooted themselves to work at the nearby Goose Bay airport. She could hardly have managed her multitude of duties without the daily backup of her redoubtable assistant and foreman of outdoor work, Jack Watts. My mother was infinitely grateful to Jack, and together they made an amazing team, weathering many a desperate crisis together.

W. Paddon 1989

My mother was given an OBE for what she did in the war years between her husband's death and my return from the war—with no doctor at all and only her own clinical competence—and she certainly deserved it.

W. Paddon 1971

fears—that he might catch fire in the ether-filled atmosphere of the operating room—were never realized.

Dr Curtis took on every case that came his way, for there was no way to transfer a patient to St. John's after freeze-up. Nor was there much need for such transfers: the hospitals there were no better than his own, and the practices and standards—thanks to the renowned specialists who volunteered their services there every summer—at St. Anthony were on occasion even better. Off duty, Dr Curtis was a great entertainer. A gifted raconteur and mimic, he had a fine sense of humour, loved company and was the life of any party.

There was a large farm at St. Anthony, where most of the poultry, pork and fresh vegetables for the hospital were produced. Dr Curtis was passionately fond of his twenty-four beautiful Holstein cows, and they seemed to feel the same way about him. I think he enjoyed rescuing a cow in obstetrical trouble almost as much as he did a human patient. He told me that he was happy with the cows, who simply got on with their work, were always productive, and never, never gossiped about each other or complained about their salaries. He used to wish his staff were more like cows. (In point of fact, he had little reason to complain about his staff, most of whom were devoted to him and gave him the very best they could.)

There is no doubt in the minds of those who knew him that Dr Curtis did indeed care for the people of the northern peninsula and the straits—his immediate district—and devoted his life to improving their lot. He had the deep respect of everyone in the area, and never expressed a wish to be anywhere but where he was. His wife, Harriet [*sic*, Harriot] was the perfect partner, a woman of considerable charm, sensitive to the feelings of others (as her husband sometimes was not) and a natural diplomat. He was wise enough to be greatly influenced by her opinions, and whenever I found myself at odds with him—as I frequently was—it was invariably Mrs Curtis who smoothed things out. Dr Curtis, to me, was a fine surgeon, whose teachings I would value all my life, but he could also be a source of great frustration and unhappiness.

To put it in the simplest terms, Grenfell had founded his organizations as a mission because he was deeply concerned with the plight of Newfoundland, including Labrador. He saw the societies of Labrador and Newfoundland as a whole, and realized that the difficulties of its people stemmed from a variety of causes: ignorance, bad diet, lack of confidence, attrition from disease, even loss of will. The hospital; the operating room—medicine itself—were only some of the ways of treating the larger malaise. On occasion, Grenfell said that education alone might do more for the overall health of the people than any number of doctors—a view which my father was to reach on his own. Dr Curtis was in no way insensitive to the social and economic ills that abounded, but he was first and foremost a surgeon and administrator. He seldom understood requests from outlying stations for the means to attack the ignorance, poverty, and even despair that caused inertia and apathy. Such men as Grenfell himself, my father, Dr Donald Hodd of Harrington, Dr Garth Forsyth of Cartwright and Doctors Moret and Harry Mount of Mary's Harbour [formerly St. Mary's River] felt that too much emphasis, and too many resources, were centred in St. Anthony. To be fair, we did have to maintain one first-class hospital, and no one wanted its programs curtailed in any way, but ensuring the continued health of the hospital did not seem to explain why Dr Curtis had never even visited northern Labrador, let alone my father's area. As far as I can ascertain, Dr Curtis was not to visit the northern stations until 1950, twenty-six years after he had assumed the superintendency....

I settled into the routine of the hospital quite contentedly thereafter, and took every opportunity to learn anything which might be of value when I returned to Labrador. I learned how to take and read X-rays, and became familiar with the practical aspects of orthopaedics, which made it easy for me to become increasingly proficient in making plaster casts, managing fractures in adults and children, and learning to make the most of available equipment. Dr Curtis went to considerable trouble to teach me as much as possible about the Grenfell mission, its relationships with the government and the people of northern Newfoundland, its financial structure and much else of importance.

We never settled the differences in our opinions, but when I finally left on the *Maraval* in 1946 for a Labrador cruise—the first of two I would make each summer—his handshake was warm and sincere, and I felt that if he disagreed with my views, he might at least come to respect them. I felt that we would somehow come to terms and work together. And indeed we did, until Dr Curtis was succeeded by Dr Gordon Thomas in 1959.

It was perhaps a very good thing that we had a staff and board of directors who were often at odds as to our first priorities, for it now seems clear that the International Grenfell Association did in fact achieve a most admirable mix of the two philosophies represented by my father and Dr Curtis.

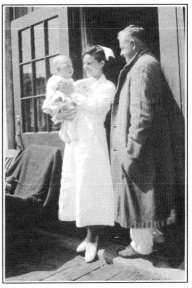

Dr Charles Curtis and a nurse at St. Anthony

His wife Harriot took over from Anne Grenfell responsibilities for the educational fund and arrangements for volunteer workers.

IT NEVER ENTERED MY HEAD*

On 31 March 1949, Newfoundland became the tenth province of Canada. The battle for Confederation had been waged long and in earnest, entailing some uneasy adjustments, as Dorothy Jupp explains.

In the second week in April [1949] an incident occurred which, in itself, was to have far reaching effects. In the preceding fall the merchants locally had not stocked up as fully as usual, and so in April there was a great shortage of food. So much so that both the doctor [Forsyth] and I made requests to the local government authorities that they should do something about it. Our requests were ignored, or forgotten, and accordingly I took matters into my own hands, and sent a message to the prime minister of Newfoundland [Joseph R. Smallwood] stating the case and asking him to do something about it.

It never entered my head for one moment that the prime minister would broadcast the text of my message; had I thought so, I would have worded it differently. However, he got things moving, and soon planes were landing and flying over, dropping foodstuffs which we distributed—so much to each family.

The first plane arrived the day after the message went through; and our doctor at St. Anthony came with the pilot. The landing was very bad, and the take-off was even worse; in fact it was dangerous, as there had been a temporary thaw.

Next day was a real dirty day, but teams came from ten miles away though the blizzard to get some food stuffs; the snow-fall was so thick that at times we could not see out of the window.

During the storm we heard an American plane flying over, but it flew off again as the clouds were too thick. Next day it came back and dropped a great deal of food. For the next week we were rushed with giving out food to men asking for it for their families; we had to do it on our own, as no official came to help us.

[In 1948] Dr Curtis was made Commander of the British Empire. This was one of the last such honours given in Newfoundland by the British government and certainly the last to an American citizen. Typically, Dr Curtis refused to go to England to accept it from the king.... A local committee ... organized a ceremony in which a large copy of the king's address to Dr Curtis was hung in the hospital, together with a bronze plaque commemorating the occassion.... Curtis accepted it and went back to work.

G. Thomas 1987

---

* Dorothy M. Jupp, *A Journey of Wonder and Other Writings* (New York: Vantage 1971)

Newfoundland's entry into Confederation in 1949 gave its people a chance to make up for the long years of inadequate education, health services, welfare and much else. Suddenly, life in both Newfoundland and Labrador began to change in countless ways. We now had real money to pay for clothing, school books, food, pension plans— a hundred things we had not even imagined.... [W]e received funds for the construction of schools, and for nurses' and teachers' salaries, all of which had previously been borne by the International Grenfell Association.

W. Paddon 1989

I had read about the work of Sir Wilfred Grenfell when I was a young boy. My parents ... were deeply committed Christians. They read me stories of missionary heroes from an early age. At 10 I had received a copy of Basil Mathews' *Wilfred Grenfell, the Master Mariner* as a prize at Sunday school. At McGill University I switched from pre-law to medicine, with the thought that I might one day become a medical missionary.

G. Thomas 1987

At the end of that week, an ice-breaker got into Cape Charles and landed tons and tons of food which was distributed by a ranger [a government official] who came down on the ice-breaker; and so our part in the matter ended.

As I said, there were some far-reaching repercussions, and one of them was the fact that a rumour got around that this was just a political gambit, staged at the time of the election. This rumour did not reach me until months later, and I was staggered by it; such a thing had never entered my head. So I emphatically state here that there *was* a food shortage, and it was left to us—the doctor and I—to do something about it after our appeal to local government authorities had failed, and that it had nothing to do at all with the election issue.... As usual, the radio and press made a great deal out of the matter; and I was snowed under with requests for information, and offers of help.

BABIES STARVING TO DEATH*

In 1946, at the age of twenty-six, Dr Gordon W. Thomas joined the Grenfell staff as assistant to Dr Charles Curtis. Thomas was a Canadian, a graduate of McGill University and a former member of the Royal Canadian Army Medical Corps. He took charge of the St. Anthony Hospital in 1954 and succeeded Curtis as IGA superintendent in 1959, Curtis becoming chairman of the board. Both men, Curtis and Thomas, steered the Mission through the difficult period when it began working closely with two levels of government, federal and provincial, and lost the splendid isolation it had once enjoyed.

In the following selection Thomas tells much the same story as Jupp, but from his point of view.

In the winter of 1948-49, politics compounded the normal uncertainties. Newfoundland's negotiations to join Canada left the wholesale business in some confusion; the merchants who supplied their posts in Labrador delivered far too little food that fall, perhaps in fear of being left with a costly inventory when Confederation brought lower wholesale prices the next year.

In any case, places like Fox Harbour, Battle Harbour, George's Cove, and Port Hope Simpson ran out of food by spring. The Newfoundland ranger at Battle Harbour reported the situation to headquarters, but nothing happened. As things got worse, Dorothy Jupp, our nurse at Mary's Harbour, sent an urgent appeal to Joey Smallwood stating that people would starve if authorities did not act soon.

The Royal Canadian Air Force base at Goose Bay tried to bring a load of supplies, but a prolonged period of mild weather had made the ice treacherous and the landing impossible for a large plane. At Premier Smallwood's order, Newfoundland Airways sent a bush plane to St. Anthony with instructions to take a doctor and a load of food into the area. I set off with Capt. Freeman Flemming, the pilot, in a de Havilland Rapide, carrying 900 pounds of food. Banks of fog lay over the straits, but we reached Mary's Harbour and landed safely.

The situation was critical. At Fox Harbour, residents were out of milk, butter, rolled oats, vegetables, and meat, and had only a little flour. Four infants were living on flour and water and were close to death. At George's Cove, nine families were destitute, feeding their children molasses and water. At Seal Bight, four families were destitute and one old man was starving in his bed.

* Gordon W. Thomas *From Sled to Satellite: My Years with the Grenfell Mission* (Toronto: Irwin Publishing 1987). Reprinted by permission of the author. Copyright, Gordon W. Thomas

Dorothy Jupp had seen children bloated with starvation and young men crippled with beriberi. It was hard to believe.

We distributed the food as fairly as we could and returned to St. Anthony, flying at 200 feet to stay under heavy cloud. I reported the situation to the premier and recommended that he send a boat immediately. The ice in the harbours was too weak to bear the weight of a large plane, and would very soon not support a small one. Joey arranged for a shipment of food on the *Sorrel*, an icebreaker, which put an end to the crisis.

This was my first direct contact with the new premier, and it came at a good time for both of us. He had barely scraped into office, campaigning on what Confederation could do to relieve desperate conditions in the outports. Now he had a drama worthy of his talent for media grandstanding, and he played it to the hilt. An editorial from the Ottawa *Evening Journal*, ten days after Confederation, gives the flavour of the attention this incident drew.

Babies Starving to Death

This headline is not describing conditions behind the Iron Curtain, nor among the desperate millions in China. It tells of conditions not only right here in North America but in a section which became part of Canada a scant week ago—the coast of Labrador …

From looking at the map and reading the reports of the Grenfell and other missions, one would wonder why people ever ventured to settle on that harsh and inhospitable coast. The answer is that it is adjacent to some of the finest fishing grounds in the world, that there are pulpwood and lumber to be cut in some of the river valleys and white foxes and other fur-bearing animals to be trapped in winter and sold in the spring.

For decades past the Grenfell Association has accepted the responsibility of looking after the Labrador fold, caring for the sick and injured, finding food supplies for the hungry and educating the children. The heroism and self-sacrifice of the Mission workers is a glorious page in the history of the desolate Labrador coast.

It is to be hoped that the Grenfell teams will continue the work of mercy they have done so courageously and well for upwards of half a century. At the same time, it would ill-become Canada to leave the care of its newly-acquired citizens in Labrador as the responsibility of private charity. High in the lists of projects of the Department of Health and Welfare should be a survey of conditions in Labrador and the taking of measures to ensure that in the future abies will no longer face death by starvation in Canada's newest province.

This incident began what was to prove a rewarding association with the premier; from now on I had ready access to his office.

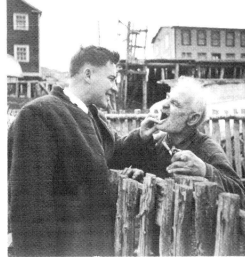

A quick check—Dr Gordon Thomas and Elihu Pilgrim at St. Anthony Bight

Dogteam driving seems romantic, and it is for the first five minutes or on a fine day. Similarly, trying to get around a tough, rugged, barren ice-bound coast by schooner or ship may be adventurous but is not the most efficient way of practising medicine.… The answer was radio-telephones plus aircraft.

G. Thomas 1975

Aircraft landing at Cartwright

By 1957 the IGA had two air ambulances working full time.

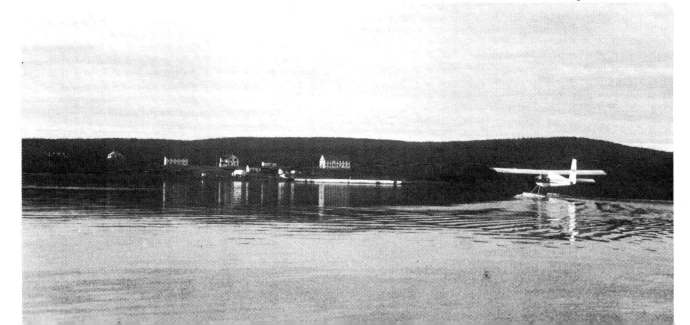

A SUMMER'S WORK ON SPOTTED ISLANDS*

Lesley Diack was a British army nurse who served in France, Iceland, North Africa, Italy and India, and discovered that she enjoyed a fulfilling job and the roving life. Like so many other nurses, she began her IGA career after a thorough vetting by Betty Seabrook, Katie Spalding's successor, the Grenfell secretary in London.

In the following selection Diack and her companion Anne, an American volunteer, are being taken by Dr Tony Paddon on the Maraval *to the Mission's station on Spotted Islands, where they have been assigned for the summer of 1950. They see patients as they go. Anne's job at Spotted Islands was to cook, teach school and work with the children, while Diack was to concentrate on public health and cope with minor medical work. At the end of that summer Diack filled in for Jupp at St. Mary's River, relieved Miss Hewitt at Mutton Harbour for the winter, and then worked for two years at Forteau.*

I never became a navigator, as [my father] had, for the nature of the medical work was changing and a more elaborate medical service was being evolved. X-ray equipment was built into the [*Maraval's*] dispensary, and we went after the problem of tuberculosis in Labrador hammer-and-tongs, X-raying everyone annually and treating all the cases we found as vigorously as possible. I was my own X-ray technician, and doing several hundred chest plates a trip in the tiny dark-room required much time.... Pending the arrival of the medical aircraft we used to have to transport our own TB cases, since the public carriers refused to accept them as passengers on the coastal boats, and sometimes there would be a half a dozen or more cases of active TB overflowing and sleeping on the deck and in the dispensary, while every bunk was being shared by two or more patients. On one occasion we arrived at North West River hospital with 41 persons aboard.

W. Paddon 1975

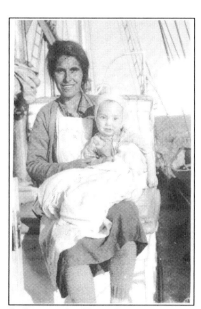

Patients on the *Maraval*

We cruised along, doctoring as we went, stopping at every settlement, almost at every house. Generally the *Maraval's* rigging would have been recognised from afar, so as soon as the siren blew and we anchored, boats would converge on us from every direction, bringing patients to see the doctor. They all came out, men, women and children; wanting pills or treatment or medicine for their 'wonderful sickness' or 'wonderful headache,' or to have their teeth pulled, or get their chests X-rayed; or just to see the doctor because he was a friend of theirs and they wanted to hear the news from down the shore. The deck swarmed with them all, as that was the only waiting room; the men in their oil-clothes, straight from fishing, unshaven and weather-beaten, and with those clear, bright eyes so typical of all seamen; the women shy, and many looking far too old for their years; the small children shy, too, mostly clinging to their mothers, but some of the older children quite the reverse, clambering in and out and all over the ship....

The settlements varied; some were poor, the houses just wooden shacks built haphazardly on the rocks; others more prosperous; everywhere, there were fish-stages, with wooden wharves perched precariously on stilts; and always, everywhere, the smell of fish....

By 7:30 that night we were ashore on Spotted Islands; the long awaited moment had arrived. The house was utterly delightful, which came as an agreeable surprise. Tony Paddon had ragged us about it so mercilessly that we should have accepted it quite calmly had it been in the very last stages of decay. We entered by a small porch straight into a long low pine-walled living room; it was very welcoming and cosy with a crackling wood fire in the old-fashioned black-leaded kitchen stove. There were brightly coloured hand-made rugs on the floor and on the simple home-made wooden furniture. There were a large dispensary and two tiny bedrooms all leading off the living room, and upstairs a long loft, with one end divided off for the ward with its two hospital beds. Most welcoming of all were [caretakers] Minnie and her husband, Tom, and they were full of pride in the care they had taken of the station.

Minnie was an absolute treasure; she was part Eskimo, short in stature, and round and plump in build; she never hurried, but somehow everything got done.... Tom was thin-faced, and *such* blue eyes looked at us from under the peak of his cap, and with such a twinkle in them; nothing was ever a trouble to him, and he was always ready to give us a hand....

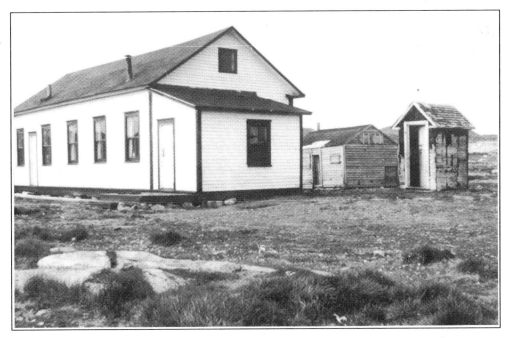

Nursing station at Spotted Islands, 1960

All [next] day we were busy unpacking and getting organized, Anne in the kitchen, and I in the dispensary. There were one or two callers with boils and bad fingers, but on the whole we felt a little redundant, not that the weather was fit even for the husky dogs which all day roamed around us in packs, like wolves. As we watched them lift up their heads to howl, or bare their teeth in a snarl, we remembered some of the gruesome stories with which Tony Paddon had regaled us, and felt inclined to believe them after all.

During the afternoon, two boys came and asked if they could split some wood for us; later they returned with a third. They just lifted the latch and marched in and sat themselves down without a word. That apparently was the custom, just knock on the door, come in, and sit; nothing else. Later, from the dispensary, I heard Anne telling them stories, and rich chuckles coming from the boys, and gradually they found their tongues....

We adapted very quickly to the simple life ... Our days started early, when, taking turns, we lit the kitchen stove; and finished late, as with curtains snugly drawn, and doors securely locked against intruders, we proceeded to bath ourselves beside the kitchen stove. We looked forward to these last few precious moments of the day when we could feel safe from interruption. This was the time snatched for letter-writing, or a brief pause for reading, or discussion between us about plans for the morrow, or for improvements, or just generally on the way things were going. Otherwise we were never alone, though after a while we had to stipulate that we must have time to eat. The children adored Anne. She had them in school all the morning, and in the afternoon they flocked into the house, for games and puzzles and the perpetual gramophone. On fine days they would have games outside, but they really preferred being in; it was probably the novelty of the bigger, better furnished house, and all the exciting things to do there. They had so few possessions of their own....

In the early evening the women would often come to call, to talk over the children, or their babies, or their problems. Sometimes they would bring their babies with them, sometimes they would sit and knit and talk, but mostly they were content just to sit. It is a very peaceful, placid existence, theirs. The farewell salutation from a Labrador householder is "There's lots of time," to which the correct reply is "Thank you." At first the newcomer from the modern world begins feverishly to make excuse, or sits down for a little longer. Later, judicious

The Labrador people have much to teach us and most of all in regard to hospitality and the welcome they give to strangers. I remember once hearing one of our doctors preach a sermon to the children on the Good Samaritan. During it he told the story of a little unwanted child begging from door to door, outcast and cold and hungry, for no one would take him in. At last he is taken in by an old peasant woman who shares her last crust with him and in sharing it discovers that it is the Christ-child whom she entertains. I remember thinking that those children wouldn't understand, the implication would be lost on them, because there isn't a door of a house on the Labrador on which a child, or any stranger for that matter, could knock and not instantly be taken in and given shelter, and not only shelter, but a share of the best that was in that house.

L. Diack 1950

147

questioning reveals that this farewell is an abbreviation for "There's lots of time to come again." Meanwhile perhaps the lesson of that abbreviation has been learned, and some of the peace of their philosophy absorbed into one's inner being.

After supper, the adolescent youth would assemble, to play the same games and gramophone records as their younger brothers and sisters had earlier, with less grace and charm and more awkwardness and noise, but who doesn't know the problems of a Youth Club anywhere?...

Anne and I had several long days out on the water doing the immunizations in the distant settlements. We could pick our weather for such trips and it was glorious to set off early on a shining morning with a whole day before us. The sea really *does* shine down north, on calm, still days, especially in late summer and in spring, and it has a brilliance and a shining beauty peculiarly its own.

A bag of candies, we found, was essential to a happy and successful immunizing trip. Our team work was good; Anne popped the candy in the mouth opened in protest as I rammed the needle home. There was a diphtheria epidemic that summer among the Eskimos further north, so we were anxious to get the immunizing done. We used the usual combined vaccine against diphtheria, whooping cough and tetanus. The thought of a possible large-scale epidemic was always rather a nightmare out there, the lack of sanitation, poor ventilation and overcrowding in many of the houses would all make for a wild-fire spread.

... All through the summer, instead of paying cash, we'd given out clothing slips in exchange for produce, or for labour; to the boys for splitting wood, to the various women who had done our laundry or baked our bread, and to the men from whom we'd hired the boats. Then, on certain days, they'd bring their slips and spend them in the [clothing] store. Anne ... had the attic all set out like something on Fifth Avenue ... all their shopping ordinarily was done through mail-order catalogues. They took hours picking and choosing and trying things on ... a very good time was had by all.

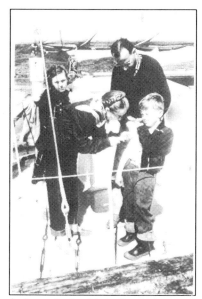

An immunization trip: polio vaccine

Small girl with hooked mat at
Harrington Harbour, 1938

THE CROTCH PARTY*

After completing a four-year fine arts program at the Nova Scotia College of Art, Anne Carney spent from June 1952 to August 1953—her 'year of adventure'—in charge of the handicraft unit at Harrington Harbour. Though hired primarily as a designer, she spent much of her time preparing the raw materials, still coming from the United States and other parts of Canada, to go out to her workers. She allocated the orders for hooked picture mats, floor mats, evening bags and the like that continued to come in from the Canadian and American shops still selling Grenfell crafts. She bought the finished products as they came in, paid her workers, balanced her books, wrote reports and assisted Dr Donald Hodd and nurse Helen Simpson at the hospital and in the operating room.

Carney's work had some bizarre aspects, as she explains below.

Raw materials for use of Grenfell hand-craft workers were supplied by Ladies' Aid groups in churches all over North America. Although I knew this fact perfectly well, I had never tried to visualize exactly what it would look like. So, the first time I had a message that a shipment of raw materials was coming in on the next trip of the *North Pioneer*, it held no particular significance for me.

* Anne E. Carney, *Harrington Harbour—Back Then* (Montreal: Price-Patterson 1991). Reprinted by permission of Price-Patterson Ltd., copyright, Anne E. Carney

A day or so later, I saw that the ship was in. But my big surprise came later in the day. One of the men drove up in the hospital jeep, and began to unload four huge wooden boxes on our doorstep. I rushed out to ask what was going on—and he said, "Here's a load a' undies to keep you out of mischief for awhile, Miss." I asked, "Do you mean there is a parcel for us, in that box?" "Oh no, Miss," he laughed—and began to wrestle the first of the boxes into our doorway.

By the time all four boxes were in the room, we could barely move. Una [my assistant] had been with one of our hookers, picking rags to use in her next hooked mat, when the boxes had arrived. Now she joined me, saying, "We has to decide when we wants to have the girls in, they wants to know." "What girls?" I asked her. "Why, look out there (pointing out the window) those girls are waitin' for you to decide." "What is it I'm supposed to decide for them?" I asked. "Well," said Una, "they wants to know when is the *Crotch* party, so they kin be sure to come."

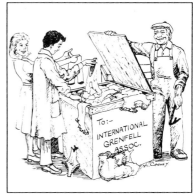

'Keep you out of mischief for awhile ...'

Seeing my bewilderment, she explained that when a load of undies came, all the panties had to have the crotches cut out, at once, for several reasons. "First of all," she said "there was likely one not washed. We has to dig out all the stinkers, first." Then, with storage space so limited no sense keeping what we could not use. "Also, the workers is not supposed to waste time cutting out the crotches. But, most important reason is the dogs. We can't carry much weight on dog teams (komatiks), so we only take what the workers will really use." "But what about the girls? Where do they fit in?" I asked. Then Una threw back her head and laughed. "How do you think all them crotches gits cut out? Do you want to cut them all? Well, we usually sets a time and pays two cents a crotch, and all them little girls gits a chance to earn a little bit of money— and we all has lots of fun, and we makes a pot of tea at the end, and has some cookies, and that's a *Crotch Party*!"

Well, I wanted those boxes out of my way double quick, so I went to the door and asked the girls when would be a good time for them. They all looked about nine or ten years of age—and all went to school. Some grades finished earlier than others—and no one wanted the later finishing ones to feel cheated. So that same day, at half past three, about a dozen of them arrived for the party.

Una brought out the big scissors, used for these occasions. We had some cookies ready, so we were all set. Things started out very solemnly. I whispered to Una, "I thought you said these sessions were fun?" She said, "They is all shy with you, you is new here. But I kin get them goin' real easy, I kin, if it's okay with you?" "Sure," said I, "I always like to have some fun." Una's face lit up—she scrabbled into the pile of panties—all dumped out in the middle of the floor by this time—and found a colossal pair. She quickly pulled them on, held them out from her sides, and asked, "Does you think these would be a good dress for the weddin' next week?" I started to laugh, grabbed up a bigger pair, and said, "Maybe these would look nicer!" Within seconds, every one of those little girls was into the spirit of the occasion, and we did have fun. But the basic purpose of our time was not lost, and piles of crotches soon built up. When we stopped for supper, each girl counted out her pile of crotches for me. I wrote carefully in our ledger how much I paid each of them, and they went happily away. Since they never had any other occasion to earn cash, they took their thirty or forty pennies with delight. Later I learned that all the local shop keepers ... could tell by the run on penny candies when the IGA had had a crotch party. We needed about four parties to finish the job, and as word spread, we had increasing numbers of girls each time. As we chopped, we chatted, and they forgot to be shy. Giggling, they told me all about their teachers and some of the

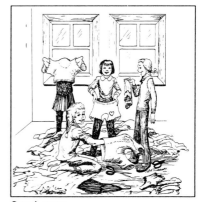

Crotch party

boys in their classes—more giggles—and all sorts of stories about their lives. We all had fun, and a tiresome job got done.

Another day I had another surprise when, answering a timid knock on the hand-craft door, I found a small solemn girl there. She asked me, "Do you want your feet cut off?" I backed up hastily and called Una, "This girl is asking about cutting feet off…" Una said, "Oh, the stockings for the braided mats!" then she told the girl that we would probably get to stockings in a few days, and she and some of her friends could come back.

PROPERTY OF NORTH WEST RIVER*

As part of the IGA's massive program of construction that began at the end of World War II, and despite perceived reservations on the part of Dr Charles Curtis, a new hospital was opened at North West River in 1954. Tony Paddon was in charge.

Around 1955, I became aware that some of our fractures could not be reduced without surgical intervention, and a requisition was sent to Dr Curtis for some bone screws and an assortment of plates. These were made of special metals which provoked no reactions in the tissues. The firm reply was that I was not qualified to use such material, and that I was to send to St. Anthony any patients whose fractures I could not reduce externally. The trouble was that the captains of coastal boats preferred not to carry patients; and even when they agreed to take them, the navigating season was only five-and-a-half months. A patient could well wait for a year to get a fracture reduced. The next suggestion was that I send the patients to the air force hospital at Goose Bay, but the military refused to accommodate or operate on civilians in their hospital except in extreme emergency. They might be flown to Montreal if necessary, but this would not be easy.…

As I thought all this over, it seemed cowardly to knuckle down to bureaucracy. The new hospital had beautiful stainless-steel hardware on doors and windows. Feeling rather foolish, I unscrewed a variety of sizes of stainless-steel screws and replaced them with good old brass. Plates were easily made from the curved edge of a food pan from our new stainless-steel kitchen. The plates required only cutting to length and width; the curve was reduced or eliminated as the fracture dictated; and we drilled and counter-sunk the plates to recess the heads of the screws. Admittedly, they didn't look quite orthodox, but they were nicely finished and the threads on the screws were coarse enough for bone—all in all, they were roughly comparable to professional products.

Shortly afterward, a young lad with the formidable name of Lucas Okuat-siaijoak arrived from Nutak with a fracture of both bones on his forearm, acquired from cranking an engine. It was not the usual cranking fracture, but involved both bones of the forearm at mid-point. One fractured bone looked easy to plate, the two ends being more or less intact, but the other was reduced to two sharp pointed ends and a few chips—highly unstable. Neither would stay in position for a minute. A bit of the open ether we were using then, and a bit of carpentry with the pilfered plates and screws, and we had one of the two bones firmly held in position by the plate and six screws. The other we left alone, for we knew that the plated bone would serve as a splint, and so it did. We put the patient in plaster, and healing was rapid and solid; we then sent him back

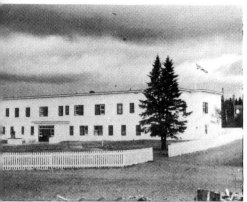
New hospital at North West River: the IGA and provincial government split the cost

After the opening of the new hospital, we really attacked tuberculosis on a large scale; there were two six-bed wards for acute cases. Early ambulation speeded up the recovery and made a hospital stay much more endurable, and on good drug regimes, the majority soon became free of the TB bacilli and contagion.… The in-hospital patients were composed of three roughly equal groups: Innu, Inuit and settlers. They were all obviously at ease and on excellent terms with each other, and the native people showed no signs of the shyness they had experienced elsewhere.

W. Paddon 1989

* W.A. Paddon, *Labrador Doctor: My Life with the Grenfell Mission* (Toronto: James Lorimer 1989). Reprinted by permission of James Lorimer Limited, copyright W.A. Paddon

home, where he soon returned to fishing with his father. Unfortunately, an aircraft from St. Anthony stopped in Nutak for some reason, and the people aboard were told that the boy had tuberculosis. This was an error—the result of a language problem—for at St. Anthony he was dismissed, as we had dismissed him, with a few flecks of calcification from a healed lesion in his chest. Someone there noted the scar on his arm and X-rayed him; shortly afterward, we received a frigid telegram asking what on earth might be the revolting object they had removed from the arm of Lucas Okuatsiaijoak. We had planned to remove it at the next opportunity, but this message was offensive in the extreme, so we sent back a reply that this beautiful example of skilful improvisation was the property of North West River, and that we would like it back intact. There was no answer at the time, but, later in the summer, I received a nice assortment of the commoner plates and appropriate screws, and the matter was dropped.

THE TRANSFORMATION OF A MISSION

The transformation of the Grenfell Mission into Grenfell Regional Health Services was a process that essentially began in 1939, with the outbreak of World War II followed by Grenfell's death. With Confederation in 1949, it gathered momentum. In the years that followed, a philanthropic, paternalistic and remote organization involved in the running of health, educational and social services for a group of needy people became an anachronism. There were economic and other factors involved.

During the war Labrador became central to Allied defence efforts. The Canadian and American armed forces each built bases at Goose Bay, where many Labradorians moved for well-paid jobs. Canadian and American bases constructed on the Island employed so many Newfoundlanders that unemployment problems were for the time being solved. Confederation came next, bringing family allowances, old age pensions, veterans' benefits, increased public services and much more. The construction of a chain of radar sites along the northern coast in the early 1950s, followed by the development of vast iron ore deposits in Labrador West and the harnessing of the giant hydroelectrical potential of Churchill Falls, transformed the northern economy. Both federal and provincial governments began to take up their proper responsibility for health, education, justice and social services within the IGA district. Under these circumstances, people were no longer willing to tolerate a mission in their midst.

In the following pages, Doctors Tony Paddon, Gordon Thomas and Peter Roberts each bring their own perspective to bear on these events.

No Market for Pioneers*

Tony Paddon remained the IGA's principal doctor in Labrador until he retired in 1978, bringing to an end his family's record of sixty-six years' continuous service in the north. From 1981 to 1986 he was Newfoundland's lieutenant-governor. He speaks first.

By the early 1970s, it was becoming obvious that the days of the Grenfell mission—the cause to which I and my father before me had devoted our lives—were numbered. We had reached this point not because of any failures on our part, but, ironically, because of our successes.

After Newfoundland became part of the Canadian Confederation in 1949, we had suddenly been able to complete our attack on the enemies of the

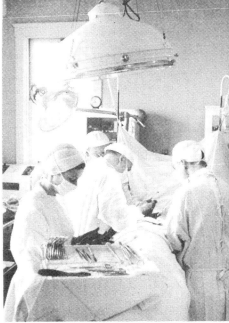

Thoracic surgery

Dr G.W. Thomas was the acknowledged master of new thoracic techniques performed at the St. Anthony Hospital, where between 1927 and 1937 there had been 900 tuberculosis admissions. By 1954 the hospital had a new 55-bed sanatorium attached.

Power too often corrupts, but the heads of the Grenfell Mission, autocrats that they were, were idealists whose affection for the people of the coast was unbounded.
Ruth Keese Little in a 1977 interview Quoted in Badger 1977

---

* W.A. Paddon, *Labrador Doctor: My Life with the Grenfell Mission* (Toronto: James Lorimer 1989). Reprinted by permission of James Lorimer Limited, copyright W.A. Paddon

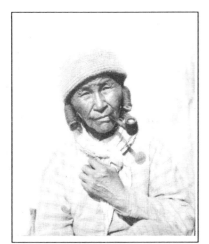

Innu woman with pipe

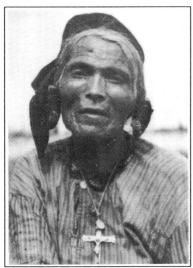

Innu man

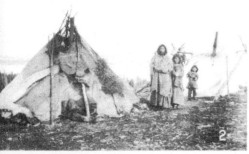

Innu trading at Cartwright

These photographs were taken in the 1930s, when the Innu as well as Inuit were riddled with tuberculosis.

past—tuberculosis, malnutrition, illiteracy and much more—and I believe we made good use of the money the provincial government provided us. As for the government, it scrupulously left us to run our own affairs, perhaps because of a realization that, without us, it would be unable to attract well-qualified medical staff for the northern part of the province. The Grenfell name was well known in Britain, and British nurses, many of whom were very well trained, were strongly drawn to northern Newfoundland and Labrador, which they considered a fascinating setting. In general, we had enough staff for our needs—nurses, technicians and doctors—most from Great Britain, and many prepared to stay for years, or even for life. These people adapted easily to life in Labrador and northern Newfoundland, and won respect and affection; and, although there were occasional grumbles about 'foreigners' in Newfoundland, the department of health was pleased with the work of the mission.

During the 1970s, the hospital at North West River was at the peak of its efficiency; it had recently been enlarged and was well equipped. Innu and Inuit people, who represented a sizeable percentage of the hospital's patients, were happy with its services and eager to keep using them. Our other facilities—the high school, the Infants' Home, and the school residences—were also flourishing; as well, we had a substantial public-health program. The government had gladly provided the money for facilities and programs, and it seemed pleased with the results.

Yet the very fact that the government was bearing nearly all the costs of our hospitals and nursing stations, as well as our dormitories and schools, spelled the end of the mission. In short, given our dependence on the government, it was inevitable that the mission would be completely absorbed into the educational and health apparatus of the provincial government. I realized this was so—and I also thought it right and proper.... The time for missions, I concluded, was long past.

... Personally, I did not want to see the Grenfell organization tarnish its reputation in any way by waiting too long to dissolve itself. I was proud to have been the son of a Grenfell doctor and to have followed in his footsteps, but this was a different era, and it was time to retire gracefully. I did precisely that, some three years later, retiring at the age of sixty-four in 1978. I planned to be utterly idle for a year or two, and then try to do something useful but unrelated to medicine. I had no inkling of what was to happen to me in 1981, when I was appointed lieutenant-governor....

When I look back on my years with the Grenfell mission, I think of the people whose names are now nearly forgotten, the nurses and teachers, the long-term volunteers, the house parents of the schools and dormitories, who during much of the mission's existence worked for a pittance and made Labrador their first love. The work they did was incalculable, and it was often based on a real understanding of the people they served. They never had an opportunity to save any money, nor did this concern them as long as they had the bare necessities. Many of them had difficult retirements for the pensions the association could provide were small, and some required help from their friends to manage at all. This situation was later much improved by Dr Gordon Thomas, and our workers were able to enter government pension schemes after Confederation, but many of those who had spent their lives in work on behalf of the people of Labrador would have done so regardless. A nurse like Dorothy Jupp, who worked nearly forty years with us, had no family except the people of Labrador ... Some of the house mothers in the school dormitories never had children of their own, but lavished their love on their charges and were content....

The hospital at North West River had endeavoured to meet the special needs of the native people ... Such people regarded the Inuit and Innu with affection and respect....

The mountains across Lake Melville from our home have not changed since my mother and father came to love them. The bay is still as broad and shining; sometimes as calm as water can ever be; sometimes a fury, driven by strong winds. Its waters are only a few yards beyond the sandy beach and our scrubby northern lawn; waters which are ice-covered and silent more than half the year, and alive with activity the rest of the time. In my lifetime, the trees around our clearing have grown very large and tall; no doubt many of them will succumb to autumn gales, but for now they make a beautiful setting.

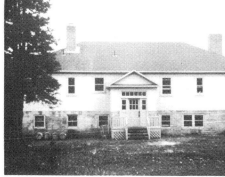

Nursing station at Nain

The primitive early days of my family's life here are long past, as are the improvisations that met our equipment shortages and the increasingly complex needs of our patients. Today, the people of North West River travel in large cars between their homes and Goose Bay; indeed, they drive to Toronto or Vancouver to visit their sons and daughters. The Inuit and Innu increasingly run their own affairs, and with much confidence. There is no longer any market for pioneers.

The Final Transition*

Gordon Thomas, IGA superintendent from 1959 to 1978, spanned an era in northern medicine stretching from dog-sled to satellite, as did Tony Paddon. More than anyone else, it was Thomas who hastened the IGA's inevitable withdrawal from running medical services in the north. He retired 1 January 1979 after thirty-two years on the coast.

The Grenfell organization had a long succession of remarkable staff members, but there was only one Grenfell. After his death, the various national associations and their supporting branches ran for some time on their own considerable momentum; but the charitable side of the work, particularly the fund-raising, was so fundamentally an expression of Grenfell's own fame and personality that some decline was inevitable after his death.

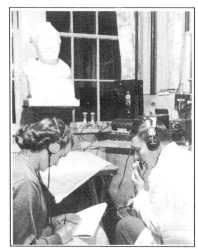

The radio-telephone (RT) room at St. Anthony

G.W. Thomas contacts a nursing station while Dorothy Erb makes notes. The RT room became the nerve centre of a regionalized health system.

A shortage of funds and staff during World War II sharply curtailed the plans of Grenfell's successor, Dr Curtis, who stoutly refused to have much to do with fund-raising himself, but the IGA maintained its basic character as an international charity throughout this time. It was Confederation and the gradual, somewhat reluctant provision of normal public services that brought fundamental change to the quality of life in our area, the scope of our work, and the source of our funding. Gradually, as the need for charity declined, the fund-raising branches ceased to function, until by the mid 1970s the only active branches were those in Montreal, Ottawa, and Toronto. There, lively and resourceful women continued to support our work through the Grenfell Labrador Mission in Ottawa, raising large amounts of money and gifts of toys, clothing, and hospital equipment.

In the United States, where branches fell largely dormant after Confederation, the Grenfell associations in Boston and New York lived on, managing endowment funds established during the hey-day of the mission's life as a charity. They sent us the annual income from these endowments but continued to control the funds. For the most part, we used this income to supplement our governments grants and to finance dental care, which got very little govern-

---

*   G.W. Thomas, *From Sled to Satellite: My Years with the Grenfell Mission* (Toronto: Irwin Publishing 1987). Reprinted by permission of the author. Copyright Gordon W. Thomas

[In the 1950s and 1960s,] via large government grants becoming available to us through participation in various programs of the Canadian system, such as hospitalization and Medicare, we were able to reorganize and develop a regional medical service covering the whole area. It was built on a system of small community health centres or nursing stations under the immediate control of subregional community hospitals, all connected with a new 170 bed regional hospital at St. Anthony which provided full consultation services.

We now have a chain of five hospitals and fourteen nursing stations or community health centres and this year are building two more.... Each regional centre is affiliated with Memorial University in St. John's and is part of the teaching program of the University for medical students, interns, and residents.

We have developed a program for teaching midwives through Dalhousie University School of Outport Nurses, and we provide for the intern training of nurse interns with special training in midwifery. This enables them to serve in remote areas as highly qualified outpost nurses. Such trained personnel have revolutionized the practice of obstetrics in the north....

Through the regionalization of health services ... our emphasis has gradually shifted from acute emergency care to a total health care service with an emphasis on public health and preventative medicine.

G. Thomas 1975

Linwood Brown, a social worker with an industrial arts background, and his wife Rachel, a nurse, ran the St. Anthony children's home from 1936 to 1945. Dedicated to the children in their care and to the community in which they worked, their influence at St. Anthony remained long after they left.

ment support until later. We also used the endowment revenues to improve staff housing and benefits, so that we could more easily attract the calibre of personnel we needed.

The international association, whose board represented the various supporting groups, became a kind of 'old boys' club,' meeting annually in the board room of a New York bank, then later twice a year in the splendour of the Union Club on Park Avenue. As I argued the logic of an air ambulance service and a modern hospital, and later the inevitability of a major role for government, I sometimes felt that the underlying purpose of this body was to keep itself in existence, to survive the fundamental erosion of its role....

Arthur Bingham, who had succeeded Dr Curtis as board chairman, died suddenly in 1967 and was in turn replaced by Bill Maier, a prominent Quaker from Bryn Mawr, Pennsylvania. Maier had been on the coast as a volunteer in his youth and had maintained an interest in the mission ever since. His feeling for the coast ran deep, and he was a good ally on the board. Sadly, on one of his trips north he contracted trichinosis from eating infected bear meat ... [and soon it] became obvious that he would have to resign as chairman.

This was of urgent concern to me, because it was clear that we needed a strong, progressive chairman who was willing to come to terms with new realities, one of which was that Newfoundlanders were no longer content to have medical service in a vast area of their province run by a well-meaning but sometimes insensitive board of directors who had little real knowledge of the area. Our annual operating budget was more than $17 million, and taxpayers by now were putting up 99.9% of it. The IGA was benevolent and efficient, but inherently paternalistic. Its contribution over the years had been magnificent, but it was run by outsiders and this would no longer do.

In Quebec, our responsibility for health care on the Lower North Shore had been taken over by the provincial government in 1972. IGA continued to provide consulting service to the hospital at Blanc Sablon and assisted in recruiting staff for the region, but medical service was now a full public responsibility.

On a speaking trip to Boston in 1975 I told members of the New England Grenfell Association that the time had come for IGA to withdraw completely from operating health services for the people of northern Newfoundland and Labrador. Further, the association should consider turning over its endowment funds to some trust organization, to be given to the appropriate government body. This was not a popular speech.

I requested a meeting with Dr Ted Badger and Dr Ed Neuhauser, two very prominent directors from New England. I told them that Bill Maier's health was so poor that he was undoubtedly considering resignation, and that his successor must be a strong personality willing to hand over health services to the Newfoundland people. I urged them to consider appointing Dr Linwood Brown, another New England director. He had been in social work for years but had spent his earlier years on the coast with his wife Rachel, running the St. Anthony orphanage. He knew the systems of health and welfare in New England and Canada, and had direct personal experience of our operations. Later that year Maier did resign and Brown replaced him.

Soon after that, Brown and I met to discuss the future. We agreed that it was our responsibility to phase out the Grenfell Mission, yielding way to government, and that we must do this regardless of the personal cost in popularity with many friends and supporters of the IGA in Canada, the U.S., and Britain. At an early board meeting, Brown appointed a task force to develop a five-year plan to achieve this transition. The group included the chairman of each supporting association, plus the IGA executive, [controller] Harold Mack and myself....

The task force met regularly—usually quarterly ... divisions were evident right from the start. Some directors, especially those from Boston and New York, totally unfamiliar with the Canadian health system and fired with Yankee enthusiasm, envisioned selling our assets to the province of Newfoundland for between $18 and $20 million. With these funds they could set up a charitable foundation, which they would continue to manage in future, thus maintaining a major presence in the north.

Officials from the [Newfoundland] departments of public works, justice, and health met on several occasions with the task force. They listened politely but it was obvious they had no intention whatsoever of paying any money over to the IGA. The government felt that our extensive land holdings and other physical assets, especially the nursing stations and hospitals, properly belonged to the people of Newfoundland. Even the facilities built or purchased entirely with donations had been gifts from benefactors to the people of the area, and many of the later facilities had been acquired through direct government grants.

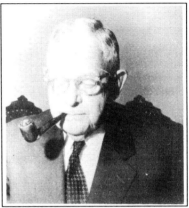

Dr Charles Curtis shortly before his death in 1963

Linwood Brown, Harold Mack, Peter Roberts, and I, with the help of some of the Canadian and British directors, were finally able to persuade the task force to forget the idea of selling IGA's assets to the people for whom they had already been given. This decision did not come easily and took many meetings as a number of the American directors were reluctant to give up control and were determined to be paid for IGA assets. They never fully appreciated the health system of Canada and continued to be influenced by private enterprise philosophy.

In the end, however, the task force and later the complete board of the IGA agreed to turn over to the Newfoundland government for the sum of one dollar all assets relating to health care. This included the hospitals, nursing stations, and their associated lands and buildings, and in addition the Piper Chieftain aircraft. The provincial health department then set up a regional hospital board that replaced the IGA and was responsible to the minister of health. The department of public works and the justice department agreed to carry out the surveys of these properties and provide the necessary documents for transfer.

The supporting associations located in Newfoundland, Ottawa, and Great Britain [sic] all agreed to disband and to turn their assets over to a newly constituted IGA. This they did and these assets gave the IGA a working capital of approximately $1 million so that it could continue to function as a corporate body.

The New England Grenfell Association in Boston, and the Grenfell Association of America in New York, each of which held large endowment funds, were not willing to disband or turn their assets over to the new IGA in Newfoundland for management, nor were they willing to amalgamate. Part of the reason for this might well have been that these substantial funds were controlled and managed by consulting banking firms in Boston and New York whose responsible officers were on the IGA board. No doubt the substantial management fees that these firms were receiving influenced their attitudes. In any case they continue to exist and appoint members to the newly constituted IGA board.

When this was all agreed, but before it was formally concluded, Brown suggested that Paddon, Mack, the financial comptroller, and I should consider retiring before the transition took place. Though I had lobbied for a strong chairman, this came as something of a shock. On reflection I recognized that he was right. We had all spent our careers under the old system and could find it difficult to adapt to the major changes that would undoubtedly follow. Paddon

There was a time in my own life when I thought it very important to perform surgical feats in isolation under adverse conditions. However, philosophically, I now think that I would prefer to be remembered as a pioneer in health care delivery.

G. Thomas 1975

resigned first in 1977. Mack and I retired in 1979, but Mack died of a heart attack later the same year.

Various honours came to us. Paddon and I were co-recipients of the Royal Bank Award and we both received honorary degrees from Memorial University. In 1970, I was invested into the Order of Canada, and in 1978 Tony became a member of the Order of Canada. Pat received the Queen's Jubilee Medal. The IGA board formally honoured Pat and me together in September 1978, when the first board meeting ever held on the coast took place in St. Anthony. In 1981, Paddon was appointed lieutenant-governor of the province, a fitting tribute to this son of Labrador. Donald Hodd received the Order of Canada shortly before he died. If anyone deserved it, he did.

The final transition to the government took place at a ceremony at St. John's early in April 1981. The responsibility for the operation of health care services went to a new regional health board appointed by the provincial government called the Grenfell Regional Health Services Board, while the ownership of much of the IGA property went to the provincial government. The IGA retained only those lands, mainly at St. Anthony, that had no direct bearing on health services. These tracts of land are fairly substantial and give the IGA a continued capital resource in the province.

The ceremony was held at a luncheon meeting at the Arts and Culture Centre in St. John's. Members of the IGA executive and task force attended, as well as senior executives. The premier at the time, Frank Moores, didn't bother to attend, although a formal luncheon was provided by the provincial government. He did not appreciate the historical significance of the event and sent along a deputy as well as the minister of health, senior officials from the department of health, and the minister of public works. When the document was signed, no one from the government could find a dollar bill to turn over to the IGA. Linwood Brown, the chairman of the IGA board, found a Canadian dollar in his pocket-book and gave it to the health minister, who in turn gave it back to him. We then all signed the dollar bill.

Grenfell pilot Tom Green

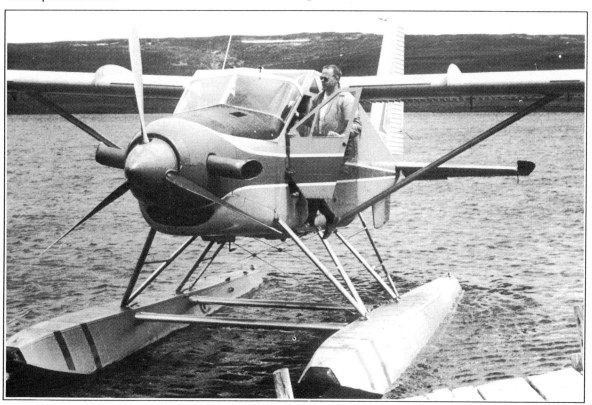

No Heroes, No Villains*

Peter J. Roberts was born in St. John's in 1944 and came first to St. Anthony as a medical student from Dalhousie University. In 1973 he returned to Roddickton as an MD. Moving to St. Anthony in 1975, he undertook a series of administrative positions. Roberts became executive director of the IGA in January 1979 and executive director of Grenfell Regional Health Services (GRHS) in April 1981.

The last word is his.

Peter J. Roberts

I am often asked to 'pronounce on the Mission'—to explain why change has come and why there is now a Grenfell Regional Health Services Board responsible for health services in this area. Now, I am not sure I can answer these questions, but there seems to be an idea about that I have some personal responsibility for all this change, or at the very least, I have some particular understanding of it. In fact, neither is true and there is no doubt in my mind that issues involved here are far bigger than I am. The process of change is far greater than any one of us and there are no heroes or villains.

Finding a perspective on this change has been eased greatly by a recent trip through time aboard the Mission plane. Really, it was a trip along the Northern Peninsula, but within that single passage I was able to rapidly review many earlier passages, indeed the substance of several years. At its most mundane, it was a visit to Roddickton and Harbour Deep—a routine visit to an area which is reasonably familiar to me. We flew south overland and coming back north; we did the pilot's tour, a low level flight along the coastline which brings the landmarks flying by at close proximity and great speed. It's a striking experience, one which can't help but recall many things to mind—the memories of people, places and events of earlier times—a spectacular rapid fire review of many personal experiences. And it couldn't have happened at a better time because it has given me a necessary perspective.

In the mellow afterglow it is, of course, all too easy to remember the good, to focus selectively on many wonderful memories I have—memories of passages with fair winds and quartering seas, good holding grounds and secure harbours; memories of stalwart Newfoundlanders born and bred to the sea and somehow restlessly reconciled to it. One thinks, too, of communities of people—the pairings and groupings which allow men and women to live peacefully and to aspire and achieve beyond mere survival. These things, and more, came immediately to mind as we flew along the coast and I could not help but conclude how good it all was.

My flight into the past was indelibly marked with reference to the IGA and that, too, is a very happy thought. One cannot consider life in this area without knowing 'the Mission.' Undoubtedly, there was life here before the Mission and there will be life here after it is gone, but as long as it existed the IGA was an essential part of the life of Northern Newfoundland and Labrador.

Without it, life in these parts would have been, I believe, far less fulfilling. One thinks primarily of the Mission people—call them missionaries if you will—who were so willing to work with the people of this coast in the hope that together they might all, both worker and people, know a better life. Some of the workers spent a lifetime here, more did not. Some were Christian and some were not. Some were doctors and nurses and there were countless more who served in other ways. This trip through time clearly isolates the essential fact that people have served with, and for, their fellows, and that no matter how

Peter Roberts, 46, executive director of GRHS since 1979, is a tall, hefty native of St. John's with ... a shock of dark hair and eyes that occasionally make him look possessed. He's a student of lighthouses, painter of bold landscapes, cross-country skier, player of old boys' hockey and builder of his own steel schooner. He and his wife, Betty Lethbridge, keep two Newfoundland dogs and live in a house, much of which he built himself, on a slope above the hospital.

Though a better administrator than Grenfell, Roberts has certain Grenfellian characteristics. He can be blunt and likes to see things done his own way.

H. Bruce 1991

---

* Peter J. Roberts, "The Process of Change" appeared originally in *Among the Deep Sea Fishers* 78, no. 2 (1981): 1-4. This was its last issue.

While no one doubts that the establishment of GRHS as a government-funded regional health authority was beneficial, veteran members of the Grenfell staff sometimes miss the hominess of the old organization. Still, much of the Grenfell spirit remains; GRHS inherited a history of toughness, heroism and independence, and when Roberts compares his organization with other regional health authorities in Newfoundland, he says, "We're more self-reliant, more aggressive, kinkier. We're less likely to toe the company line." Behind his own pushiness lies a crucial conviction: "I don't buy the theory that because you're in the boonies you should accept lower standards of health care."

... He talks of staff members who put in 15-hour days, nurses who not only attend to patients' medical needs but cook meals for them in their homes, and ambulance pilots who answer calls at all hours of the night.

H. Bruce 1991

A sense of both service and adventure brings doctors, dentists and nurses to GRHS from all over Canada and the United States, from Scotland, Ireland and England and, after medical training in Britain, from Africa and Asia as well.

Some come to stay but soon quit. The region is so cold in winter, so tough to get around and so remote from such routine pleasures as movie theatres, fine restaurants and big-league newspapers. Others, however, join GRHS for only a spell but succumb to the Grenfell obsession.

H. Bruce 1991

grand or menial their work may have been, they have contributed to this worldly life. No mere detail must obscure this fact for herein lies the greatest achievement: the Mission provided the means for all these people to serve their fellow man.

It would be less than honourable for us to ignore the fact that our selective recall fortunately does much to obscure many of the less pleasant aspects of earlier times. One doesn't wish to belabour the point at times like this, but who can deny that behind every piece of medical heroism there lies human discomfort and unhappiness—often tragedy. How often do we marvel at our ability to cope in times of trouble without properly recognizing the prevailing misery which has, in the first place, caused the problem? Is it not too much to say then that most of us who have cared to look have seen much that we would not choose for ourselves? Of course not and, in fact, we have spent the better part of our time working to improve the life of the people of this area. The 'good old days' weren't always that good and there were many times when people could reasonably have prayed for a more equitable fate.

Now, I suppose the really good news is that the Northern Newfoundland of the 1960's and 1970's, and now the 1980's, is a far different place than the Northern Newfoundland of earlier times, especially pre-Confederation Newfoundland. Changes have been incredible and there has been a constant improvement in living conditions. The people of the area now know a prosperity previously unthought of. There is no poverty, and although there may often be failed expectations, there is none of the hardship so characteristic of earlier times.

The health of the people in this area has improved as well. Advances in the standard of living—better housing, more employment, extended public utilities, government income support and supplements—all of these things have combined to do much to overcome the ill health which prevails in their absence. Our own efforts have been important and we have been able to do our fair share by developing greatly improved primary services, a dental service, health prevention and promotion, and active and modern facilities for the care of the acutely ill. Undoubtedly, much remains to be done, but these deficiencies do not alter the fact that the people of this area are now better off than at any time in history and they are much more healthy.

For the IGA, there were two significant changes. The first was the general improvement in the standard of living throughout the area. Secondly, there was a tremendous improvement in the level of funding available to the IGA. At the time of Confederation, all aspects of the Mission were costing less than one half million dollars. In 1980 this amount had become something in excess of seventeen million dollars for health services alone. Obviously, much more could be done with the increased amounts of money available. And again, it was the people of the province, through government, who decided that money was needed to improve services for the people of this area.

From there, it is only a short step to the realization that in this democracy of ours, the people themselves must participate in the management of health services. We now consume nearly twenty million dollars of public funds. Is it too much to ask that people be responsible for what is theirs and that we, the workers, be responsible to those whom we serve? Is there any point in asking if the Toronto General Hospital, the Massachusetts General Hospital, or St. Thomas' Hospital in London would be interested in a board of directors composed of the esteemed and successful people of Northern Newfoundland and Labrador? The point hardly needs discussion. Just as the people of Newfoundland and Labrador have willingly altered life throughout this province,

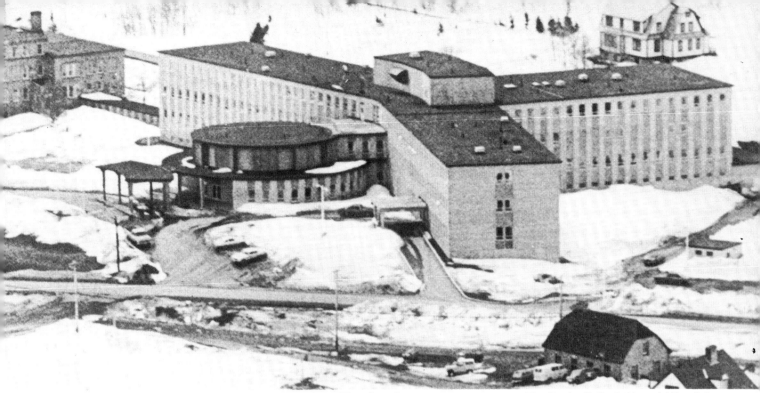

The Charles S. Curtis Memorial Hospital, St. Anthony, the old hospital at left

we must now wilfully determine our own fate. The time has come to accept responsibility and accountability.

All of this is not to say that the newly established Grenfell Regional Health Services Board is going to be problem-free. It isn't. It will face the standard set of problems that the IGA has been coping with for years. A change in our corporate structure is unlikely to change these.

What is different is simply this: each generation must develop its own solution to the problems of its age. Old responses are always that, and although they may have worked in former times and although they may partially meet a current need, they rarely answer the problems of today and those of the future. Life and survival demand constant renewal. Organizations and human institutions are not exempt from the laws of nature. The successful response of one generation may well be the failure of another and it is only through intelligent adaptation that we can hope for and aspire to continued successes in our work.

I have every reason to believe that this generation will do every bit as well as the preceding one. The way has been shown clearly and the problems are known to us all. There is no reason to think that we will be any less successful in our time than our predecessors were in theirs. We will show this generation to be just as capable as any other has been; in fact, were we transposed to an earlier time, we would undoubtedly solve the problems of that age just as did those who actually were there at work. Similarly, were a generation of earlier workers to face today's situation, I have no doubt that they would respond much as we do today.

In short then, one can only conclude that all those dire predictions cannot be substantiated in fact. There is no disruption of the mission. We have not lost our integrity. Our commitment is just as great as ever and our work is even better. After all is said and done, the people of this area are becoming more healthy and they continue to look forward to a more fulfilling life. What we've changed is an organization which has outlived its age. In truth, we have lost nothing. To the contrary, we have gained something very essential. We now have an organization which is managed by representatives of those we serve—more accessible and more accountable. All else remains the same. We have prospered in the past and will do so in the future as long as there is good work to be done and as long as there are good people willing to do it. It was so in Grenfell's time and it is so today.

The International Grenfell Association remained responsible for the delivery of health and other services initiated by Grenfell until Grenfell Regional Health Services (GRHS) was formed in April 1981. Established under the provincial Hospitals' Act, GRHS is now responsible for health services in northern Newfoundland, coastal Labrador and the Lake Melville region. The board's membership is comprised of representatives from the areas served, as well as two members nominated by Memorial University.

GRHS operates an integrated regional health service consisting of two hospitals, seventeen primary health centres and nursing stations, public health and dental services, and currently employs more than 800 people. The 100-bed Charles S. Curtis Memorial Hospital at St. Anthony provides service in the major medical specialities and is affiliated with Memorial University's Faculty of Medicine. It has full support services in nursing, physiotherapy, occupational therapy and laboratory work.

In 1981, the role of the IGA changed to that of a foundation. Its board of directors consists of a maximum of twelve: two from each of the supporting associations (the Grenfell Association of America, the New England Grenfell Association and the Grenfell Association of Great Britain and Ireland) and six directors at large. The IGA continues to promote health, education and other services in northern Newfoundland and Labrador.

Bibliography

Badger, Theodore L. "Grenfell Vignette: Mrs. John Mason Little." *Among the Deep Sea Fishers* 74, no. 3 (1977): 5-6

Banfill, B.J. *Labrador Nurse*. London: Robert Hale 1954

Barbour, Florence Grant. *Memories of Life on the Labrador and in Newfoundland*. New York: Carlton Press 1973

Berton, Pierre. "The Adventures of Wilfred Grenfell" in *The Wild Frontier: More Tales from the Remarkable Past*. Toronto: McClelland and Stewart 1978

Briggs, S. Edgar. "Dr. Grenfell, Premier of the Labrador." Reprinted from *Record of Christian Work*. *Among the Deep Sea Fishers* 2, no. 2 (1904): 3-7

Brinton, Mary Williams. *My Cap and My Cape: An Autobiography*. Philadelphia: Dorrance 1950

Bruce, Harry. "Care in a Cold Climate." *Imperial Oil Review* 75, no. 403 (1991): 2-9

Burry, Lester. "Memories of Labrador" in *The Book of Newfoundland*, Vol. 4., J.R. Smallwood, ed. St. John's: Newfoundland Book Publishers 1967: p. 59

—. "Reminiscences of a Clergyman in Labrador." *Newfoundland Medical Association Newsletter* 17, no. 4 (1974): 20-2

Carney, Anne E. *Harrington Harbour—Back Then*. Montreal: Price-Patterson 1991

Corner, George W. *Anatomist at Large*. New York: Basic Books 1958

—. "Hospital Work of the Labrador Mission." *Modern Hospital* 3 (1914): 72-8

Devine, P.K. *In the Good Old Days! Fishery Customs of the Past*. St. John's: Harry Cuff 1990

Diack, Lesley. *Labrador Nurse*. London: Victor Gollancz 1963

Duncan, Norman. *Dr. Grenfell's Parish: The Deep Sea Fishermen*. New York: Fleming H. Revell 1905

—. "Grenfell of the Medical Mission." *Harper's Magazine* 110 (1904): 28-37

Durgin, George Francis. *Letters from Labrador*. Concord, N.H.: Rumford Printing 1908

Forsyth, C. Hogarth. "Cartwright Today." *Among the Deep Sea Fishers* 41, no. 1 (1943): 12-14

—. "Life and Work in Labrador." *Medical Press Circular* 204 (1940): 398-402

Gordon, Henry. *The Labrador Parson: Journal of the Reverend Henry Gordon, 1915-1925*. F. Burnham Gill, ed. St. John's: Provincial Archives of Newfoundland and Labrador 1972

Gosling, W.G. *Labrador: Its Discovery, Exploration, and Development*. London: Alston Rivers 1910

Goudie, Elizabeth. *Woman of Labrador*. David Zimmerly, ed. and intro. Agincourt, Ontario: Book Society of Canada 1983

Grenfell, Anne and Katie Spalding. *Le Petit Nord, or, Annals of a Labrador Harbour*. Boston and New York: Houghton Mifflin 1920

Grenfell Association of Great Britain and Ireland. *A Brick for Labrador*. London: [1930]

Grenfell, Wilfred T. (1903 [1]) "Among the Deep-Sea Fishermen." *Outlook* 74 (1903): 695-701

— (1903 [2]). "Among the Vikings of Labrador." *Missionary Review of the World* 16, no. 7, new series (1903): 481-2

—(1907 [1]). "The Close of Open Water." *Among the Deep Sea Fishers* 4, no. 4 (1907): 8-11

—(1905 [1]). "The Deep Sea Mission: Dr. Grenfell's Lecture on his Labrador Labors." *Evening Herald* 12 December 1905

—. *Down North on the Labrador*. New York: Fleming H. Revell 1911

—. *Down to the Sea: Yarns from the Labrador*. New York: Fleming H. Revell 1910

— (1906 [1]). "Dr. Grenfell's Log." *Among the Deep Sea Fishers* 4, no. 3 (1906): 9-11

—. "Dr. Grenfell's Log." *Among the Deep Sea Fishers* 6, no. 2 (1908): 21-2

—. (1903 [3]). "Extracts from Dr. Grenfell's Letters to 'The Toilers.'" *Among the Deep Sea Fishers* 1, no. 1 (1903): 6-10

—. *Forty Years for Labrador*. Boston and New York: Houghton Mifflin 1932

— (1930 [1]). "Industrial Work and Clothing." *Among the Deep Sea Fishers* 28, no. 3 (1930): 128-32

—. *A Labrador Doctor: The Autobiography of Wilfred Thomason Grenfell, M.D. (Oxon.), C.M.G.* Boston and New York: Houghton and Mifflin 1919

—. "Labrador: Lesson in Humanity." *Rotarian* 53, no. 6 (1938): 22-5

—. *Labrador's Fight for Economic Freedom*. Self and Society Booklet No. 19. London: Ernest Benn 1929

—(1905 [2]). "Leaves from the Log of the Lend-a-Hand." *McClure's Magazine* 24, no. 6 (1905): 624-32

—(1903 [4]). "The Log of the S.S. Strathcona." *Among the Deep Sea Fishers* 1, no. 3 (1903): 6-8

—(1905 [3]). "The Log of the S.S. Strathcona." *Among the Deep Sea Fishers* 2, no. 4 (1905): 5-19

—(1906 [2]). "The Log of the S.S. Strathcona." *Among the Deep Sea Fishers* 3, no. 4 (1906): 8-17

—(1930 [2]). "Medicine in the Sub-arctic: The Mary Scott Newbold Lecture. Lecture 22." *Transactions and Studies of the College of Physicians of Philadelphia* 52 (1930): 73-95

—. *The Romance of Labrador*. New York: Macmillan 1934

—. *Vikings of Today, or, Life and Medical Work among the Fishermen of Labrador*. Frederick Treves, pref. London: Marshall Bros. 1895

—. "Warm Hearts in Labrador." *Rotarian* 47 (1935): 6-10

—(1907 [2]). "Why I am against Liquor." *Among the Deep Sea Fishers* 5, no. 1 (1907): 18-9

Grenfell Worker. "Labrador Answers." *Newfoundland Quarterly* 34, no. 2 (1934): 33-6

[Hodd, Donald.] *Doctor of the Snows: Dr. Donald Hodd, M.D.* Questions by Dan Mauger. Sept-Iles: Editions Le Musée des Sept-Isles 1979

Johnson, Donald McI. *A Doctor Regrets ... Being the First Part of 'A Publisher Presents Himself.'* London: Christopher Johnson 1949

Johnston, James. *Grenfell of Labrador*. London: S.W. Partridge 1908

Jupp, Dorothy M. *A Journey of Wonder and Other Writings.* New York: Vantage 1971

Kelloway, Warrick F. "Memories of Labrador and Dr. Wilfred Grenfell." *Newfoundland Quarterly* 70, no. 2 (1973): 11-4

Kerr, J. Lennox. *Wilfred Grenfell: His Life and Work.* New York: Dodd, Mead 1959

Kingman, Rufus A. "Personal Observations." *Among the Deep Sea Fishers* 1, no. 4 (1904): 5-6

Kivimaki, Anna. "Nursing with the Grenfell Mission." *American Journal of Nursing* 37, no. 6 (1937): 593-8

Little, John Mason. "Beriberi." *Journal of the American Medical Association* 63, no. 15 (1914): 1287-90

— (1908 [1]). "Medical Conditions on the Labrador Coast and North Newfoundland." *Journal of the American Medical Association* 50, no. 13 (1908): 1037-9

— (1908 [2]). "A Winter's Work in a Sub-arctic Climate." *Boston Medical and Surgical Journal* 158, no. 26 (1908): 996-7

Loder, Millicent Blake. *Daughter of Labrador.* St. John's: Harry Cuff 1989

Luther, Jessie. "Development of the Industrial Work in Dr. Grenfell's Mission at St. Anthony." *Among the Deep Sea Fishers* 4, no. 4 (1907): 11-4

—. "In Retrospect," *Among the Deep Sea Fishers* 28, no. 3 (1930): 112-24

Mayou, Edith. "Sketch of Dr. Grenfell's Work on the Labrador and Northern Newfoundland." *Among the Deep Sea Fishers* 6, no. 1 (1908): 12-5

McGrath, Judy, comp. "Indian Harbour Hospital" in *Them Days: Stories of Early Labrador* 4, no. 1 (1978): 5-41

Merrick, Elliott. *Northern Nurse.* New York: Charles Scribner 1942

Morton, Rosalie Slaughter. *A Woman Surgeon: The Life and Work of Rosalie Slaughter Morton.* New York: Frederick A. Stokes 1937

New England Grenfell Association. *Post-War with the Grenfell Mission.* Boston: 1946

Paddon, Harold G. *Green Woods and Blue Waters: Memories of Labrador.* St. John's Breakwater 1989

Paddon, Harold L. "Labrador Today: A Lecture to the Medical and Physical Society." *St. Thomas Hospital Gazette* 35 (1936): 283-87

—. "Vale, Indian Harbour." *Among the Deep Sea Fishers* 27, no. 3 (1929): 108-11

Paddon, W. Anthony. "Life in Labrador with My Famous Father" in *The Book of Newfoundland,* Vol. 5, J.R. Smallwood, ed. St. John's: Newfoundland Book Publishers 1975: pp. 489-93

—. *Labrador Doctor: My Life with the Grenfell Mission.* Toronto: James Lorimer 1989

—. "Medicine in Northern Labrador: The First Years." *Newfoundland Medical Association Newsletter* 16, no. 3 (1971): 26-31

Peacock, Doris. "Mina (Gilchrist) Paddon" in *Remarkable Women of Newfoundland and Labrador.* Presented by St. John's Local Council of Women. St. John's: Valhalla Press 1976: pp. 48-9

Peacock, F.W. with Lawrence Jackson. *Reflections from a Snowhouse.* St. John's: Jesperson 1986

Peattie, D.C. "Man of the Month." *Review of Review* 96, no. 1 (1937): 25-6, 58

Richards, J.T. "Doings in the North." *Among the Deep Sea Fishers* 6, no. 2 (1908): 23-4

—. *Snapshots of Grenfell.* Irving Letto, intro. St. John's: Creative 1989

Roberts, Peter J. "The Process of Change." *Among the Deep Sea Fishers* 78, no. 2 (1981): 1-4

Rowland, John T. *North to Adventure.* New York: Norton 1963

Sayre, Francis Bowes. *Glad Adventure.* New York: Macmillan 1957

Scott, J.M. *The Land that God Gave Cain: An Account of H.G. Watkins' Expedition to Labrador, 1928-29.* London: Chatto and Windus 1933

Sears, Fred C. "The 1933 Labrador Garden Campaign." *Among the Deep Sea Fishers* 32, no. 1 (1934): 8-12

Simms, George "I Remember One Time in Particular." *Among the Deep Sea Fishers* 73, no. 3 (1976): 12-3

"Sir Wilfred Grenfell—a True Knight." *Newfoundland Quarterly* 27, no. 2 (1927): 25-7

Smallwood, Joseph R. "The Co-operative Movement in Newfoundland" in *The Book of Newfoundland,* Vol. 1, J.R. Smallwood, ed. St. John's: Newfoundland Book Publishers 1937: pp. 276-8

Spracklin, Dulcie Lear. "Samaritan of the North." *Newfoundland Stories and Ballads* 9, no.1 (1962): 46-7

Thomas, Gordon W. *From Sled to Satellite: My Years with the Grenfell Mission.* Toronto: Irwin Publishing 1987

Thomas, Gordon W. "Surgery in the Sub-Arctic." *Journal of Thoracic and Cardiovascular Surgery* 70, no. 2 (1975): 203-13

Wakefield, R.W. "Mrs. A.W. Wakefield." *Among the Deep Sea Fishers* 74, no. 1 (1977): 16-7

Waldo, Fullerton L. *With Grenfell on the Labrador.* New York: Fleming H. Revell 1920

Wells, H.G. *Marriage.* New York: Duffield 1912

Willcox, Hilton L. *Beneath a Wandering Star.* Edinburgh: Pentland Press 1986

Withington, Alfreda. *My Eyes Have Seen: A Woman Doctor's Saga.* London: Robert Hale 1941

Additional Reading

Kennedy, John C. "The Impact of the Grenfell Mission on Southeastern Labrador." *Polar Record* 24, no. 149 (1988): 199-206

Moore, Tom. *Wilfred Grenfell.* Don Mills, Ont.: Fitzhenry and Whiteside 1980

Rompkey, Ronald. *Grenfell of Labrador: A Biography.* Toronto: University of Toronto Press 1991

—. "Elements of Spiritual Autobiography in Sir Wilfred Grenfell's 'A Labrador Doctor.'" *Newfoundland Studies* 1, no. 1 (1985): 17-28

—. "Heroic Biography and the Life of Sir Wilfred Grenfell." *Prose Studies: History, Theory and Criticism* 12, no. 2 (1989): 159-73

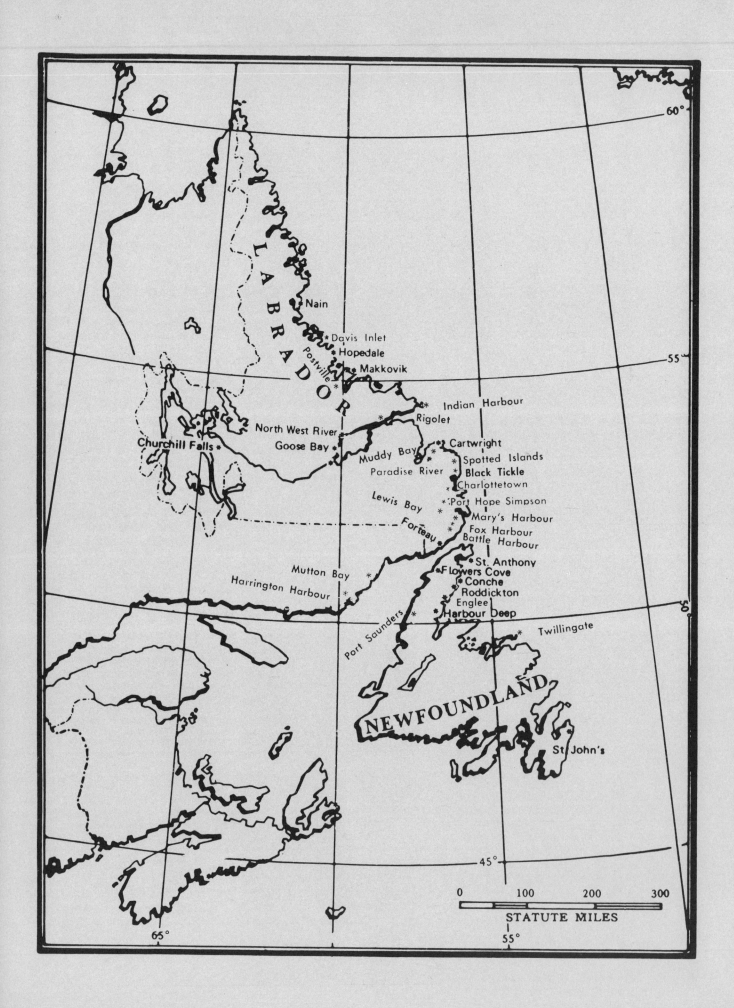